Diagnostic Tests in Nephrology

Edited by
John Bradley
and
Ken Smith
Department of Renal Medicine
Addenbrooke's Hospital
Cambridge
UK

A member of the Hodder Headline Group
LONDON · SYDNEY · AUCKLAND
Co-published in the United States of America by
Oxford University Press Inc., New York

First published in Great Britain in 1999 by
Arnold, a member of the Hodder Headline Group,
338 Euston Road, London NW1 3BH

http://www.arnoldpublishers.com

Co-published in the United States of America by
Oxford University Press Inc.,
198 Madison Avenue, New York, NY10016
Oxford is a registered trademark of Oxford University Press

British Library Cataloguing in Publication Data
A catalogue record for this book is available from the British Library

Library of Congress Cataloging-in-Publication Data
A catalog record for this book is available from the Library of Congress

ISBN 0 340 740 85X

1 2 3 4 5 6 7 8 9 10

Typeset in 11/13 Adobe Garamond by Photoprint, Torquay, Devon
Printed and bound in Great Britain by the Alden Press, Oxford

Diagnostic Tests
in Nephrology

This book is dedicated to the memory of Dr David Evans

Contents

Contributors

Stephen Alexander
Division of Nephrology
Children's Hospital and Harvard
    Medical School
300 Longwood Avenue
Boston
MA 02115
USA

John Bradley
Department of Renal Medicine
Addenbrooke's Hospital
Cambridge
CB2 2QQ
UK

David Briscoe
Division of Nephrology
Children's Hospital and Harvard
    Medical School
300 Longwood Avenue
Boston
MA 02115
USA

Patricia Campbell
Department of Medicine
Division of Nephrology and
    Immunology
University of Alberta Hospitals
Edmonton, AB
T6G 2B7
Canada

Les Culank
Department of Biochemistry
Addenbrooke's Hospital
Cambridge
CB2 2QQ

Linda De Luca
Division of Nephrology
University of British Colombia
St Paul's Hospital
1081 Burrard Street
Vancouver
V6Z 1Y6
Canada

Vikas Dharnidharka
Division of Nephrology
Children's Hospital and Harvard
    Medical School
300 Longwood Avenue
Boston
MA 02115
USA

Lukas Foggensteiner
Addenbrooke's Hospital
Cambridge
CB2 2QQ
UK

Siân Griffin
Department of Renal Medicine
Addenbrooke's Hospital
Cambridge
CB2 2QQ
UK

Matthew Hand
Pediatric Nephrology
Maine Medical Center
Portland
ME 04702
USA

Terence Kealey
Department of Biochemistry
Addenbrooke's Hospital
Cambridge
CB2 2QQ
UK

David Lomas
Department of Radiology
Addenbrooke's Hospital and
    University of Cambridge
Cambridge
CB2 2QQ
UK

Simon McPherson
Department of Radiology
Jubilee Wing
Leeds General Infirmary
Great George Street
Leeds
LS1 3EX
UK

Peter Mathieson
Department of Renal Medicine
Southmead Hospital
Bristol
BS10 5NB
UK

Allan Murray
Department of Medicine
Division of Nephrology and
    Immunology
University of Alberta Hospitals
Edmonton, AB
T6G 2B7
Canada

David Oliveira
St George's Hospital Medical School
Tooting
London
SW17 0RE
UK

Aram Rudenski
Department of Biochemistry
Addenbrooke's Hospital
Cambridge
CB2 2QQ
UK

Richard Sandford
Department of Medical Genetics
University of Cambridge
School of Clinical Medicine
Addenbrooke's Hospital
Cambridge
CB2 2QQ
UK

Ken Smith
Department of Renal Medicine
Addenbrooke's Hospital
Cambridge
CB2 2QQ
UK

Sathia Thiru
Department of Pathology
Addenbrooke's Hospital
Cambridge
CB2 2QQ
UK

Philip Wraight
Department of Nuclear Medicine
Addenbrooke's Hospital
Cambridge
CB2 2QQ
UK

Preface

Although history-taking and examination remain the principal tools of medicine, many patients with renal disorders do not present with clinical features until their disease is advanced. Even when symptoms and signs are present, clinical evaluation can prove misleading. Nephrologists have learnt to depend heavily on investigations from many disciplines in the management of patients with renal disease.

Diagnostic Tests in Nephrology provides a detailed review of these investigations from the perspective of laboratory-based clinicians, radiologists and nephrologists. The book is aimed at postgraduate doctors, but the diversity of topics covered means that, in addition to nephrologists, it should be useful to doctors practising in a number of specialties including immunology, radiology and pathology, and other health professionals, such as nurses and dietitians, working in renal units.

The book is divided into two parts. The first part contains a detailed description of tests used in nephrology, including the principle underlying the test, how it is performed and the interpretation of abnormal results. The second part describes how these tests are used in the investigation of specific renal disorders.

John Bradley and Ken Smith
Cambridge, UK
April 1998

Part One
Diagnostic Tests

The biochemical investigation of renal disease

Aram Rudenski, Les Culank and Terence Kealey

The cellular and molecular processes that underlie renal function are becoming clearer every year, and their investigation during pathological conditions contributes to scientific knowledge. Yet the tests used to diagnose and monitor kidney disease continue to be those based on the understanding of the nephron elucidated by the early physiologists.

Epithelial physiology

The genitourinary system is an epithelium, and shares the properties of other epithelia. As illustrated in Figure 1.1, epithelia are characterized by polarity. Epithelial cells provide the interface between the body and the external environment: luminally they face the outside world, while basolaterally they sit on a basement membrane that separates them from, but physically connects them to, the underlying mesenchyme. The basement membrane is composed of specialized glycoproteins such as laminin, fibronectin and collagen IV. These are variously secreted by the epithelial and mesenchymal cells, but their cross-linking at specific molecular sites by specific enzymes during embryonic development directs the formation of the basement membrane at the epithelial/mesenchymal interface.

Epithelial cells are themselves polar. Each epithelial cell membrane is discretely but continuously joined to its neighbours in an unbroken ring of so-called 'tight junctions'. These junctions, which result from the fusion of discrete lengths of adjacent cell membranes, divide the luminal from the basolateral membranes. These two membranes contain very different complements of lipids and, more importantly, transporting proteins. Lipid

Fig. 1.1

Characteristic transport proteins in an idealized epithelium. The 3Na$^+$/2K$^+$ ATPase exchange is inhibited by ouabain and digoxin. The Na$^+$/K$^+$/2Cl$^-$ co-transporter is frusemide-inhibited. The Na$^+$ channel is amiloride-inhibited. Epithelia may also express K$^+$, Cl$^-$ and H$_2$O channels, either luminally or basolaterally.

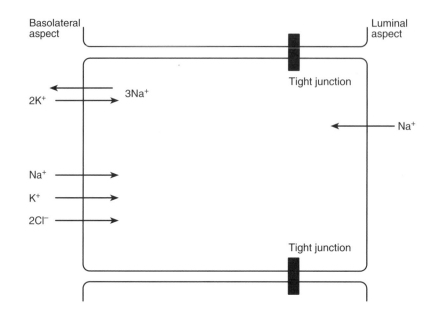

bilayer leaflet membranes are poorly permeable to water, and the flux of ions, solutes and solvent is protein-mediated.

Polar transport is a characteristic of epithelia unless crucial layers are dead or modified by disease. An epithelium may be either secretory (basolateral → luminal ion or water flux) or reabsorptive (luminal → basolateral). Whatever it is, it invariably expresses 3Na$^+$/2K$^+$ ATPase, and this is basolateral in its location. It is this protein that by its Na$^+$/K$^+$ transporting properties, establishes the high internal [K$^+$] and low internal [Na$^+$] that cells then exploit to drive the secondary movement of other ions and molecules.

Other important transporting proteins whose properties have been characterized include the Na$^+$/K$^+$/2Cl$^-$ co-transporter (basolateral, inhibited by the frusemide class of diuretics; it exploits the Na$^+$ and K$^+$ electrochemical gradients to direct Cl$^-$ efflux luminally), the Na$^+$ (and sometimes H$^+$) amiloride-sensitive channel (luminally) and the H$^+$, K$^+$Cl$^-$ and H$_2$O channel families (members of which might be found luminally or basolaterally, depending on the particular epithelium). The H$_2$O channels, or aquaporins, have only recently been discovered.

It should be noted that there are different classes of transporting proteins within cell membranes, including those that are simply channels. (These provide ion-specific but unmediated 'holes' through the membrane, which allow particular ions to pass passively down their electrochemical gradient; they obey first order kinetics.) Mediated transport proteins include those that allow the passage of only one ion in one direction, those that exchange ions in different directions, and those that co-transport more than one species of ion in the same direction. These mediated transport proteins may simply conduct ions down the sum of their electrochemical gradients, or they may be linked to the action of an enzyme such as the ATPase of the $3Na^+/2K^+$ ATPase. In either case, mediated transport ultimately obeys Michaelis–Menten kinetics.

The so-called 'tight' junctions are, in fact, variably tight. Some, like those of the glomerulus, are extremely permeable indeed to water and ions (see below). Others, like those of various parts of the distal convoluted tubule and collecting duct, are extremely impermeable. Ions, solute and water molecules may therefore traverse an epithelium by either the transcellular or paracellular route, depending on the variation in permeability of different epithelia. The tight junctions do not, however, seem to possess much specificity in their variable permeability to ions and water. They are either tight or loose, but they are probably not 'tight' to some species and 'loose' to others. The passage of water is solute-driven, either through channels or tight junctions. Such solute-mediated forces include osmosis and so-called solvent drag.

Renal glomerular physiology

Each kidney contains about one million nephrons, each made up of:

- a glomerulus
- a proximal convoluted tubule
- a loop of Henle (not all human nephrons have one of these; see below)
- a distal convoluted tubule
- a collecting duct.

Each nephron is also intimately associated with:

- an afferent (glomerular) arteriole
- an efferent (glomerular) arteriole
- the (tubular) vasa recta
- the juxtaglomerular apparatus.

The glomeruli and proximal and distal convoluted tubules are found in the cortex of the kidney. The loops of Henle and collecting duct are medullary.

GLOMERULAR FUNCTION

The glomeruli are organs of filtration. Some 20% (increasing to 30% in pregnancy) of the normal cardiac output of approximately 5 l/min flows through the kidneys, most of it passing through the glomerular afferent arterioles. Within the kidney, the distribution of blood flow is subject to minute-to-minute control. Among other functions, the juxtaglomerular apparatus plays a crucial role in sensing inadequate sodium delivery and responding by the release of renin to stimulate angiotensin production. The importance of this regulation is highlighted in cases of renal artery insufficiency, when renal failure can be precipitated by inhibitors of angiotensin converting enzymes such as captopril.

Of the 1 l/min of glomerular blood flow, about 12–14% is filtered, generating some 200 l of plasma ultrafiltrate entering the tubules each day. Most filtration occurs across the glomerular filtration membrane, which is composed of the endothelial cells of the arteriole, a basal lamina, and the epithelial cells of the visceral layer of Bowman's capsule, the so-called podocytes. These specialized cells develop a network of interdigitating foot processes which contain slit diaphragms. These are tight junctions that are modified for filtration.

The cut-off molecular weight (MW) for filtration is around 60–70 kilodaltons (kDa), which coincides with the MW of albumin (65 000). However, relatively little albumin is normally filtered, despite its size, because highly sialylated glomerular epithelial proteins such as podocalyxin interact electrostatically with plasma proteins such as albumin to exclude them. Most of what little albumin is filtered is reabsorbed in the tubules. Consequently, the composition of the glomerular filtrate is almost indistinguishable from that of plasma, with the obvious exception of the proteins, and the filtration force is opposed by a small but insignificant colloid osmotic or so-called oncotic pressure.

Renal tubular physiology

PROXIMAL TUBULAR FUNCTION

This is dominated by isosmotic transport consequent upon active Na^+ reabsorption. Thus, around 90–95% of all filtered Na^+ is reabsorbed by the proximal tubule, accompanied by almost all of the filtered Cl^-. Since the proximal tubule is a very 'loose' epithelium and rich in water channels known as aquaporins, 90–95% of the filtered water is also reabsorbed, following the NaCl isosmotically. Almost all of the filtered K^+, Ca^{2+} and Mg^{2+} are actively reabsorbed by the proximal tubule, as are all of the filtered glucose, amino acids, and uric acid. Glucose reabsorption obeys Michaelis–Menten kinetics, and transport is saturated at around 11 mmol/l. If plasma, and hence glomerular filtrate, levels exceed this, then glucose will appear in the urine (glycosuria). Uric acid is both secreted into, and reabsorbed from, the tubule in an apparently futile cycle that results in its near-complete reabsorption by the proximal convoluted tubule.

Almost all the HCO_3^- is reabsorbed in the proximal tubule (see below). Phosphate is variably reabsorbed, partly depending on the level of parathyroid hormone (PTH). The net consequence of proximal tubule activity is therefore to reabsorb about 95% of the Na^+, 95% of the filtered water, effectively all of the reusable nutrients, and the bulk of the other electrolytes. The remaining flux provides the substrate for homeostatic adjustment by the distal parts of the nephron. Filtered metabolic waste products such as urea and creatinine, however, remain in the luminal fluid (some urea leaks back, and there is a small active tubular secretion of creatinine).

THE LOOPS OF HENLE

The ascending (efferent) limb of the loop, which is closely apposed to the descending (afferent) limb, contains chloride pumps that actively pump Cl^- into the descending limb. Na^+ follows electrochemically. Because the descending limb receives chloride and sodium all the way down, the concentration of these ions rises all the way down, so the osmolarity of the descending limb, which is isosmolar at entry (approximately 300 mosmol/l); rises to around 1300 mosmol/l at the tip. Because the descending limb and tip of the loop of Henle are loose epithelia, the osmolality of the interstitial fluid around the tips of the renal papillae may also approach 1300 mosmol/l; but the ascending limb is a tight epithelium, and so the fluid that leaves it is hypo-osmolar (Figure 1.2).

This so-called countercurrent multiplication within the loops of Henle is an efficient way of creating a zone of high osmolarity because at any one time, in any one place, the chloride pumps are only moving chloride across relatively small electrochemical gradients, but the cumulative effect of the chloride pumping along the descending limb is to create a zone of high absolute osmolarity at the tips of the renal papillae. It should be noted, however, that only about 20% of nephrons in humans possess a loop of Henle, so the capacity of humans to concentrate urine is limited. The human cannot, for example, survive on sea-water because human urine cannot match its osmolarity, whereas desert rats, all of whose nephrons possess long loops of Henle, can survive on sea-water.

Fig. 1.2
Countercurrent
multiplication. All units are
in mosmoles/l.

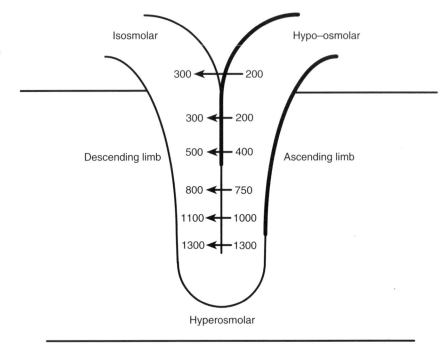

THE COLLECTING DUCT

This duct has two functions. First, it acts as a conduit to the renal pelvis, and secondly it is variably permeable to water. Under the influence of antidiuretic hormone (ADH), water channels will open to allow the selective passage of H_2O into the interstitial fluid down its concentration gradient in response to osmotic forces. From the interstitial fluid, it will be transported into the circulation by the vasa recta.

Renal electrolyte and acid-base handling

SODIUM EXCHANGE

The bulk of filtered Na^+ is reabsorbed isosmotically with H_2O and Cl^- in the proximal tubule, but sodium reabsorption in exchange for hydrogen ions also occurs in both the proximal and distal convoluted tubules and in the collecting duct (Figure 1.3). In the proximal tubules, Na^+ exchange results in the reclamation of filtered HCO_3^- (see below). In the distal convoluted tubules and collecting duct, the process is generally associated with the generation of HCO_3^- and the regulation of pH (see below).

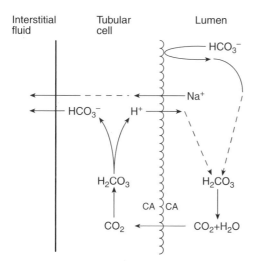

Interstitial fluid   Tubular cell   Lumen

Fig. 1.3
Na^+/H^+ exchange and HCO_3^- reclamation/ generation. CA, carbonic anhydrase. The luminal membrane is impermeable to HCO_3^-.

Potassium and hydrogen ions compete for secretion in exchange for sodium ions. It appears that this Na^+ exchange for either K^+ or H^+ can be regulated by two distinct mechanisms.

- Aldosterone stimulates the exchange, which is why Conn's syndrome, for example, is associated with hypernatraemia, hypokalaemia (or whole body potassium deficiency) and a metabolic alkalosis.
- The exchange can also, however, be directly stimulated by high levels of intracellular $[H^+]$, which therefore acts as a pH-stat. (see below).

H^+ SECRETION, HCO_3^- REABSORPTION AND THE RENAL TUBULAR ACIDOSES

Both the proximal and the distal convoluted tubules secrete H^+ in exchange for sodium. Their different actions reflect the different overall workings of the two structures, as the function of the proximal tubular secretion of H^+ is primarily the reabsorption of filtered HCO_3^-, while distal tubular secretion is involved in whole body acid-base fine-tuning and, in general, this involves bicarbonate generation.

The proximal tubule
The mechanism here is relatively straightforward. H^+ is pumped into the tubular lumen where it can combine with the bicarbonate ion to form carbonic acid:

$$H^+ + HCO_3^- \leftrightarrow H_2CO_3.$$

Equilibration is reached almost instantaneously, and depends upon pH and bicarbonate concentration.

Carbonic acid can dissociate to form water and carbon dioxide:

$$H_2CO_3 \leftrightarrow H_2O + CO_2.$$

This reaction is relatively slow, but is accelerated by the enzyme carbonic acid anhydrase, which is normally found in the brush border of the renal tubules. Whereas the luminal membrane is impermeable to HCO_3^-, it is permeable to CO_2, which enters the luminal cell to recombine with water, again under the action of carbonic anhydrase (CA), to form carbonic acid, which can then dissociate to yield bicarbonate and hydrogen ions. The H^+ is then pumped back into the lumen of the tubule, whereas the HCO_3^- is reabsorbed (probably accompanied by Na^+).

The activity of CA is increased by a raised intracellular concentration of H^+ and CO_2. It is likely that the increased CA of intracellular K^+ deficiency is due to increased intracellular H^+. This explains the classical combination of systemic metabolic alkalosis with aciduria in patients with potassium depletion.

The distal tubule

The 10–15% of filtered HCO_3^- that escapes titration with H^+ in the proximal tubule is then reabsorbed by H^+ titration in the distal convoluted tubule by H^+ luminal secretion in exchange for sodium. However, the system is regulated at this point because the Na^+/H^+ exchange is $[H^+]$-sensitive.

It is this $[H^+]$-sensitivity that explains why the luminal membrane is impermeable to HCO_3^-. This complex system of HCO_3^- reclamation/ generation is thus rendered pH-sensitive. For example, in the event of an alkalosis, distal tubular H^+ secretion is inhibited and HCO_3^- is then lost in the urine, helping, of course, to correct the body alkalosis. Generally, however, it is a metabolic acidosis that the renal acid-base homeostatic mechanisms are required to prevent. Metabolism normally creates acids (apart from the production of CO_2, which is normally expired, and lactic acid, which reaches a steady state and recycles) from the catabolism of phosphate- and sulphate-containing amino acids, which leads to the production of phosphoric and sulphuric acids. The total quantity of these acids (referred to as the net acid) excreted daily by the kidneys is normally equal to the total daily synthesis of about 50–100 mmol of these fixed acids, and is the source of the metabolic acidosis of chronic renal failure.

Under the normal circumstance of the body metabolism generating acid, all the filtered HCO_3^- is reabsorbed. In addition, the tubule itself can utilize respiration-derived carbon dioxide which, after combination with water to form carbonic acid, can generate further H^+ to be lost in the lumen, with the generation of HCO_3^- to be retained in the body as a buffer. Secretions of additional H^+ are then buffered by urinary HPO_4^{2-} to form $H_2PO_4^-$. While ammonium secretion has a role to play in acid-base balance, the mechanism of its regulation and its importance are disputed. During acidosis, glutaminolysis is accelerated, leading to generation of additional ammonium ions. Ammonium ions would normally be converted in the liver to urea, with the generation of acid and the loss of ammonium base, providing further ways in which secretion of ammonium can enhance acid secretion.

Tests of glomerular function

Serum urea and creatinine are the most commonly used measures of glomerular function. The production rate of urea is more variable, making it a less useful measure of renal function than creatinine.

Creatinine is mostly derived from muscle breakdown and turnover. A 50% loss of renal function is needed before the serum creatinine rises above the normal range; it is therefore not a sensitive indicator of mild to moderate renal injury. Serum levels are low in the young, the elderly, and those with small muscle mass, including sick patients after several weeks in bed. It should be noted that such patients may have an apparently normal serum creatinine even if their clearance is markedly reduced. (NB Some methods of measuring creatinine may be subject to interference by bilirubin, drugs, or ketones, which falsely elevate measured creatinine levels. Physicians should familiarize themselves with the limitations of the assays used in their own hospitals.)

Urea is a product of the hepatic metabolism of amino acids derived from dietary and catabolic protein. Poor diet, malabsorption, or liver disorders may lower the serum urea. Urea production increases with cellular catabolism (infection, trauma, steroid therapy) or following protein load (dietary or following gastrointestinal haemorrhage). Serum urea rises faster than creatinine in dehydration, and falls faster in overhydration.

GLOMERULAR FILTRATION RATE

As noted above, the glomeruli filter about 120 ml/min of fluid. The glomerular filtration rate (GFR) can be determined by measuring the rate of clearance of a substance that is filtered. For a compound, C, passing into the tubules with the filtrate and then passing into the urine, given the concentration of that compound in the blood and the amount appearing in the urine every minute, one can calculate the amount cleared by the glomerulus every minute because 118 ml or so of the 120 ml of fluid filtered each minute at the glomerulus is returned by the tubules, compound-free, to the circulation. This is the GFR. The formula is:

$$\text{GFR} = \frac{\text{urinary [C]} \times \text{urine volume per unit time}}{\text{serum or plasma [C]}}$$

The ideal test compound C would be of low molecular weight to optimize filtration, and would be neither actively secreted nor reabsorbed by the tubule (to remove tubular activity from the measurement of GFR). Such a compound is the polysaccharide inulin, but inulin is not endogenous and so it has to be infused or injected. It is not used in clinical practice. The standard endogenous compound used clinically is creatinine. Some creatinine is secreted by the tubules, so that creatinine clearance is marginally higher than that of inulin. Urea is freely filtered by the glomerulus, but approximately 50% is reabsorbed so urea clearance is less than GFR.

CREATININE CLEARANCE TESTS

An exact 24-hour collection of urine is made, and a blood sample is taken during the collection, theoretically midway through it, but a sample taken within a day of the urine collection will usually suffice (except in patients with rapidly changing renal function). The creatinine clearance is most reliably calculated as follows:

$$\text{Creatinine clearance (ml/min)} = \frac{\text{urine creatinine (mmol/24 h)} \times 694}{\text{serum creatinine (}\mu\text{mol/l)}}$$

The normal adult clearance is about 100–120 ml/min, but increases in pregnancy and tends to decrease with advancing age, particularly over 60 years. The clearance can be related to body surface area, which may be helpful for small children.

Errors

The commonest error is a failure to collect timed urine accurately. For this reason, some laboratories and some nephrologists do not measure creatinine clearance. On the other hand, where reliable collection does occur, such as in intensive care units, creatinine clearance is still the best routine measure of a patient's GFR.

Serum creatinine as a surrogate for clearance

Within individuals, there can be a close inverse relationship between serum creatinine concentrations and GFR; thus serum creatinine concentrations can be used clinically to monitor the rate of fall of GFR in individuals. However, variation between individuals rules out the use of serum creatinine levels as a screening test for relatively small losses of GFR, as there may be a quite significant impairment of GFR without a rise of serum creatinine concentrations above the normal range.

Some physicians use the inverse of the serum creatinine concentration, and they may also correct for age, sex, and weight in their search for a surrogate for a full GFR estimation in monitoring the progress of an individual patient on a long-term basis.

OTHER CLEARANCE STUDIES

[^{99m}Tc] DTPA (diethylenetriamine pentaacetic acid) and [^{51}Cr] EDTA (ethylenediaminetetraacetic acid) are among the substances used in routine clinical practice when a clearance result is essential but an accurate creatinine clearance is not feasible. ([^{99m}Tc] DTPA can allow simultaneous kidney imaging.) The substance is injected intravenously. Time is allowed for equilibration into the interstitial space, blood samples are taken at intervals, and the rate of fall in the circulation is used to calculate GFR.

GLOMERULAR FILTRATION OF PROTEINS – ASSESSING GLOMERULAR DAMAGE

In the normal state, up to 150 mg of protein is lost in the urine per day, of which half is Tamm–Horsfall mucoprotein derived from the renal tubules. Less than 30 mg of the daily urine protein loss is albumin. There are smaller amounts of other proteins, both blood- and renal-derived.

When the glomeruli are damaged, their efficiency at retaining plasma proteins is impaired. Since albumin has a molecular weight at the threshold of glomerular filtration and is the most abundant protein in serum, it is the main protein lost into the filtrate when glomeruli are damaged.

Among the methods available for studying proteins in the urine of patients are the following.

- Stick tests are, in practice, a screening test for albumin. They are subject to errors such as false-positives in alkaline or infected urine, or false-negatives in boric acid preservative.
- Sensitive and specific methods such as immunoassay for albuminuria, either as a 24-hour excretion or expressed as an albumin to creatinine ratio in a spot or overnight urine. (Note that in an ideal world all such measurements would be performed on 24-hour urine collections, but a number of tests, including this one, are often performed on untimed urine samples. The analyte concentration is reported as a ratio to that of

creatinine as the rate of appearance of creatinine in the urine is relatively constant, irrespective of volume.)
- Colorimetric and turbidimetric methods for protein (i.e. more than just albumin) are largely used in monitoring nephrotic syndrome, pre-eclampsia, and renal diseases in general, even though albumin is the dominant protein species. These assays are ideally performed on accurate 24-hour urine collections.
- Electrophoresis with immunofixation to detect the presence of light-chains (p. 37) in place of the classic Bence Jones test, which is no longer employed.

The upper normal limit of urinary albumin and total urinary protein is around 30 mg/l and 100–150 mg/l, respectively.

Microalbuminuria

Excretion of albumin that is below the 300 mg/l detection limit of stick tests but above the upper limit of normal of 30 mg/l is called micro-albuminuria. The albumin detected is of normal structure but small in quantity. It is used to monitor the developing nephropathy in patients with diabetes mellitus, in whom microalbuminuria predates the onset of overt renal disease. Detection may allow the early use of angiotensin-converting enzyme inhibitors to slow progression of the nephropathy.

Albuminuria

If a stick test for albumin is positive, an accurate measurement of 24-hour urine protein should be confirmed by a laboratory method.

Large rates of albumin loss in the urine lead to the nephrotic syndrome. This is the triad of proteinuria that is heavy enough to cause hypoalbumin-aemia and oedema. The aetiology can be identified on biopsy (Chapter 7), so quantitative selectivity of proteinuria is now rarely of help, except in children when selective proteinuria can support a diagnosis of minimal change disease, obviating the need for renal biopsy. Oedema only becomes apparent when gram quantities of albumin are lost per day, though a frothy urine may be seen earlier on (p. 34). As well as low serum albumin, the patient typically has high serum haptoglobins and lipoproteins. There is great individual variation in the levels of albumin loss that can be tolerated before these signs are seen.

Tests of tubular function

The concentrating power of the tubules provides the best screen for tubular function. Conventionally, a urine osmolality in excess of 600–850 mosmol/kg excludes significant tubular disease or diabetes insipidus, when further investigation of generalized tubular dysfunction is not necessary unless specific defects such as renal tubular acidosis are being sought.

In the oliguric patient passing well under 100 ml/hour urine, a urine osmolality of more than double serum osmolality with a spot urine sodium below about 20 mmol/l suggests prerenal hypovolaemia needing treatment, particularly if the central venous pressure is low. A less concentrated urine with higher sodium suggests incipient renal failure.

Other tests of tubular function, including urine tests for glucose, amino acids and acidity, may all be abnormal in Fanconi's syndrome-type generalized tubular defects, whether inherited or acquired. Glycosuria in pregnancy is not necessarily abnormal, and it is important that screening for diabetes in pregnancy is based on blood glucose assessment.

FLUID DEPRIVATION TESTS

These are rarely performed, being potentially dangerous, unpleasant and labour-intensive. The monitoring of the progression of chronic renal failure, for example, is best done through the GFR. Fluid deprivation tests are generally only indicated to distinguish between the polyurias of diabetes insipidus and psychogenic polydipsia, but often fail to do so.

Diabetes insipidus may be posterior pituitary in origin, resulting in inadequate ADH secretion, or may be associated with inherited or acquired kidney diseases, which may lead to a lack of response to ADH. Any cause of tubulointerstitial disease may lead to diabetes insipidus, though more specific defects can occur congenitally or as a result of toxicity from drugs such as lithium or some forms of tetracycline. In patients with true diabetes insipidus, an increased fluid intake is required to keep up with the urine water loss and to keep plasma osmolality within normal limits. Fluid restriction can lead to life-threatening cardiovascular collapse.

Psychogenic polydipsia is a psychiatric disorder in which the patient drinks an excessive quantity of water. Patients will often seem indifferent and seek to disguise it, drinking surreptitiously from flower vases, for example. The results of fluid deprivation may be equivocal in patients with psychogenic polydipsia because their renal medulla is not as hyperosmolar as that in the normal subject, so that ADH is less effective. Nonetheless, urine osmolality does rise slowly.

The physiological purpose of the fluid deprivation test is to show that the kidney cannot concentrate the urine in the face of a increasing serum osmolality. Different authors quote different lower limits of normal urine osmolality under these circumstances, ranging from 600 mosmol/kg to 850 mosmol/kg.

The test is contraindicated when serum osmolality is already high and the urine osmolality is not elevated as Nature has already reproduced the test conditions. Moreover, the test is potentially dangerous as fluid restriction can lead to life-threatening cardiovascular collapse. For this reason, fluid deprivation should be carried out under close supervision, with hourly monitoring of urine volume, urine osmolality, serum osmolality, and weight. The test is ended if 5% of body weight is lost. Close supervision also ensures that the patient does not cheat and drink, which will give misleading results.

A rise in plasma osmolality without an adequate rise in urine osmolality indicates diabetes insipidus. If the results indicate this, the subject should be given ddAVP, a synthetic ADH analogue, to check whether the problem is due to lack of ADH secretion or is truly nephrogenic. If the results are unhelpful but the patient needs an unequivocal diagnosis, then a saline infusion test is indicated. This causes a gradual rise in measured serum osmolality, during which plasma ADH and urine osmolality are also serially measured.

RENAL TUBULAR ACIDOSIS (RTA)

There are at least three types of acidosis caused by disorders within the renal tubules. They generally give rise to low actual, standard and total blood bicarbonate levels, and a negative base excess. This is also the pattern seen in chronic renal failure. (Most laboratories no longer assay chloride with the standard venous urea and electrolyte profile, nor do they use the anion gap, but in the renal tubular acidoses the serum chloride is generally high and the anion gap normal because the conditions involve direct derangement of the body's usual bicarbonate buffer system.)

Distal renal tubular acidosis (RTA-1)
This may present in either childhood or adult life. Some cases are inherited (autosomal dominant), but some are sporadic. Others are apparently transient and may correct in later life. A number of cases of RTA-1 are acquired, either secondary to autoimmune diseases (especially Sjögren's syndrome) or to any renal medullary condition.

The pathophysiology is that the distal tubular H^+ pump is only partially effective, thus failing to generate the 800–900:1 H^+ gradient between the tubular lumen and blood that normal subjects can achieve. The mechanism of that pump failure is currently unclear, but it is worth noting that two rare aetiologies have been described. Some rare inherited cases have been attributed to carbonic anhydrase deficiency, and one acquired cause is amphotericin B therapy. This antifungal agent acts as an ionophore for protons, and in some patients it negates the action of the H^+ pump by allowing immediate H^+ back-leakage. Thus, even in the presence of severe acidosis, the urine pH cannot be reduced to below 5.5.

RTA-1 is associated with marked hypokalaemia, which can be explained by the fact that H^+ and K^+ compete for Na^+ exchange and, since the H^+ pump (which is an Na^+ exchange protein) is ineffective, K^+ is preferentially exchanged for Na^+. In addition, mild impairment of sodium reabsorption leads to secondary hyperaldosteronism. A reduction in citrate secretion is said to be the factor that promotes calcium stone formation in the urinary tract, although the mechanism of nephrocalcinosis is not clear.

Treatment first involves correction of the low potassium level with supplements, before the long-term treatment of sodium bicarbonate is given. Otherwise, correction of the acidosis will precipitate a further fall in extracellular potassium as it re-enters the intracellular compartment.

Proximal renal tubular acidosis (RTA-2 or bicarbonate-wasting RTA)

This is usually associated with a generalized disorder of the proximal tubule, Fanconi's syndrome, in which there is glycosuria, amino-aciduria, and hyperphosphaturia (leading to rickets or osteomalacia) and RTA-2. Fanconi's syndrome may be genetic or acquired. Urine tests for glucose, amino acids, phosphate and pH give the diagnosis. The syndrome has many causes, including most causes of tubulointerstitial disease. A rare familial autosomal dominant isolated RTA-2 has also been described. Acquired causes include vitamin D deficiency and exposure to toxic heavy metals such as mercury or cadmium.

The basic lesion in RTA-2 is a loss of the capacity of the proximal tubule to secrete H^+. The distal tubule is therefore flooded with bicarbonate, which spills over into the urine. Interestingly, however, the bicarbonate-wasting so lowers plasma $[HCO_3^-]$ that the distal tubular flooding is arrested, under which circumstances the distal tubule can be shown to retain fully the capacity to reduce urinary pH to between 4.5 and 5.3. The failure of the H^+ pump leads to a failure of Na^+/H^+ exchange, and Na^+ is lost in the urine, leading to secondary hyperaldosteronism. This, in turn, leads to excessive K^+ loss in the urine, whole-body K^+ deficiency and polyuria.

Therapy centres on K^+ supplementation, and although potassium bicarbonate salts are the preferred treatment, active replacement of all the lost HCO_3^- is not called for as it will merely aggravate the natriuria and kaluria. The loss of bicarbonate is so great that, by comparison with RTA-1, it usually is not possible to reverse the acidosis.

Hyperkalaemic renal tubular acidosis (RTA-4)

This is a consequence of failure of the mineralocorticoid system. The secretion may fail, as in Addison's disease, or deficient renin production can lead to the condition of hyporeninaemic hypoaldosteronism. This can be found in conditions where there is renal damage, such as in patients with diabetic kidney disease.

A lack of the aldosterone effect, pseudohypoaldosteronism, has been described, in which the inherited defect is in the amiloride-sensitive epithelial sodium channel. Iatrogenic causes include K^+-sparing and anti-mineralocorticoid diuretics and prostaglandin synthase inhibitors, which block renin production. In the absence of effective mineralocorticoid activity, circulating $[K^+]$ and $[H^+]$ rise, and $[Na^+]$ falls. The above may respond to treatment with the mineralocorticoid fludrocortisone, unless there is a failure of sensitivity.

Tests for RTA

There are many causes of acidosis. Diabetic ketoacidosis, poisoning, and lactic acidosis, as well as rare inherited metabolic disorders in children, should be excluded first. Of the renal causes of acidosis, the commonest is renal failure, acute or chronic, which should be apparent and does not usually require further investigation of the acid-base disorder. It is only in the remaining patients, who will present with other signs of renal tubular acidosis, such as hypokalaemia, renal stones, or osteomalacia, that the diagnosis may need to be made. In such patients, a systemic metabolic acidosis is present, and the urine pH gives a further clue to the diagnosis in that it is inappropriately unacidified.

Hypokalaemia occurs with RTA-1 and RTA-2, while hyperkalaemia accompanies RTA-4. In RTA-1, urine pH is usually above 6, and always above 5.5, while in RTA-2, the urine pH will have fallen to between 4.5 and 5.3.

Ammonium chloride loading test

This test is now used only rarely to test tubular capacity to excrete acid under an induced systemic acidosis, except for in a few atypical RTA-1 patients. It is potentially dangerous and should be undertaken only in specialized practice.

TESTS FOR TUBULAR DAMAGE

An early marker of tubular damage may be the increased secretion of tubular proteins such as *N*-acetylglucosaminidase or retinol-binding protein. Their use is not, however, well established in clinical practice.

MISCELLANEOUS TESTS

Urine light-chains

Excess production of immunoglobulin light-chains in multiple myeloma can lead to impairment of renal function, and, ultimately, renal failure, as well as to general systemic complications of amyloidosis. Electrophoresis of urine with immunofixation is usually used to look for the condition.

Stones

Urine and plasma should be analysed for excessive metabolites that predispose to stone formation (p. 43). Analysis of the stone itself is also of value, with analysis by thermogravimetric analysis or infrared spectroscopy being particularly useful if the stone consists of oxalate, cystine or uric acid. In paediatric urolithiasis, it is important to exclude RTA-1 and primary hyperoxaluria. Measure parathyroid hormone (PTH) if any stone patient is hypercalciuric.

Tubular reabsorption of phospate (TmP)/GFR

This can be calculated from simultaneous serum and urine creatinine and phosphate. This used to be employed in the diagnosis of parathyroid disease, but is now redundant.

1,25 Dihydroxyvitamin D

This rarely needs to be measured in practice, even though its reduced rate of synthesis is important for pathophysiology and treatment (p. 200).

Renal failure

The final section of this chapter examines the role of biochemical investigation in acute and chronic renal failure. These aspects are dealt with in detail in Chapters 9 and 10. The principles do not differ from those related to kidney physiology already discussed, but the conditions are characterized by damage to overall renal function, rather than derangements in a single aspect of renal physiology, and a more holistic approach to the patient is required.

ACUTE RENAL FAILURE

The mechanisms of the syndrome of acute renal failure are complex and still being investigated. The many causes ultimately seem to lead to a final common pathway involving cytokines, free radicals, and vascular and metabolic dysfunction, but it is often preventable, and usually reversible if limited to acute tubular necrosis. A simple model that assumes that both kidneys cease to function is, however, useful in understanding the clinical chemistry of the situation. Because cell turnover (which involves cell destruction) and protein and DNA turnover are ongoing processes throughout the body, their waste products will accumulate. These processes are accelerated in acute renal failure. Thus K^+ accumulates in the blood and interstitial fluids (intracellular $[K^+]$ is in excess of $100\,mM$), urea and creatinine (the nitrogenous metabolic products) accumulate in the body and blood, and H^+ accumulates in the blood. The acidosis further aggravates hyperkalaemia by promoting intracellular potassium loss. Uric acid, resulting from degradation of purines from nucleotides and DNA, also accumulates in the blood.

Acute renal failure is therefore characterized by catabolism and renal shutdown leading to a metabolic acidosis with elevated serum levels of potassium, urea, creatinine and uric acid. Following removal of metabolites by dialysis or filtration, their reaccumulation is rapid in patients with renal failure.

The hydration state and the $[Na^+]$ in the blood will depend largely on intake. If the anuric patient's intake is greatly in excess of insensible losses, then haemodilution and fluid overload may develop. If the patient is ingesting or being infused with significant quantities of NaCl, then hypernatraemia may also develop. In the critically ill, haemofiltration may cope with such volume excess better than dialysis.

Biochemical investigation of acute renal failure

Investigations contribute to diagnosis and to preventing the consequences, which are life-threatening: cardiac arrhythmia and dysfunction due to hyperkalaemia and severe acidosis; pulmonary oedema from fluid overload; hypertension; and uraemic encephalopathy. Thus, fluid balance, which may require weighing of the patient, and monitoring of serum urea, creatinine, sodium, potassium, and bicarbonate or arterial pH are crucial.

Early on, measurement of urine osmolality and sodium may give a clue to the presence of prerenal failure, allowing prophylaxis, which may prevent actual damage to the kidney. Any urine produced should be examined by microscopy for red cells and casts, and should have its protein concentration measured; imaging techniques will help exclude obstructive uropathy.

Biochemical clues to aetiology

A very high serum creatine kinase level may suggest a diagnosis of rhabdomyolysis as a cause of acute renal failure, though this may be clinically obvious. A stick test for haemoglobin in the urine will be positive for myoglobin. Further distinction between the two proteins calls for laboratory investigation.

The presence and concentrations of certain nephrotoxic drugs can be determined in the laboratory: these include lithium, gentamicin, and cyclosporin A. Nephrotoxic drugs not routinely analysed for include amphotericin, morphine and tetracyclines.

CHRONIC RENAL FAILURE

The easiest way of understanding this insidiously developing syndrome is to invoke the so-called 'one nephron' hypothesis. Imagine that a patient only possessed one nephron, what would happen? Well, first, the glomerular filtration rate will be very low, so circulating concentrations of urea will rise dramatically. Consequently, urea will act as an osmotic diuretic because, after the iso-osmotic reabsorption of water and solutes by the proximal convoluted tubule, the remaining high urea solute load will counteract any ADH-driven urine concentration. Paradoxically, chronic renal failure is therefore associated with a diuresis, one of relatively fixed osmotic strength. (In reality, of course, a patient with a single active nephron would be anuric. Blood levels of urea start to rise when about 60–70% of nephrons have been lost. Polyuria would be maximal at around 80–90% nephron loss, but further nephron loss would lead to a progressive oliguria and, terminally, anuria). The net result is that patients are unable to regulate their fluid volume, so cannot tolerate increases in fluid intake, or dehydration resulting from decreased intake or increased extrarenal losses.

The remaining biochemical features of chronic renal failure become easy to understand. A metabolic acidosis ensues because the remaining nephrons, and the urine into which they are pumping $[H^+]$, are saturated: their capacity is insufficient for the excretion of the normal daily metabolic generation of H^+. If the original disease process is primarily tubulointerstitial, the capacity of the tubular cells to excrete acid will already be suboptimal.

K^+ is almost completely reabsorbed in the proximal convoluted tubule, to be resecreted in exchange for Na^+ at the distal convoluted tubule. Hyperkalaemia is therefore usual in chronic renal failure, because, in a situation analogous to that of H^+, the capacity of the remaining terminal convoluted tubules to secrete K^+ is exceeded. (In reality, however, chronic renal failure rarely leads to a clear loss of nephrons, and the remaining nephrons may sometimes possess damaged convoluted tubules. If the damage is predominantly proximal, then the early reabsorption of K^+ is incomplete, and the patient loses K^+ in the urine to develop hypokalaemia and/or a total body deficiency of K^+.)

Among other substances excreted at a reduced rate in chronic renal failure are drugs that may need to be given in smaller or less frequent doses and, in a few toxic examples such as gentamicin and digoxin, will require monitoring of the serum concentration.

Further findings in chronic renal failure

Serum calcium concentrations As the kidney becomes more damaged, its capacity to convert 25-hydroxy vitamin D to its active form by 1α-hydroxylation becomes increasingly impaired. As a result, calcium absorption and bone mineralization decrease, and serum calcium concentration may tend to fall. To some extent, the acidosis counters this effect by causing an increased amount of the total calcium to be ionized, and by favouring bone demineralization, but the main factor is the secondary hyperparathyroidism.

Corrected calcium, allowing for serum albumin, is accepted clinically as being more reliable than measured serum total calcium. Although ionized calcium seems a theoretically attractive analyte, and is measured by some machines, its routine place is unestablished.

Serum phosphate concentrations Phosphate excretion is promoted by the action of PTH, but when the glomerular filtration rate falls below 40 ml/min, the capacity of the kidney to excrete phosphate is limited, even under maximal stimulation of PTH, so serum phosphate rises. The hyperphosphataemia itself leads to increased secretion of PTH. These changes are further affected by other factors, including vitamin D status, dialysis, acidosis, and aluminium therapy.

Renal bone disease is thus contributed to by many causes, but there is no doubt that its severity can be reduced by remedying the deficiency of 1α-hydroxylated forms of vitamin D, thereby correcting calcium deficiency. Further, serum phosphate levels can be controlled by phosphate-binding agents taken orally. In conjunction, both manoeuvres can reduce the degree of hyperparathyroidism.

Serum uric acid concentrations Uric acid is reabsorbed by the proximal convoluted tubule, where some is then resecreted. The resecretion appears to be the rate-limiting step, so in chronic renal failure serum uric acid levels rise in parallel with those of urea, for the same reason that serum $[K^+]$ and $[H^+]$ rise.

The biochemical monitoring of chronic renal failure

As in acute renal failure, the primary aim is to prevent life-threatening complications by assessing when end-stage renal failure has developed and when intervention in the form of dialysis or transplantation needs to be considered. Depending on the nature of the renal disease and on factors related to the individual's physiology and lifestyle, electrolyte imbalance, fluid balance or uraemia, any one alone or in combination, may be the predominant feature that signals end-stage renal disease.

The basic routine tests include serum creatinine, urea, Na^+, K^+, Ca^{2+}, and albumin, 24-hour urine protein and creatinine clearance where possible. Serum bicarbonate is mainly used for patients being treated conservatively. Serum PTH is monitored with the aim of keeping it as low as is achievable in such patients, and where relevant to assess the degree of tertiary hyperparathyroidism.

DIALYSIS

Monitoring of patients on dialysis is much the same as that for patients with chronic renal failure, although more intense. Various tests have been developed to assess the adequacy of dialysis, usually by measuring the amount of urea removed during the procedure. These tests are discussed in detail in Chapter 10. Aluminium is also monitored as aluminium toxicity has been shown to be a factor that contributes to renal bone disease, particularly osteomalacia. Nowadays aluminium levels in the dialysate are therefore closely monitored to ensure they are low, and there is a reluctance to prescribe aluminium antacids and phosphate-binders. Nevertheless, dialysis is inefficient at removing aluminium, so serum levels are measured in patients given these drugs. Care is needed to avoid contamination of the blood and serum samples.

TRANSPLANTATION

Blood concentrations of the immunosuppressive drugs such as cyclosporin A and tacrolimus are monitored because metabolism is so variable between and even within individuals. The purpose is to ensure that levels are adequate to counter rejection, but not so high that toxicity, including nephrotoxicity, results. Creatinine clearance measurements provide a useful indicator of graft function. Most of the other routine monitoring tests may also apply to transplanted patients.

Further reading

Clague, A. and Krause, H. (1997) The diagnosis of renal tubular acidosis. Broadsheet No. 40, *Pathology*, **29**, 34–40.

Krepper, M.A., Verbalis, J.G. and Nielsen, S. (1997) Role of acquaporins in water balance disorders. *Curr. Opin. Nephrol. Hypertens.*, **6**, 367–78.

Preuss, H.G. (ed.) (1993) *Clinics in Laboratory Medicine: Renal Function*, W.B. Saunders, Philadelphia (**13**,1).

Wells, M. and Lipman, T. (1997) Pitfalls in the prediction of renal function in the intensive care unit. A review. *S. Afr. J. Surg.*, **35**, 16–19.

Haematology

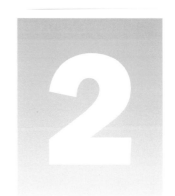

John Bradley

Anaemia

In chronic renal failure, anaemia is associated with inappropriately low plasma levels of the hormone erythropoietin, which is synthesized and secreted predominantly, by the peritubular cells of the renal cortex. Although other factors such as reduced red cell survival, iron deficiency and retained inhibitors of erythropoiesis may all contribute to the low haematocrit, more than 90% of patients respond to treatment with erythropoietin, suggesting that deficiency of this hormone is the principal cause of the anaemia. The blood film in chronic renal failure is usually normochromic and normocytic. 'Burr' cells, with a characteristic spiked surface, are commonly seen in severe anaemia.

In normal individuals circulating levels of erythropoietin are 5–25 mU/ml, whereas in patients with severe haemolytic anaemia levels may reach 2000 U/ml. In chronic renal failure, as plasma levels of erythropoietin decrease, the haematocrit falls. Although there is considerable variation in the severity of anaemia associated with chronic renal failure, a significant correlation does exist between degree of renal impairment and the haemoglobin concentration. Patients with polycystic kidney disease often continue to produce erythropoietin and have a higher haemoglobin level than might be expected from the degree of uraemia, whereas anephric dialysis patients produce none and usually suffer from marked anaemia.

The increase in haemoglobin that occurs after administration of erythropoietin is associated with decreased fatigue, increased exercise tolerance, and a reduction in the need for blood transfusion. In patients with predialysis advanced renal failure, erythropoietin has been reported to correct anaemia and improve well-being, without affecting the rate of decline in renal function.

Before starting to administer erythropoietin it is necessary to:

- consider other causes of anaemia
- ensure adequate blood pressure control

- check iron stores to exclude iron deficiency and predict patients requiring iron supplements.

Iron deficiency is a frequent component of anaemia in haemodialysis patients, and is the commonest cause of failure to respond to erythropoietin. However, assessment of iron status is notoriously difficult in haemodialysis patients, as the usual markers of iron deficiency may not be present. A serum ferritin level of less than 100 µg/ml, transferrin saturation less than 20%, or the presence of hypochromia in more than 10% of red cells on a blood film have been identified as useful criteria.

Failure to respond to erythropoietin may result from:

- iron deficiency
- blood loss
- infection
- inflammatory conditions
- hyperparathyroidism
- aluminium toxicity
- malignancy
- vitamin B_{12} or folate deficiency

INVESTIGATION OF THE POOR RESPONDER TO ERYTHROPOIETIN

Assuming the patient is compliant and is receiving at least 200 U/kg/week (most patients respond to 75–150 U/kg/week), re-assess iron status. If there is any doubt about the iron status of a patient who has failed to respond to erythropoietin, a trial of intravenous iron should be considered. If iron deficiency has been excluded, the following investigations should be performed.

- Reticulocyte count – a reticulocytosis (of at least 3–4%) occurs in haemolysis or blood loss. Increased serum bilirubin, reduced haptoglobins, or fragmented red cells on a blood film suggest the presence of haemolysis. Otherwise a reticulocytosis that is not accompanied by a rise in haemoglobin suggests blood loss, usually from the gastrointestinal tract. The finding of faecal occult blood provides supportive evidence for this, and strengthens the case for investigation of the gastrointestinal tract to exclude peptic ulceration, angiodysplasia, diverticular disease and malignancy.
- Serum vitamin B_{12} and folate levels. Macrocytosis may not be present due to concurrent iron deficiency. Folate losses are rarely a problem in dialysis patients, and can be readily replaced by dietary or oral folate supplementation.

- C-reactive protein – provides the best measure of underlying infection or inflammatory disease as the erythrocyte sedimentation rate is unreliable in renal disease (p. 31).
- Aluminium level – aluminium overload causes a microcytic anaemia that is resistant to treatment with erythropoietin, possibly by interfering with iron utilization. Even in the absence of severe anaemia or microcytosis, aluminium may contribute to the poor response to erythropoietin. The presence of aluminium staining on > 30% of trabecular bone surface appears to provide the best marker for haematopoietic toxicity from aluminium. In such cases, chelation therapy with desferrioxamine to reduce the aluminium burden improves the anaemia.
- Parathyroid hormone level – the presence of secondary hyperparathyroidism is associated with a poor response to erythropoietin. This effect may predominantly be consequent upon bone marrow fibrosis.

Polycythaemia

Polycythaemia accompanied by increased plasma erythropoietin levels occurs in a number of renal conditions. It occurs in 2–10% of patients with hypernephroma, although anaemia is a commoner finding, occurring in one-third of patients. Increased erythropoietin production may occur within the tumour, or in surrounding ischaemic tissue. Renovascular disease may be complicated by polycythaemia, presumably as a consequence of renal ischaemia. Simple renal cysts, polycystic disease and medullary cystic disease have all been associated with polycythaemia. Hydronephrosis and renal parenchymal disease are rare causes of polycythaemia.

Polycythaemia complicates 15–20% of cases of renal transplantation. Although it can occur in the presence of normal renal transplant function, it often complicates rejection, renal artery stenosis or hydronephrosis of the transplanted kidney. Venesection and cessation of diuretic therapy correct the polycythaemia and reduce the risk of thromboembolism. Theophyllines or angiotensin-converting enzyme inhibitors reduce the haematocrit in some cases.

Leucocyte abnormalities in renal failure

Total neutrophil and monocyte counts are usually normal in patients with chronic renal failure, but there is often a moderate lymphopenia. However, functional abnormalities can be demonstrated in all leucocyte populations, and are likely to account for the increased incidence of infection in uraemic patients.

NEUTROPHILS

In vitro neutrophils from uraemic patients demonstrate reduced chemotaxis to a number of stimuli including *Escherichia coli*, C5a and immune complexes. Phagocytic function is impaired, and oxidative metabolism is diminished, reducing the capacity of neutrophils to produce free radicals. These impaired functional responses *in vitro* contrast with the neutrophil activation that occurs in patients undergoing haemodialysis. Complement activation following contact of blood with dialysis membranes is thought to trigger this neutrophil activation. Neutrophil aggregation and adhesion to endothelial cell surfaces, particularly in the lungs, occurs within 30 minutes of starting dialysis, leading to neutropenia, and possibly accounting for the breathlessness experienced by some dialysis patients.

MONOCYTES

Chemotactic and phagocytic capacities are reduced in monocytes from uraemic patients. In addition, monocyte Fc receptor function is impaired in uraemic patients. During dialysis, monocyte activation similar to that observed in neutrophils, is thought to occur.

LYMPHOCYTES

A reduction in both the number and function of lymphocytes is associated with impaired cellular immunity in patients with chronic renal failure. Cutaneous anergy, delayed rejection of allografts and impaired immuno-globulin production in response to vaccines have all been demonstrated. Only 50% of dialysis patients mount an antibody response to hepatitis B vaccination.

Coagulation

PLATELETS

Platelet number is characteristically normal in patients with renal failure, although platelet adhesiveness and aggregation are both reduced, resulting in a prolongation of the bleeding time. Clinically this manifests itself as a bleeding tendency with bruising, bleeding from operative sites and gastro-intestinal blood loss.

Several factors may contribute to the platelet defect.

- Uraemic toxins – *in vitro* uraemic platelet function can be restored to normal by incubation in normal serum. Furthermore, the prolonged bleeding time can be partially corrected by dialysis.
- Qualitative and quantitative abnormalities of factor VIII:von Willebrand factor (FVIII:vWF) multimers, which serve to cross-link platelets to exposed surfaces. 1-deamino-8-D-arginine vasopressin (DDAVP) transiently corrects the prolonged bleeding time, probably through the transient release of FVIII:vWF complexes from storage sites in endothelial cells. Cryoprecipitate, which contains FVIII:vWF multimers is also effective.
- Altered prostaglandin metabolism – serum thromboxane B_2 is reduced in patients with renal failure, reflecting a reduction in platelet thromboxane B_2 synthesis.
- Anaemia – correction of anaemia by transfusion or erythropoietin frequently corrects the bleeding time.

COAGULATION FACTORS

Acquired abnormalities of coagulation factors in patients with renal disease can result from urinary loss, renal sequestration, or abnormal distribution of extracellular fluid. They are rarely associated with bleeding problems. Most commonly, factors involved in the intrinsic pathway are reduced (Figure 2.1), leading to prolongation of the activated (kaolin) partial thromboplastin time (APTT or KPTT). The APTT is the time taken for the patient's citrated plasma to clot when phospholipid (a platelet substitute), kaolin (activates factor XII) and calcium are added. It measures deficiencies of factors V, VIII to XII and fibrinogen.

HYPERCOAGULABILITY IN RENAL DISEASE

Hypercoagulable states occur most commonly in patients with the nephrotic syndrome. Alterations in antithrombin III, protein S and fibrinolysis are thought to be the most important abnormalities.

Antithrombin III is a **ser**ine **p**rotease **in**hibitor (**serpin**) that inhibits the actions of factors VII, IX, X, XI, XII and thrombin. Protein C is a vitamin K-dependent coagulation factor that inhibits the effects of factors V and VII by limited proteolysis. Protein C activity is dependent upon the presence of protein S, which forms a calcium-dependent complex with protein C and phospholipid.

Low levels of antithrombin III occur as a result of urinary loss in patients with heavy proteinuria. Low protein S levels may also result from urinary loss, although levels of free protein S may also be reduced in renal disease as

Fig. 2.1

The coagulation cascade.

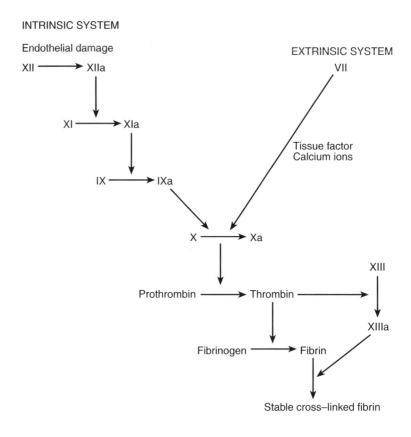

INTRINSIC SYSTEM

Endothelial damage

XII → XIIa

EXTRINSIC SYSTEM

VII

XI → XIa

Tissue factor
Calcium ions

IX → IXa

X → Xa

XIII

Prothrombin → Thrombin

XIIIa

Fibrinogen → Fibrin

Stable cross–linked fibrin

a result of elevated levels of C4b, which acts as a binding protein for protein S. Protein C is highly negatively charged, and heavy urinary losses are unusual. Levels of protein C vary in renal disease, but protein C activity is often reduced.

Reduced fibrinolytic activity in renal disease may result from urinary loss of plasminogen, or accumulation of fibrinolytic inhibitors such as plasminogen activator-inhibitor. Triglyceride levels are often increased, and correlate inversely with fibrinolytic activity.

HAEMOLYTIC URAEMIC SYNDROME AND THROMBOTIC THROMBOCYTOPENIC PURPURA

Acute renal failure in the haemolytic uraemic syndrome (HUS) and thrombotic thrombocytopenic purpura (TTP) results from occlusion of intrarenal arteries and arterioles by platelets and fibrin thrombi. There is thrombocytopenia due to platelet consumption, but coagulation factors are normal. This contrasts with disseminated intravascular coagulation in which prothrombin and partial thromboplastin times are increased, and fibrinogen and factor V levels are reduced. Elevated levels of fibrin degradation products in HUS and TTP may result from breakdown of fibrin thrombi. The rupture of red cells as they pass through regions of intravascular coagulation causes a microangiopathic haemolytic anaemia. The laboratory features are those of a haemolytic anaemia with reticulocytosis, increased plasma unconjugated bilirubin and decreased plasma haptoglobins. The diagnostic feature of microangiopathic haemolytic anaemia is the presence of red cell fragments on a blood film.

ERYTHROCYTE SEDIMENTATION RATE

The erythrocyte sedimentation rate (ESR) is a widely used measure of the acute phase response. It is a measure of the rate of sedimentation of red cells in a vertical tube of citrated blood. Sedimentation is increased by erythrocyte aggregation, which is enhanced by the presence of large molecular weight plasma proteins, including fibrinogen, α_2-macroglobulin and immunoglobulins. The ESR is elevated in over 90% of patients with end-stage renal disease, and measurement has little clinical usefulness. Possible reasons for the raised ESR in patients with chronic renal failure include age, anaemia, increased fibrinogen levels and hypocalcaemia, either through a direct effect of the reduced calcium level, or as a result of increased parathyroid hormone levels.

Further reading

Bathon, J., Graves, J., Jens, P. *et al.* (1987) The erythrocyte sedimentation rate in end stage renal failure. *Am. J. Kid. Dis.*, **10**, 34–40.

Bauer, C., Koch, K.M., Scigalla, P. and Wieczorek, L. (eds) (1994) *Erythropoietin: molecular physiology and clinical applications*, Marcel Dekker, New York.

Bia, M.J., Cooper, K., Schnall, S. *et al.* (1989) Aluminium induced anemia: pathogenesis and treatment in patients on chronic haemodialysis. *Kid. Int.*, **36**, 852–8.

Descamps-Latscha, B. and Herbelin, A. (1993) Long term dialysis and cellular immunity: a critical survey. *Kid. Int.*, **43**, S135–42.

Eberst, M.E. and Berkowitz, L.R. (1994) Hemostasis in renal disease: pathophysiology and management. *Am. J. Med.*, **96**, 168–79.

Rao, D., Shih, M. and Mohini, R. (1993) Effect of parathyroid hormone and bone marrow fibrosis on the response to erythropoietin in anaemia. *N. Engl. J. Med.*, **328**, 171–5.

Examination of the urine

Peter Mathieson

As a young house physician on a renal unit in London, the author was indoctrinated with the idea that as well as the usual history and physical examination, a full medical assessment of a new patient should incorporate an analysis of the urine, including microscopy of the urine sediment. To present a patient to the consultants without including such information was asking for trouble. This was sound advice, and it is indeed important to have an understanding of the usefulness of examining the urine, while also having an awareness of its limitations. Using fast, simple methods, additional information about the patient with known or suspected renal disease can often thus be obtained. Occasionally, management may be radically affected. With the current emphasis on screening and preventive medicine, analysis of the urine should form part of good general clinical practice, enabling earlier diagnosis of kidney disease and thus offering the opportunity for more effective intervention.

Taking the history

QUANTITY AND TIMING

Patients will usually notice if there is a sudden change in the volume of urine they pass, although this more often applies to an increase in urinary volume rather than to a severe **reduction** in urine output, which may in fact be of more urgent clinical importance. Patients are particularly likely to report nocturia since this disturbs normal sleep patterns. The thirst reflex is powerful, and the need to take a drink to the bedside table at night is often a useful indicator that the power of urinary concentration may be abnormal. Nocturia is a common and non-specific symptom in chronic renal failure, especially if the primary disease affects the tubulo-interstitium, but may also result from a more specific defect, for example in diabetes insipidus when it will usually be associated with polydipsia (excessive thirst) and daytime urinary frequency.

When there is frequency of micturition, associated dysuria (pain or discomfort on passing urine) may indicate the presence of urinary infection, although this symptom can occur with particularly concentrated urine or as a result of blood, chemicals or other irritants being present in the urine. The passage of frequent small volumes of urine may also indicate infection, but can be due to bladder dysfunction or disease, including neurological disease, or to psychological factors.

Incomplete bladder emptying, or double micturition, where the patient has to pass urine twice or more in rapid succession in order to achieve a feeling of complete emptying, may indicate bladder pathology. Double micturition is said to have some specificity for the presence of a bladder diverticulum or vesico-ureteric reflux since, in both these situations, when the bladder contracts to empty, some urine will travel in the 'wrong' direction and then return to the bladder once the initial voiding is over.

When the only symptom of renal dysfunction is oliguria (defined arbritrarily as excretion of less than 400 ml of urine in a 24-hour period, which is insufficient urine to allow adequate excretion of the waste products of metabolism), it may take several days for the patient and/or carer to notice. Unfortunately, this failure to appreciate the presence and/or significance of oliguria often applies to health care professionals as well as to patients, leading to frustrating delays in referral to a nephrologist and/or correction of the underlying problem.

APPEARANCE

Urine (and indeed any other water-based liquid) that contains a significant amount of protein will tend to form froth when agitated vigorously. The patient will notice this when voiding into a toilet bowl, and since males tend to do this from a greater height than females, usually facing forwards, there may be a gender influence on reporting of this observation! Patients often look surprised when asked if their urine is frothy (beer drinkers usually appreciate the analogy if you ask them whether their urine has a 'head' on it!), but occasionally this is a useful sign. For example, a patient who has had a remission of his/her nephrotic syndrome and then notices that the urine has become frothy again should seek medical attention.

Discoloration of the urine causes alarm and will usually lead to a visit to the doctor. Ironically, this is particularly the case if the urine is a vivid colour, when the cause is usually innocent such as food colouring, beetroot, or drugs (e.g. rifampicin). More subtle alterations in colour, particularly a reddish-brown tinge due to red blood cells, may be more sinister but are often ignored, at least initially. If this symptom **is** reported, it is important to establish any antecedent events, e.g. trauma, fever/intercurrent viral illness (associated with haematuria especially in IgA nephropathy, see pp. 107–108), or vigorous physical exertion (exercise-induced haematuria). Medical rarities may present with abnormalities of the appearance of the urine. Examples are intermittent acute porphyria, when excess porphobilinogen may give the urine a red-brown discoloration that darkens further on standing; and alkaptonuria, which is characterized by urine that goes black on standing due to the oxidation of the homogentisic acid that is excreted in excess by individuals with this inborn error of metabolism.

The urine

SPECIFIC GRAVITY

This is rarely informative when taken in isolation, but every student knows the specific gravity of the urine in chronic renal failure (1.010, isosmolar with plasma). A dilute urine (specific gravity closer to 1.0) first thing in the morning is unusual and should raise the suspicion of a failure of urinary concentration (e.g. diabetes insipidus).

pH

This varies widely in health, but the pH of an early morning sample should usually be acid. If it is not, renal tubular acidosis is possible (failure to acidify the urine) or a systemic alkalosis may be present (in which case the alkalinity of the urine is appropriate). If renal tubular acidosis is suspected, the patient can be given ammonium chloride (0.1 g/kg body weight) and the urine pH be measured again. Unfortunately, ammonium chloride commonly causes vomiting, but if the drug is ingested successfully and the urine is not rendered acid then a defect of urinary acidification has been proved.

TASTE

The enthusiasm of nephrologists for examination of the urine does not usually extend to tasting it, and this is certainly not advocated as a clinical routine! This section is included merely to stress that the original diagnostic test for diabetes mellitus was to taste the sweetness of the urine. Glycosuria can occur without elevation of the blood glucose, such as, for example, because of a reduced renal 'threshold' for glucose (e.g. in pregnancy), or because of renal tubular damage leading to glucose leakage. Nevertheless, it should always be regarded as an indication for simultaneous measurement of blood glucose and, if in doubt, for formal assessment of glucose tolerance.

Dipstick testing

This is useful both for screening and for serial assessment in patients with known renal disease. Sticks are available to test for a specific substance such as albumin, or to perform multiple tests, e.g. for protein, blood, glucose, bilirubin and ketones on one stick. Stick tests for protein are semi-quantitative: a 'trace' of protein may be normal but any more than a trace is not, and protein excretion should then be quantified (see below). 'False-positive' tests for protein may occur when large amounts of blood or pus are present in the urine, but these should be evident on urine microscopy. Dipsticks that test for leucocyte esterase are now available as a simple screening test for pyuria, but the usefulness of these is influenced by the fact that false-negatives and false-positives have been reported in association with the use of various antibiotics. Positive stick tests for blood should always be an indication for urine microscopy, and many urologists now feel that a single positive sample for haematuria should be an indication for investigation (pp. 41–42). False-positives occur with haemoglobinuria (e.g. associated with intravascular haemolysis, which is rare) or myoglobinuria (e.g. with overt rhabdomyolysis or with lesser degrees of muscular damage, such as following vigorous physical exertion). As mentioned above, glyco-suria should always lead to an assessment of glucose tolerance. Ketonuria is normal in fasting samples but assumes greater significance in diabetes mellitus, especially if associated with glycosuria.

Further analysis of proteinuria

The finding of positive stick tests for protein should be followed by formal quantification of protein excretion, and ideally by further characterization of the nature of the proteins (p. 37). Quantification requires either collection of all urine passed in a defined time period, usually 24 hours, or analysis of the protein concentration in a single urine sample. In the latter case, correction is required to take account of variability due to varying degrees of concentration of the urine. This is usually performed by expressing the ratio of albumin excretion to that of creatinine, giving an albumin:creatinine ratio. This may be particularly accurate on early morning samples, and gives a reasonable prediction of the daily albumin excretion, although this would seem to be true mainly at low levels of proteinuria.

Timed collections have advantages for serial measurements, especially in patients with nephrotic-range proteinuria, but human error is always a possibility when these are used, most commonly because of inadequate explanation of what is required rather than poor compliance. It is important to explain that urine present in the bladder at the start of the time period should be discarded, but urine present in the bladder at the end of the period must be included. The author usually explains that the aim is to collect all the urine that the body has 'made' during the set period. Patients should pass urine at a defined time of day and discard it, then collect all subsequent urine passed until the same time the next day, when they should pass urine and this time include it. Overnight samples are more convenient than 24-hour samples, and probably just as good. These have the added advantage of avoiding being misled by orthostatic proteinuria, a phenomenon seen in some apparently healthy adolescents or young adults in whom proteinuria is postural, being present in the upright posture but absent when recumbent.

When urinary protein is predominantly albumin, the proteinuria is said to be 'selective'. When there is a more generalized protein leak, the proteinuria is 'non-selective'. Protein selectivity is usually expressed as the ratio of IgG (molecular weight 160 000) to transferrin (molecular weight 80 000, similar to albumin which is 70 000). Highly selective proteinuria with a ratio of IgG:transferrin below 0.1 is typical of minimal change nephropathy and said to be a good prognostic sign, at least in childhood nephrotic syndrome.

When urinary total protein excretion is markedly elevated (above 3 g per day), it will usually indicate excessive albumin excretion and be suggestive of glomerular disease (Chapter 7). For lower levels of total protein excretion, it may be important to analyse further the constituent proteins. The main protein excreted in normal urine is Tamm–Horsfall glycoprotein, which is synthesized by renal tubular cells. Renal tubular damage from any cause leads to excessive excretion of low molecular weight proteins such as α_2- and β-globulins, especially β_2-microglobulin: when these predominate in the urine the proteinuria is said to be 'tubular'.

Bence Jones proteinuria is the term given to the excretion of free light-chains and is indicative of a plasma cell dyscrasia such as myeloma, when light-chains are typically synthesized in excess of heavy-chains. The excess light-chains are of sufficiently low molecular weight (20 000 to 40 000) to be filtered at the glomerulus, and since no mechanism exists for the efficient reabsorption of such large quantities of light-chains by the renal tubule, they are excreted in the urine. Bence Jones protein is best detected by electrophoresis of the urine, when it appears as a narrow band. The urine should ideally be artificially concentrated before electrophoresis to improve the diagnostic yield. The type of light chain can be identified by specific antisera, and if the source is a monoclonal proliferation of plasma cells, the light-chains should all be of the kappa or lambda type. Simple screening tests for Bence Jones protein include gentle heating (the protein precipitates at about 45°C then redissolves on boiling) and Bradshaw's test, where urine is gently layered on to a few millilitres of concentrated hydrochloric acid in a test tube and a thick white precipitate forms at the interface. Bradshaw's test will not give a positive result with albumin, but excess intact globulin will give a precipitate, so that if there is non-selective proteinuria in a patient with the nephrotic syndrome, leading to excretion of IgG, this test will be positive.

Detection of low levels of albuminuria, so-called 'microalbuminuria', has been widely used for the early detection of diabetic nephropathy. Specific assays for albumin are available, and the albumin excretion rate can be calculated from a timed urine sample. Normal is less than 20 µg/min (equivalent to 28.8 mg in 24 hours); 20–200 µg/min is the range referred to as microalbuminuria; albumin excretion rates in excess of 200 µg/min (so-called 'macroalbuminuria') are associated with dipstick-positive proteinuria and, in the context of diabetic renal disease, are taken to indicate established ('overt') nephropathy. It is generally accepted that measures aimed at halting the progression of diabetic nephropathy should be directed at those individuals with microalbuminuria, since the renal lesion at this stage may be reversible. Since these levels of albuminuria will not, by definition, be detectable by conventional dipstick testing, screening strategies for early detection of incipient diabetic nephropathy require sensitive and specific assays for albumin.

Urine microscopy

This is ideally performed on a freshly voided sample, although delays of an hour or two make little difference. The urine should be briefly centrifuged (1000 rev/min for 2–3 minutes) or left to stand for approximately an hour. (Routine urine microscopy in diagnostic laboratories usually uses un-centrifuged urine, and this largely explains the lower detection rate of abnormalities of the urinary sediment in such samples.) Most of the urine is then poured away, and the sediment resuspended by gentle shaking or flicking. A drop of urine is placed on a microscope slide, a cover slip placed over it, and the urine examined by microscopy. Phase-contrast microscopy is best, but a simple optical microscope will suffice. Staining is not essential. It is usual to start by scanning the sample at low power ($\times 10$), and then to examine any areas of interest at higher power ($\times 40$). Casts are often best studied by moving the focus up and down to visualize the different planes of the tubular structure of the cast. Examination of the urine in a haemocytometer allows easy quantification of red and white cell numbers, which can be useful for monitoring disease progression or response to therapy.

RED BLOOD CELLS

These are biconcave discs without nuclei and appear brownish in colour in unstained urine. They may appear as smooth, regular cells of uniform size, or they may vary in size and shape (Plate 1). The latter, so-called 'crenated' or 'dysmorphic' red cells, are generally more suggestive of a glomerular origin for the bleeding, and the former usually indicate bleeding from more distal sites in the urinary tract. Using phase contrast microscopy, it is usually possible for experienced observers to make this distinction. Various techniques have been proposed to distinguish 'glomerular-type' red cells from others: flow cytometry, Coulter analysis, measurements of mean cell volume, etc. can all provide objective measures of red cell size and volume and the degree of variability in a given sample. The assessment of haematuria is considered further below.

WHITE BLOOD CELLS

These are nucleated cells, larger in size than red blood cells. Lymphocytes appear as round cells with a single round nucleus and little cytoplasm, polymorphs as larger cells with multilobed nuclei and more cytoplasm. Granules can often be seen in the cytoplasm of polymorphs, but neutrophils cannot be distinguished from eosinophils without staining. This is rarely important, but simple staining techniques can be used by diagnostic laboratories to confirm or deny eosinophiluria if this is suspected, such as, for example, in association with allergic interstitial nephritis. The presence of bacteria (small refractile dots or rods, usually motile in fresh samples) suggests infection, when the accompanying white cells will usually be neutrophils. The assessment of bacteriuria is considered further below.

EPITHELIAL CELLS

These are larger polygonal cells with abundant cytoplasm. A large number suggests perineal contamination of the sample, casting doubt on the significance of any associated bacteriuria.

CASTS

Casts are cylindrical structures that are several times larger than blood cells. Excessive shaking of the sample, prolonged centrifugation or undue delay in performing microscopy may all lead to disruption of intact casts, when only fragments will be seen and distinction from debris/artefacts may be difficult. Inexperienced urine microscopists worry about their ability to identify casts, but they are usually obvious as long as low light is used and the plane of focus is moved up and down to assess the structure of any objects seen. Artefacts such as hairs, threads of fabric and so on can be easily distinguished. Casts are typically of uniform diameter along their length and fit one of the following subtypes.

- **Hyaline casts** appear as translucent structures without any formed elements within the structure (Plate 1). They may occur in normal urine but are present in increased numbers when there is proteinuria.
- **Granular casts** have discernible cellular debris within them. They may be 'finely' (Plate 2) or 'coarsely' (Plate 3) granular depending on the size of the fragments making up the structure. They are often brownish in colour. They indicate cellular disintegration within the renal tubules, where casts are believed to form, and therefore indicate renal parenchymal damage. They are not specific for any particular disease process.
- Cellular casts are made up of intact cells and are of great significance and more specific diagnostic value than other types of cast. Those containing intact red blood cells (Plate 4) are indicative of glomerular disease; casts comprising intact white blood cells (Plate 5) are seen with interstitial nephritis or pyelonephritis.

CRYSTALS

These are often seen in normal urine, and while they may be spectacular in appearance they are rarely of diagnostic use. Acid urine typically contains calcium oxalate crystals; alkaline urine may contain ammonium magnesium phosphate ('triple phosphate') crystals.

MISCELLANEOUS

Spermatozoa, which may appear in normal urine (from both males and females!), look like tadpoles and are of no pathological significance. Yeasts are small round refractile structures that are smaller than red blood cells; *Trichomonas vaginalis* are pear-shaped organisms about twice the size of white blood cells and have flagella at one pole. Various artefacts may be seen and will be easily recognized by virtue of size, bizarre structure or absence on repeated samples.

URINE CYTOLOGY

This is a specialist subject. If urothelial malignancy is suspected, fresh urine should be sent to a cytology laboratory for analysis: malignant cells can be identified by experienced observers and the presence of suspicious or frankly malignant cells is an indication for further urological investigation.

Urinary infection

If urinary infection is suspected, great attention must be paid to the techniques for obtaining a urine sample suitable for use in laboratory confirmation. A mid-stream sample of urine is conventionally suggested, but it is probably more important to make sure it is a 'clean' sample than a mid-stream one. In males, the foreskin should be peeled back; in females, the labia must be held apart and the peri-urethral area cleaned from front to back with swabs soaked in sterile water (not antiseptics). If there is continuing uncertainty, samples of urine can be obtained by urethral catheterization or by suprapubic aspiration. The latter technique may be particularly useful in young children, from whom it is difficult to obtain a 'clean-catch' sample.

Quantification of urinary bacteria is now routine in diagnostic bacteriology laboratories, and is usually expressed as colony counts or colony-forming units per ml of urine (cfu/ml). There is good evidence that a colony count of more than 10^5 cfu/ml is indicative of 'significant' bacteriuria. Of course, this does not necessarily equate with **clinical** significance: the patient's symptoms and the clinical context should always be taken into account. Furthermore, the absence of this level of bacteriuria does not exclude infection: lower colony counts or negative urine cultures may be reported, especially if there has been prior use of antibiotics.

Various methods have been employed to facilitate the rapid and reliable diagnosis of urinary infection. The 'dipslide' is a microscope slide coated in culture medium which can be dipped into the urine sample and then transported to the laboratory: the density of colonies growing on the slide after incubation at 37°C for 24 hours can be directly assessed. As mentioned earlier, dipsticks are becoming available to detect pyuria; some dipsticks include a test for nitrite, the presence of which in the urine is suggestive of infection. There is still a use for simple urine microscopy, however. The direct visualization of bacteria and the associated leucocytes is straightforward and rapid, allowing early diagnosis and treatment pending laboratory confirmation of the nature of the infecting organism and its pattern of antibiotic sensitivity.

Assessment of haematuria

If red blood cells are confirmed by microscopy and there is no evidence of trauma, stones or infection, further investigation is warranted. Urologists may undertake cystoscopy, urine cytology, imaging of the kidneys and urothelial tract; nephrologists will require blood tests for autoimmune disease and may offer renal biopsy (Chapter 7). Patients taking anticoagulants should be assessed in an identical manner: these drugs may provoke bleeding from a pathological lesion but do not in themselves provide adequate explanation for haematuria. As mentioned earlier, the origin of bleeding into the urine can sometimes be inferred from the morphology of the red cells, but more commonly the decision about whether to pursue urological or nephrological investigations is made on other grounds, e.g. the age of the patient or whether the referring practitioner knows his/her local urologist better than the local nephrologist!

Unnecessary waste of time and resources can often be avoided if attention is paid to simple clues. Again, the merits of urine microscopy must be emphasized: small and/or misshapen red cells suggest a glomerular origin; the presence of casts points to a renal lesion; the same is true when the haematuria is associated with proteinuria. Any or all of these findings should lead to a nephrological referral. The age of the patient is often used to infer the most likely cause of haematuria, and it is certainly the case that urothelial malignancy is uncommon before the age of 40, and that renal disease is more likely than cancer in children or adolescents. However, malignancies do occur at earlier ages, and glomerulonephritis can occur at any age from cradle to grave. If the initial investigations (be they nephrological or urological) fail to provide an explanation, the complementary set should be undertaken. However, in 15–20% of cases, detailed investigations fail to detect significant pathology. In such individuals, repeat urine testing for red cells is required, and investigations (especially urological) should be repeated if the problem persists.

Urinary electrolytes

These are mainly useful in the patient with acute renal failure, especially if a 'prerenal' element is suspected (i.e. a failure of renal perfusion due to hypotension, intravascular volume depletion, or reduced renal blood flow). Urinary electrolytes are underused: in selected patients this simple test can give useful prognostic information and can sometimes guide management. If a patient with acute renal failure has a low urinary sodium concentration (< 10 mmol/l) and a high urinary urea (usually expressed as the urine:plasma urea ratio, high values being greater than 10:1), this indicates avid sodium conservation by the kidneys and the ability to concentrate the urine appropriately. This is a good prognostic sign: the kidneys are still working well enough to retain sodium and excrete urea. In this situation, correction of the prerenal problem can be expected to salvage the situation. If, on the other hand, the patient with a prerenal problem has a high urinary sodium (> 40 mmol/l) and a low urine:plasma urea ratio (< 4), then established renal damage has supervened. Of course, measures should still be taken to correct the underlying prerenal problem, but the likelihood of escaping established renal failure is lower.

The one other situation where urinary sodium is useful diagnostically is when the hepatorenal syndrome is suspected (Chapter 9), when a low urinary sodium is typical because of secondary hyperaldosteronism.

Urine abnormalities in renal stone disease

The recent passage of a renal calculus will usually be obvious from the history. When there is doubt, the presence of haematuria supports the diagnosis. More important in the context of renal stone disease is a consideration of investigations that can lead to identification of predisposing factors and to intervention to reduce the risk of recurrence. If a stone can be retrieved for laboratory analysis, useful information can be obtained. Calcium oxalate-containing stones are the most common: timed urine collections should then be performed, in containers with an acid preservative, to assess urinary excretion of calcium and oxalate since increases in either will predispose to stone formation. Uric acid stones (more difficult to detect while still in the patient because they are typically radiolucent) should lead to measurement of the urinary excretion of urate, in containers with no preservative. Calcium phosphate stones form in alkaline urine, and a failure to acidify the urine, such as because of renal tubular acidosis, should be excluded. Stones made up of a mixture of calcium, magnesium and ammonium phosphate (known as 'triple phosphate', or struvite) are typically associated with alkaline urine and with persistent urinary infection, especially with urea-splitting organisms such as *Proteus*. Rare types of stones are those made up of xanthine or cystine, which occur when inborn errors of metabolism lead to excessive excretion of one of these amino acids.

More commonly, the stone is long gone and a decision must be made about how extensively to investigate the patient who gives a history suggestive of the passage of a renal calculus. The plasma calcium should be checked: hypercalcaemia requires further investigation, particularly to exclude conditions such as primary hyperparathyroidism and sarcoidosis. At least one 24-hour urine collection should usually be performed: hypercalciuria in the presence of a normal serum calcium is perhaps the most commonly identified metabolic abnormality predisposing to stone formation. Citrate is a natural inhibitor of stone formation, and hypocitraturia may be an important predisposing factor: 24-hour urine collections to quantify citrate excretion can be justified on the grounds that administration of potassium citrate may provide a simple means of reducing the risk of recurrence. Persistently alkaline urine, especially in early morning samples, is noteworthy: urinary infection should be excluded, and if none is found, renal tubular acidosis should be suspected and tests of urinary acidification undertaken. Certain further clues may be obtained from a careful history: a history of ileal disease, resection or bypass should raise the suspicion of enteric hyperoxaluria. Stones in childhood and/or a positive family history of renal calculi suggest the possibility of primary hyperoxaluria. In both situations, urinary oxalate should be measured by timed collection of urine.

Other urinary parameters

The urine is a convenient vehicle for the analysis of certain chemicals and metabolites in non-renal disease: examples are excretion of 5-hydroxyindole acetic acid (5HIAA), the main metabolite of 5-hydroxytryptamine (5HT), in carcinoid syndrome; vanillylmandelic acid (VMA) and catecholamines (adrenaline and noradrenaline) in phaeochromocytoma; phenolphthalein in suspected laxative abuse, when alkalinization of the urine gives a pink colour; and analysis for alcohol, drugs or metabolites in toxicological testing.

There has been considerable interest recently in the measurement of urinary levels of various markers of immunological activity in glomerulonephritis, mainly as a tool to avoid serial renal biopsies in the assessment of disease activity and/or in the selection of patients for immunotherapy. Examples are the soluble interleukin-2 receptor, a marker of T lymphocyte activation, in minimal change nephropathy where it is said to be an early indicator of impending relapse; interleukin-6 which may be a marker of disease activity in those forms of nephritis that feature mesangial cell proliferation, especially IgA nephropathy; platelet-activating factor, which is present at high levels in the urine in several forms of nephritis; and, perhaps most promising of all, markers of complement activation such as the C3 breakdown product C3dg or the soluble form of the membrane attack complex C5b-9, which are useful markers of ongoing immunopathological activity in membranous glomerulonephritis and possibly predictive of a good response to immunosuppressive therapy. This last example is perhaps one of the easiest to understand and is a neat illustration of the value of examining urine since the site of the tissue injury in membranous nephropathy is at the subepithelial portion of the glomerulus, i.e. on the urinary side of the glomerular basement membrane. It is therefore natural that if complement activation is occurring at this site, in free communication with the urinary space, then measurement of a product of that complement activation in the fluid that bathes the area, namely the urine, should provide an excellent surrogate marker for assessment of the disease activity.

The role of immunosuppressive treatment in membranous nephropathy remains controversial, particularly the best means of selecting patients for active therapy with potentially hazardous drugs in order to optimize the risk:benefit ratio. Analysis of urinary levels of products of complement activation may play an important part in this selection process in future.

Conclusions

Analysis of the urine can give valuable insights into the processes taking place in the organ in which it was formed. Modern technology has allowed automation of certain aspects of urine analysis, and has also allowed the production of simple standardized kits and dipsticks for rapid reliable analysis of the urine and its contents. However, no technical expertise nor any sophisticated equipment is needed for the performance of simple urine microscopy, which should remain part of the routine assessment of the patient with known or suspected renal disease. Whether by these simple methods or by more technologically-advanced procedures, it is foolish not to take the opportunity nature affords us to examine directly the fluid that has so recently left the organs we wish to study.

Further reading

Coe, F.L., Parks, J.H. and Asplin, J.R. (1992) The pathogenesis and treatment of kidney stones. *N. Engl. J. Med.*, **327**, 1141–52.

Fogazzi, G.B., Passerini, P., Ponticelli, C. and Ritz, E. (1994) *The Urinary Sediment*, Chapman & Hall Medical, London.

Kon, S.P., Couples, B., Short, C.D. *et al.* (1995) Urinary C5b-9 excretion and clinical course in idiopathic human membranous nephropathy. *Kid. Int.*, **48**, 1953–8.

Schröder, F.H. (1994) Microscopic haematuria. *Br. Med. J.*, **309**, 70–2.

Williams, J.D., Asscher, A.W., Moffat, D.B. and Sanders, E. (1991) *Clinical Atlas of the Kidney*, Gower Medical Publishing, London.

Immunological tests in nephrology

David Oliveira

Immune-mediated disease plays a significant role in nephrological disorders. The availability and interpretation of a number of different immune assays is therefore of particular significance, especially in the setting of un-diagnosed acute renal failure. The most widely used serological markers of immune-mediated renal disease are measures of complement activation and auto-antibody production.

Complement

The normal complement system (Figure 4.1) consists of the classical and alternative pathways that converge at C3. The subsequent common pathway involves the formation of the membrane attack complex. The classical pathway may be activated by the Fc portion of antibody molecules; at least

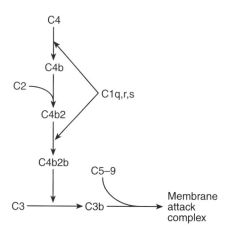

Fig. 4.1
Classical pathway and membrane attack complex.

Fig. 4.2
Alternative pathway and
amplification loop.

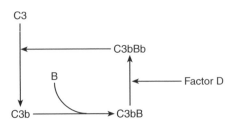

two of these are required in close proximity, and may be provided by a
single IgM molecule or two IgG molecules. Following binding of C1q, C1s
is subsequently activated and leads to the formation of the classical pathway
convertase. A similar sequence of events may also be triggered by the
binding of the mannan-binding protein to carbohydrate residues on micro-
organisms. The alternative pathway (Figure 4.2) has similarities to the
classical pathway but differs in that it is continuously being activated at a
low rate. Control of this tick-over is provided by competition between
factor B and factor H for binding to C3b. Factor H acts as a co-factor for
the enzyme factor I, which inactivates C3b. This background is important
when interpreting the various assays of complement components or function and associated antibodies relevant in nephrology.

The complement system directly lyses bacteria and cells via the membrane attack complex. Its products opsonize antigen, facilitating phagocytosis. They also act as mediators of inflammation, promoting neutrophil
aggregation and homing, chemotaxis and mast cell degranulation. In
addition to these traditional roles, it is becoming clear that products of the
complement system (e.g. C3d) interact with the acquired immune system,
directing lymphocytic responses towards pathogens, which bind complement components in an antigen-specific fashion (O'Rourke, Tooze and
Fearon, 1997).

COMPLEMENT OR COMPLEMENT-RELATED ASSAYS

An overall assessment of the classical pathway and formation of the
membrane attack complex may be obtained by assessment of total haemolytic activity in the form of the CH50 assay. This test determines the
volume of serum (as a source of complement components such as C1q)
required to produce the haemolysis of 50% of a standard quantity of red
cells presensitized with antibody bound to their surface. This lysis is
secondary to the eventual formation of the membrane attack complex.
Deficiencies in any of the components from C1 through to the membrane
attack complex (Figure 4.1) may therefore lead to a reduction in the CH50.
An important limitation is that certain components of this pathway (e.g. C3

and C4) are normally present in serum at levels well above those required for normal haemolytic activity. A normal CH50 assay will therefore not exclude reduced levels of these components. This limitation can of course be overcome by assaying the individual components, and this is usually done for C4 and C3. A reduced C3 concentration may reflect activity of either the alternative or classical pathways, whereas a reduced C4 concentration will reflect classical pathway activity only. A raised concentration of C3 or C4 is commonly found as part of an acute phase response and has little diagnostic significance.

It is possible to measure a variety of the breakdown products of complement activation. Such assays can be useful in determining a level of complement activation insufficient to result in depletion of C3 and/or C4, and also in determining whether a low level of any of these components is due to activation or decreased synthesis. However, these assays are not generally available and are usually confined to a research setting.

There is a number of different autoantibodies to a variety of complement components. C3 nephritic factor (C3Nef) is an autoantibody that binds to and stabilizes the alternative pathway C3 convertase C3bBb. This leads to continuous activation of the alternative pathway, and its presence is usually associated with profound C3 depletion. Occasionally, very low concentrations of C3Nef are compatible with a normal C3 concentration. A number of different assays for C3Nef rely on this stabilizing property. Less common nephritic factors include another autoantibody, which appears to activate the alternative pathway but differs from classical C3Nef in requiring prolonged *in vitro* incubation for activation. In addition, it also appears to be dependent on properdin. An analogous autoantibody that binds to and stabilizes the classical pathway convertase C4b2a has also been described.

In addition to the nephritic factors described above, there are at least two autoantibodies with specificity for C1q. One detects a neoantigen exposed when C1q binds to a solid phase or an immune complex. The second antibody binds to C1q in the fluid phase and is associated with profound depression of circulating C1q levels. Apart from C3Nef, antibodies interfering with the complement cascade are rarely measured in clinical practice.

INTERPRETATION OF COMPLEMENT AND COMPLEMENT-RELATED ASSAYS

As mentioned above, a raised level of complement components is not of diagnostic significance. The main issue is therefore an interpretation of hypocomplementaemia. In general, this may be due to genetic deficiencies, immune-mediated activation of the complement system, or non-immune-mediated activation.

Genetic deficiencies of all the complement components have been described. Partial deficiencies, e.g. of C4, are quite commonly represented in the population. A complete deficiency of any component will be reflected in a reduced CH50, but a partial deficiency of C4 may only be apparent from a lowered concentration of this particular component. Absolute deficiencies of components of the classical pathway have an extremely strong association with immune complex disorders such as systemic lupus erythematosus (SLE). It is very likely that such deficiencies are in fact causal, and represent a failure of the normal role of the classical pathway in the safe disposal of immune complexes. There is also a higher instance of partial deficiencies of classical pathway components in patients with SLE, and again this may well contribute to the pathogenesis of the disease. It is therefore important to be aware that a low C4 in, for instance, the setting of SLE, may reflect a partial genetic deficiency and/or increased consumption.

Hypocomplementaemia due to immune-mediated activation may occur in the setting of certain isolated renal diseases, or in some systemic diseases that may affect the kidneys (Table 4.1).

Hypocomplementaemia with reduced serum C3 concentrations is found in almost 90% of cases of post-streptococcal glomerulonephritis. Activation appears to by mainly by the alternative pathway, but in some cases raised levels of the relevant degradation products suggest some activation of the classical pathway. Other forms of infection-related glomerulonephritis, such as those found in the context of infective endocarditis, infected ventriculo-atrial shunts and visceral abscesses, are also associated with hypocomplementaemia, but this is usually due to classical pathway activation, with

Table 4.1

Renal disease and hypocomplementaemia

Disease	Complement abnormalities	Type of activation
Post-streptococcal glomerulonephritis	↓C3	Alternative pathway
Glomerulonephritis secondary to infective endocarditis, infected ventriculo-arterial shunts, visceral abscesses	↓C4 ↓C3	Classical pathway
Mesangiocapillary glomerulonephritis type I	(↓C4) ↓C3	Alternative (and classical) pathway(s)
Mesangiocapillary glomerulonephritis type II	↓C3	Alternative pathway
Systemic lupus erythematosus	↓C4 ↓C3	Classical pathway
Cryoglobulinaemia	↓C4 ↓C3	Classical pathway

depression of both C4 and C3. Activation of the alternative complement pathway has been described in infective endocarditis associated with *Staphylococcus aureus*, and may be due to non-immune interactions with bacterial products such as staphylococcal protein A.

The various different forms of mesangiocapillary glomerulonephritis are variably associated with hypocomplementaemia and a variety of nephritic factors. The most clearly defined association is between type II mesangiocapillary glomerulonephritis (dense deposit disease) and C3Nef. Nearly all cases of type II mesangiocapillary glomerulonephritis are associated with hypocomplementaemia at diagnosis, and this is nearly always due to the presence of C3Nef. As might be expected from its mechanism of action, this produces profound depression of C3 due to alternative pathway activation with normal levels of C1q and C4. C3Nef and hypocomplementaemia may also be found in association with partial lipodystrophy, with or without type II mesangiocapillary glomerulonephritis. Recent work suggests that abnormal activation of the alternative pathway in the vicinity of the fat cell may contribute to fat cell damage and therefore to lipodystrophy.

Other forms of mesangiocapillary glomerulonephritis are more heterogeneous than type II, and in turn a variety of complement activation mechanisms may be involved. In some cases, circulating immune complexes seem to be involved, activating complement via the classical pathway. The longer acting properdin-dependent C3 nephritic factor has been detected in nearly every hypocomplementaemic serum from cases of type I and III mesangiocapillary glomerulonephritis. There is a good correlation between C3 activation by this nephritic factor *in vitro* and *in vivo* C3 concentration, suggesting that the factor is of pathophysiological significance. Analysis of all these various cases suggests that the hypocomplementaemia in type II mesangiocapillary glomerulonephritis is usually due to classic C3Nef activity, in type III to the slower acting C3 nephritic factor, and that type I is multifactorial, with contributions from both types of nephritic factor as well as activation by the classical pathway due to immune complexes.

Hypocomplementaemia is commonly found in active SLE, particularly in the context of renal involvement. There is an approximate correlation, with many individual exceptions, between the concentration of anti-DNA antibodies, circulating immune complexes and evidence of complement activation as shown by low C3 and C4 on the one hand, and activity of lupus nephritis on the other. Precisely which of these variables is useful for following disease activity needs to be determined in each individual patient.

Cryoglobulinaemia (p. 59), particularly type II cryoglobulinaemia, is characteristically associated with very low C1, C4 and C2 and slightly low C3, findings suggestive of generalized activation by the classical pathway.

There is a variety of non-immune causes of hypocomplementaemia that need to be borne in mind. These include the activation of the complement system produced by foreign membranes in the context of cardiopulmonary bypass and haemodialysis, the low C3 and occasionally decreased C4 seen in some patients with haemolytic uraemic syndrome and/or thrombotic thrombocytopenic purpura, and the hypocomplementaemia occasionally found in cases of cholesterol embolization.

Finally, the two autoantibodies to C1q mentioned above are found in different situations. The antibody to C1q in the fluid phase, which is associated with decreased circulating levels of C1q, has a strong association with hypocomplementaemic urticarial vasculitis, and is also found in some patients with SLE. Antibodies to the neoantigen of C1q may be found in some cases of mesangiocapillary glomerulonephritis and may lead to false-positive reactivities in some assays of circulating immune complexes.

Antiglomerular basement membrane antibodies

Antiglomerular basement membrane (GBM) antibodies occur in the setting of Goodpasture's syndrome: the occurrence of pulmonary haemorrhage together with acute glomerulonephritis. These manifestations may occur in the setting of other diseases, and therefore it is best to refer to this particular entity as anti-GBM disease or Goodpasture's disease. Although the condition is rare (annual incidence approximately 0.5/million population), early diagnosis is important in order to avoid irreversible renal damage and potentially fatal pulmonary haemorrhage. The ready availability and correct interpretation of an anti-GBM assay are therefore of particular importance.

CHARACTERISTICS OF ANTI-GBM AUTOANTIBODIES

A number of properties of anti-GBM antibodies are relevant when considering the assay and its interpretation. The antibodies are nearly always of the IgG class although rare examples of IgA and IgM anti-GBM antibodies have been found. Furthermore, there is a restriction to particular subclasses, notably IgG1 and IgG4. This restriction may be relevant to pathogenicity as IgG1 antibodies can fix complement and bind to Fc receptors, whereas IgG4 antibodies are much less active in these respects. Evidence for the pathogenicity of the autoantibody is provided by animal transfer experiments, the almost complete association between the antibody and the disease, and the correlation between the titre of antibody and the severity of the nephritis. There does not appear to be a change in affinity of antibodies with the evolution of the disease (at least in the peripheral blood), and serial titres may therefore be helpful in following the progress of the disease and in guiding treatment (immunosuppression and plasma exchange).

The epitope recognized by anti-GBM antibodies (known as the Goodpasture epitope) has been identified as the non-collagenous domain of the alpha-3 chain of type 4 collagen. This epitope appears remarkably constant from patient to patient in that a single mouse monoclonal antibody directed against the same epitope will block the binding of the vast majority of anti-GBM antibodies from different individuals. It is interesting that this epitope appears to be absent (as judged by lack of binding of anti-GBM antibodies) from the basement membrane of patients with Alport's syndrome. This hereditary form of nephritis and deafness is known to be due to defects in the alpha-5 chain of type 4 collagen, but presumably the resultant disorganization of the basement membrane means that the Goodpasture epitope on the alpha-3 chain is either not formed or obscured in some way. A further consequence is that renal transplants in patients with Alport's syndrome represent exposure to new antigens in the form of both the alpha-5 chain and the Goodpasture epitope. Such patients are at risk of developing anti-GBM disease, and serial monitoring for anti-GBM antibodies is therefore indicated.

As with many pathogenic antibodies, the amount of tissue damage is dependent upon factors in addition to antibody binding. This needs to be kept in mind when interpreting the relationship between the serum titre of the autoantibody and the clinical manifestation of disease. For example, it is well recognized that smoking contributes to the development of pulmonary haemorrhage in anti-GBM disease, and such haemorrhage may follow exposure to cigarette smoke with no change in the titre of the autoantibody. In animal models of anti-GBM disease, it has been shown that renal injury is exacerbated by intercurrent infection or the administration of inflammatory cytokines, and it is likely that similar effects apply in humans.

DETECTION OF ANTI-GBM ANTIBODIES

In routine clinical practice the most usual method of detection of anti-GBM antibodies is via some form of solid-phase immunoassay. This was originally developed as a radioimmunoassay but is now usually performed as an ELISA (enzyme-linked immunoadsorbent assay). The antibodies may also be detected by indirect immunofluorescence on a renal biopsy specimen, but confirmation of specificity of binding under these circumstances (short of eluting the antibody from the sample, which is a research procedure) is not possible. Finally, and again a research procedure, the antibodies can be characterized by Western blotting, that is identification of a specific band produced by separating the target antigen according to size and/or charge in a gel, then transferring to nitrocellulose and probing with patient sera.

The solid-phase assay is performed in a standard manner. A preparation that contains the non-collagenous domain of type 4 collagen isolated from the glomerular basement membrane (the antigen is also now available in recombinant form) is coated on to a solid phase, usually polystyrene plates. After washing and blocking non-specific binding sites, test and control sera are applied to the plate. After a further washing step, bound antibodies are detected with either a radiolabelled or enzyme conjugated anti-immunoglobulin reagent. Results are usually expressed as percentage binding with respect to a known positive control included in the same assay; results greater than 100% are therefore possible. A normal range is produced as usual using a number of samples from normal controls. Increased specificity in the assay may be obtained by pre-incubating serum samples with target antigen in a soluble form. This will reduce specific binding in the assay, but not non-specific binding.

Indirect immunofluorescence of renal biopsies is covered in Chapter 7, but the characteristic finding in anti-GBM disease is bright linear deposition along the GBM. It is impossible to confirm the nature of the target antigen recognized under these circumstance (as can be done for the solid-phase assay described above), and occasionally similar patterns are produced in diabetes mellitus and SLE. Western blotting is highly specific in allowing the identification of antibodies binding to fragments that can be unambiguously identified as the non-collagenous region of the alpha-3 chain of type 4 collagen. It remains a research technique, however.

INTERPRETATION OF RESULTS

In the presence of a characteristic clinical picture, a strongly positive result in the solid-phase immunoassay and/or the demonstration of linear staining by immunofluorescence on the renal biopsy allows the diagnosis of anti-GBM disease to be made with some confidence. False-positives in the solid-phase assay are most commonly due to non-specific binding, which can, to some extent, be controlled as described above. Occasionally, autoantibodies are present with specificity for other components of the glomerular basement membrane. There is little evidence that these are pathogenic and they may simply represent an immune response to neoantigens exposed by the ongoing inflammatory process. False-negatives in the assay may arise if an IgG-specific detection antibody is used in the assay and one of the rare non-IgG anti-GBM antibodies is present. There are also occasional cases that clinically fit the picture of anti-GBM disease and have linear GBM staining on the renal biopsy, but in which circulating autoantibodies cannot be detected. One possible explanation for this situation is that there are circulating autoantibodies present but at too low a concentration to be detectable in the solid-phase assay. Western blotting is occasionally successful in revealing some of these antibodies. Another explanation is derived from the fact that anti-GBM disease appears to be self-limiting, in that even without treatment the autoantibody response eventually disappears. In some cases, this may have happened by the time the patient presents. Under these circumstances diagnosis really depends upon the finding of linear immunofluorescence on the renal biopsy. Possible false-positives for this particular pattern have been mentioned above. Occasionally a false-negative is produced because the glomerulus and the GBM have been so disrupted by inflammation that the characteristic pattern is no longer seen.

CO-OCCURRENCE OF OTHER AUTOANTIBODIES

As mentioned above, the autoimmune response in anti-GBM disease is really very specific and does not reflect polyclonal activation. However, there is a subgroup of patients with anti-GBM antibodies who also have antineutrophil cytoplasmic antibodies (ANCA, see below). Some of these patients appear to have a small vessel vasculitis as the primary illness and the anti-GBM antibodies are directed against other components apart from the Goodpasture antigen, as mentioned above. Other patients clearly have classic anti-GBM disease; the contribution, if any, of ANCA to pathogenesis in these cases is unclear. Of even more dubious pathogenic significance is the demonstration, in a proportion of patients with anti-GBM autoantibodies, of a low titre of anti-mitochondrial antibodies, found more usually in primary biliary cirrhosis.

Antineutrophil cytoplasmic antibodies

The discovery of ANCA and subsequent delineation of the various autoantigens involved has made an important contribution to the classification and management of the systemic vasculitides. Although this is still a somewhat controversial area, the current consensus is that these antibodies are characteristic of the forms of vasculitis that involve small blood vessels. These include Wegener's granulomatosis, microscopic polyangiitis, isolated crescentic nephritis (this can be considered as a vasculitis confined to the kidney) and Churg–Strauss vasculitis. The existence of ANCA in other conditions such as Henoch–Schönlein purpura is still the subject of investigation. Together these conditions are much commoner than anti-

GBM disease and make an important contribution to nephrological work-load in terms of both acute and chronic renal failure; this highlights the importance of ANCA assays.

CHARACTERISTICS OF ANCA

ANCA are usually of IgG class. A number of authors have found restrictions to particular subclasses, but there is some inconsistency. An important subgroup of patients has IgM ANCA. This particular class appears to be associated with a high risk of pulmonary haemorrhage. It is possible that IgA ANCA may be present in some cases of Henoch–Schönlein purpura, but this is much less clearly defined.

There has been considerable progress in defining the specificity of ANCA. As originally defined by indirect immunofluorescence (see below), two fluorescent patterns were recognized: cytoplasmic staining (c-ANCA) or perinuclear staining (p-ANCA). It now seems clear that the majority of patients with c-ANCA have autoantibodies with specificity for proteinase-3 (PR3), a constituent of the neutrophil primary granule. p-ANCA are more heterogeneous, but a major target is myeloperoxidase (MPO). Other antigens that may give a similar perinuclear pattern of staining include elastase, lactoferrin, cathepsin G and bacteriocidal permeability-increasing protein; new specificities are continually being described.

Whether ANCA contribute to pathogenesis is a controversial question. Perhaps the most powerful piece of evidence is the demonstration by a number of groups that ANCA have the capability of activating neutrophils *in vitro*. It is not difficult to see how this property could contribute to tissue injury.

DETECTION OF ANCA

The original method of ANCA detection, and one that is still in wide use, is indirect immunofluorescence. For this procedure neutrophils from a normal donor are applied to a slide and fixed. Patient serum is then layered over the fixed cells and, following an incubation period, any ANCA that are bound to the neutrophils are detected with a fluoresceinated second layer with anti-immunoglobulin specificity. The results are read under a fluorescent microscope, preferably by an experienced observer with the appropriate positive and negative controls. This method essentially gives a qualitative result in terms of the presence or absence of ANCA, with a staining pattern that is usually classified as cytoplasmic, perinuclear or indeterminate. Some quantification may be attempted by an assessment of the intensity of the fluorescence or by the application of various dilutions of the original serum to obtain a titre.

Indirect immunofluorescence has been supplemented and to some extent superseded by the development of solid-phase immunoassays. These have the advantages of objectivity, and ease of standardization and quantification. They are performed in the same way as the anti-GBM assay. A target antigen is first coated on to the solid-phase. Originally this was a crude neutrophil extract, but purified antigens such as proteinase-3 and myeloperoxidase have become available more recently. The use of the crude extract may still have some advantages in the detection of as yet undefined specificities. Following incubation of dilutions of the patient's sera with the solid-phase, bound antibodies are detected, usually with an enzyme conjugated anti-immunoglobulin reagent. As with the anti-GBM assay, results may be given as a percentage of a positive control included in the same assay. Attempts to control for non-specific binding may also be made by pre-incubation of the sera with neutrophil extract or specific antigen.

INTERPRETATION OF RESULTS

In the appropriate population in nephrological practice, most typically patients with rapidly progressive glomerulonephritis, a positive indirect-immunofluorescence or a positive solid-phase assay for either anti-PR3 or anti-MPO has a sensitivity and specificity of greater than 90% for the diagnosis of a small vessel vasculitis. The combination of a positive c-ANCA indirect immunofluorescence pattern together with PR3 positivity, or a p-ANCA indirect immunofluorescence pattern together with anti-MPO positivity, increases the specificity to 99%, with some loss of sensitivity. There are differences between the clinical pictures, in that patients with Wegener's granulomatosis will tend to be positive for anti-PR3 antibodies, whereas those with microscopic polyangiitis are usually positive for anti-MPO antibodies. Renal-limited vasculitis occupies an intermediate position. Other clinical associations include antilactoferrin antibodies (p-ANCA pattern) in some cases of rheumatoid vasculitis.

A small number of cases of patients with primary systemic vasculitis are ANCA negative. This proportion is increased in disease that is limited to, for instance, the upper respiratory tract, and in cases that have received immunosuppressive treatment.

Other autoantibodies of nephrological significance

SLE, which may effect the kidneys in a wide variety of ways, is associated with the presence of a variety of autoantibodies. The most familiar are antinuclear antibodies (ANA), which are present in over 95% of untreated cases of SLE and which are detected by direct immunofluorescence on Hep-2 cells. However, they are also present in approximately 3–4% of normal Caucasoid patients. More specific for SLE are antibodies such as anti-Sm and anti-double stranded DNA. The concentration of anti-double stranded DNA antibodies has been shown to correlate roughly with the clinical activity of SLE, and very occasionally anti-double stranded DNA antibodies may occur in the absence of antinuclear antibodies. They are usually measured by Farr assay, although ELISAs are being used increasingly. Anti-Sm antibodies are seen in 30% of patients with SLE, and if detected they are highly specific for that illness. Active SLE is also one of the causes of a glomerulonephritis associated with hypocomplementaemia (see above).

Antiphospholipid antibodies may be seen in the context of SLE or other connective tissue diseases, or may occur on their own in the primary antiphospholipid antibody syndrome. The presence of these antibodies is associated with recurrent miscarriage, thrombocytopenia and arterial thrombosis. On occasion, the latter manifestation may involve the kidney, either at the level of the glomerular capillaries or in larger blood vessels. Antiphospholipid antibodies of differing properties may be detected by a variety of assays, including tests for anticardiolipin antibodies and for the lupus anticoagulant.

A number of other connective tissue diseases that may affect the kidney are also associated with characteristic autoantibodies. Mixed connective tissue disease, which probably has a similar range of renal manifestations to SLE, may also be associated with a variety of antinuclear antibodies, but in particular is characterized by the presence of antibodies to extractable nuclear antigens, such as anti-U1-RNP. Systemic sclerosis is also associated with a variety of antibodies, including Scl.70. The presence of PM-Scl antibodies identifies a small proportion of systemic sclerosis patients with a high frequency of myositis and renal disease.

Immunoglobulins and paraproteins

The routine measurement of the total amounts of the main immunoglobulin classes is of limited diagnostic utility in nephrology, although a general depression of all classes may help to point toward a diagnosis of myeloma. Although concentrations of IgA are raised in approximately 50% of cases of IgA nephropathy, this is of limited diagnostic use. More helpful is the detection of the products of abnormal B cell clones (paraproteins), and immunoglobulins that have the ability to precipitate in the cold (cryoglobulins).

PARAPROTEINS

A variety of more or less malignant monoclonal B cell disorders may be associated with the production of various paraproteins that have the potential for renal deposition. These include Waldenström's macroglobulinaemia, light-chain nephropathy, AL type amyloidosis, various forms of fibrillary glomerulonephritis and myeloma. Myeloma may be associated with either light-chain nephropathy or renal amyloid, but can also cause the characteristic myeloma kidney associated with intratubular deposits of paraprotein. Some of these conditions can be diagnosed by electrophoresis of serum and detection of the circulating paraprotein. In other cases free light-chains may be detected in the urine in the form of Bence Jones proteinuria (p. 37). Once a paraprotein has been detected, appropriate haematological follow-up is required for further diagnosis and treatment.

CRYOGLOBULINAEMIA

Immunoglobulins that have the capacity to precipitate in the cold are identified by observing a precipitate in serum collected and transported at 37°C and then incubated at 4°C. The precipitate is washed, reprecipitated, and then analysed by electrophoresis. Cryoglobulins thus detected may be classified into three types. A type I cryoglobulin is a monoclonal product of a B cell clone. It may therefore occur in the setting of any disorder associated with the production of a paraprotein. Electrophoresis of the cryoprecipitate protein shows only the monoclonal component. Type II, or mixed cryoglobulinaemia, has a monoclonal component, usually an IgM, which has rheumatoid factor activity. This is therefore associated with captured polyclonal IgG. Electrophoresis of the cryoprecipitate shows both the monoclonal and polyclonal components. Recent work has shown that the majority of cases of type II cryoglobulinaemia without an obvious underlying cause (previously known as mixed essential cryoglobulinaemia) are associated with hepatitis C virus infection. A type III cryoglobulinaemia simply consists of a polyclonal component only and is seen in association with any disorder that leads to long-term stimulation of the immune system and consequent polyclonal increases in immunoglobulins.

All forms of cryoglobulinaemia may be associated with hypocomplementaemia, reflecting activation via the classical pathway (p. 50), and immunopathology in the form of skin rash, arthralgias, renal and liver involvement. However, these manifestations are most characteristically seen in the setting of a type II cryoglobulinaemia. In addition to measuring complement components, quantification of the cryoprecipitinable protein can be useful treatment.

Circulating immune complexes

Circulating immune complexes may be measured by a wide variety of assays such as the Raji cell' assay, C1q binding, PEG precipitation and several others. These assays have different sensitivities and specificities and can also detect different types of immune complexes. In general, the nephrologist does not need to be too concerned with these aspects as the measurement of circulating immune complexes has a very limited clinical role. Although circulating immune complexes may well be involved in immunopathogenesis, it seems likely that the vast majority are not in fact free but associated with complement receptor 1 (CR1) on red blood cells. It is therefore not surprising that free circulating immune complexes do not generally correlate at all well with disease activity. There may be the occasional patient with, for instance, SLE in whom the measurable immune complexes do correlate with disease activity. However, from the nephrological point of view, other indices such as proteinuria and serum creatinine are likely to prove more valuable. There is therefore probably little place for measuring circulating immune complexes in nephrological practice outside a research setting.

HLA typing in renal disease

As with many other diseases that have a significant immunopathogenic component, a variety of renal diseases have associations with the major histocompatibility complex (MHC). The first of these to be described was an association between DR2 and antiglomerular basement membrane disease; subsequently a number of different MHC alleles have been associated with a variety of other renal diseases (Table 4.2).

Methods for MHC typing are evolving rapidly from serological to molecularly-based methods (Chapter 11). These investigations are generally expensive and do not have a place in routine clinical practice. They do, of course, have a valuable role to play in a research setting, where correct interpretation of the results really requires a detailed knowledge of the particular methodology being used; these considerations are beyond the scope of this chapter. In addition to the MHC, a number of other genetic markers that may be linked with a variety of renal diseases are being investigated, but these are also currently solely of research interest. They include immunoglobulin receptor polymorphisms and variants of alpha-1-antitrypsin in systemic vasculitis, and the association between various allotypes of the immunoglobulin molecules and antiglomerular basement membrane disease.

Disease	MHC association	Comment
Antiglomerular basement membrane disease	DR15	DR15 is a split of DR2
Membranous nephropathy	DR3	In Caucasoid population; link is with DR2 in Japanese
Systemic lupus erythematosus	DR3	Primary association probably with C4 null alleles found on DR3-bearing haplotypes
ANCA-positive vasculitis	DR13	Association is **negative**: patients have a significantly lower frequency of the allele (a split of DR6)
Minimal-change nephropathy	DR7	

Table 4.2
MHC associations in renal disease

Effects of renal failure on immune function

Uraemia has a generally depressive effect on a number of aspects of the immune system. The assays used to demonstrate this effect are mainly of research interest.

Of the specific elements of the immune system, there is a depression of both T and B cell function. T cells show a reduced ability to proliferate to a variety of antigenic stimuli. It is unclear to what extent this is due to deficient function of accessory cells, such as macrophages, dendritic cells or B cells, and to what extent it is a primary problem with the lymphocytes. Some degree of correction can be obtained by providing exogenous interleukin-2, suggesting that defective production of this important cytokine is at least partly responsible for the defect. The defective B cell response could of course be secondary to the defective T cell response, but again there may be a primary problem with the B cell itself.

Of the non-specific elements of the immune system, a defect in macrophage function has already been mentioned above. An opposite problem may be due to activation of macrophages during haemodialysis, particularly with cuprophane membranes. This leads to the production of interleukin-1 and tumour necrosis factor, which could be responsible for some of the long-term adverse effects of haemodialysis. There is also a defect in polymorphonuclear granulocytes, which show defective chemotaxis and a variable decrease in phagocytosis and the ability to produce a respiratory burst. These cells are also affected by dialysis with cuprophane membranes, which, following complement activation, lead to sequestration of granulo-cytes within the pulmonary circulation.

The above abnormalities of the immune system are clearly of pathological significance, as it is well recognized that uraemic patients have defects in immunity as shown by increased skin graft survival, increased susceptibility to various infections, and a poor response to vaccination. This last point is of particular significance as a proportion of patients will not respond well to immunization against hepatitis B.

Reference

O'Rourke, L., Tooze, R. and Fearon, D.T. (1997) Co-receptors of B lymphocytes. *Curr. Opin. Immunol.*, **9**(3), 324–9.

Further reading

Lachmann, P.J., Peters, D.K., Rosen, F.S. and Walport, M.J. (eds) (1993) *Clinical Aspects of Immunology*, 5th edn, Blackwell Scientific Publications, Oxford.

Oliveira, D.B.G. (1992) *Immunological Aspects of Renal Disease*, Cambridge University Press, Cambridge.

Radiology

Simon McPherson and David Lomas

Introduction

A wide range of imaging techniques are available for imaging the aetiology and sequelae of renal disease.

Plain radiographs provide high spatial resolution and contrast based on the differential attenuation of X-rays by bone, air and soft tissues. They are relatively inexpensive, widely available and are useful for assessing renal tract calcification and the bony skeleton. Soft tissue contrast is relatively limited and, because of the projection nature of the technique, radiographs can be complex to interpret, making the detection of renal outlines and subtle renal calcification difficult.

Contrast radiography, i.e. the intravenous urogram (IVU), provides an overview of the renal urinary collecting system, allowing the detection of lesions of the renal pelvis and ureter. It allows a basic assessment of the renal parenchyma and a crude overview of renal function. The IVU remains widely used for general assessment of the renal tract, but has been replaced in many areas of parenchymal assessment by cross-sectional imaging techniques such as ultrasound (US), X-ray computed tomography (CT) and, more recently, magnetic resonance imaging (MRI).

X-ray angiography is now a rapid procedure, frequently performed on an outpatient or day-case basis; it provides a high spatial resolution assessment of the renal tract vasculature. Although there are competing techniques such as US and magnetic resonance angiography (MRA) for vascular assessment, X-ray angiography remains the primary technique for demonstrating renal artery stenosis and permits therapeutic procedures such as angioplasty and stenting.

Ultrasound provides good soft tissue contrast based on differential tissue acoustic impedance. Developments over the last decades have allowed increasing spatial resolution and the application of a range of Doppler methods (pulse wave, colour and power Doppler) to demonstrate renal vasculature. It is widely available, portable, relatively quick to perform and permits multiplanar sectional views of the renal parenchyma and bladder. True renal size can be measured between the upper and lower poles, but this may be underestimated if care is not taken to obtain a true long axis measurement. A normal adult kidney will measure at least 9 cm, which equates to an IVU length of 11.5 cm (due to the inherent magnification in X-ray radiography). The presence of gas impedes ultrasound and commonly prevents adequate assessment of, for example, the ureter.

CT provides global cross-sectional imaging of the abdomen and improved soft tissue contrast when compared with plain radiographs. It provides an excellent overview of the renal tract and the relationships with other internal organs and their abnormalities. Both CT and radiographic procedures involve ionizing radiation and may require the use of intravenous contrast administration – factors that must be balanced against the diagnostic benefits. CT and US are both excellent techniques for guiding renal tract interventions such as biopsy, aspiration or drainage procedures.

MRI uses static and dynamic magnetic fields combined with pulsed radiofrequency energy to generate images with excellent soft tissue contrast but relatively poor sensitivity for calcification. MRI can provide much of the cross-sectional information generated by CT but is often less readily available and is currently unsuitable for guiding interventional procedures.

Nuclear medicine techniques play an important role in the assessment of renal function and metabolic bone disease. Although spatial resolution and geometric accuracy are limited, much clinically useful renal functional information is available from both static and dynamic studies (Chapter 6).

Renal vascular disorders

RENAL VEIN OBSTRUCTION

This is most commonly due to thrombus or tumour within the renal vein but may be caused by extrinsic compression (e.g. lymphoma or pancreatic tail carcinoma). Radiological appearances depend on the speed and extent of venous occlusion and the presence of collateral circulation. Chronic cases may be relatively asymptomatic, but in acute obstruction patients present with haematuria (rupture of venules/capillaries), pain, flank mass or renal impairment (if bilateral), which may influence the initial choice of investigation.

● Ultrasound will frequently demonstrate the intrarenal vessels and may provide a clear view of the hilum and main renal vein, particularly the right one. Colour and duplex Doppler may permit an experienced operator to diagnose renal vein thrombosis by the absence of main renal vein flow and the direct visualization of echogenic thrombus in the expanded renal vein. In the acute phase the kidney is typically enlarged and hypoechoic, becoming hyperechoic over time.

- Contrast-enhanced CT may demonstrate delayed renal enhancement, perinephric oedema (the so-called renal 'cobweb') and an enlarged renal vein that fails to enhance. CT complements US by demonstrating the left renal vein more clearly than the right.

- Where available, combined MRI and MRA will provide the same information without the use of intravenous contrast medium.

- IVU is not diagnostic, but in acute venous obstruction it demonstrates smoothly enlarged kidneys with a decreased nephrogram. The collecting system is frequently not opacified, but when it is the calyces may appear compressed and elongated owing to the parenchymal oedema. In up to 25% of chronic cases the IVU may be entirely normal owing to good collateral drainage, although in some people these vessels may be seen to notch the ureter.

- Venography is now rarely required. The inferior cavagram shows absent inflow from the renal vein or a filling defect protruding from the vein. Selective renal venography will be required to detect filling defects or occluded tributaries if the cavagram is normal.

- Scintigraphy is non-specific but may be useful in assessing split renal function.

RENOVASCULAR HYPERTENSION

Renovascular causes account for approximately 5% of hypertension in adult patients. The difficulty in making the diagnosis of **true** renovascular hypertension begins after the demonstration of an anatomical lesion suggesting renal artery stenosis (RAS). Approximately half the 50-year-old patients with hypertension will have atherosclerotic stenoses of the renal arteries that do not significantly contribute to their hypertension. In addition, RAS has also been demonstrated at autopsy in 49% of patients who were normotensive in life. It remains difficult to identify those with pure renovascular hypertension or essential hypertension combined with an angiotensinogenic component. Even selective renal vein renin sampling is neither sensitive nor specific enough to detect all patients who have renovascular hypertension. Elevated renin secretion that lateralizes to the affected side does, however, have a significant positive predictive value for treatable renovascular hypertension. The decision to treat is easier in younger patients, as an anatomical lesion is more likely to be significant, and the cost and side-effects of long-term medical treatment will be much greater. Regrettably, in some cases the only way of confirming renovascular hypertension is by demonstrating a response to revascularization.

RENAL ARTERY STENOSIS

RAS or renal artery occlusion may result in renovascular hypertension (discussed above) and/or renal insufficiency. When gradual in onset it is frequently asymptomatic, whereas acute occlusion can be painful, particularly when due to arterial dissection. Atherosclerosis underlies 75% of RAS cases, and fibromuscular hyperplasia 20%; numerous rare conditions such as irradiation, neurofibromatosis, Takayasu's disease, arterial dissection and emboli account for the remainder. There is continuing debate about the best method of investigating these patients, and local practice may vary depending on imaging expertise.

- US will usually show a normal echogenicity kidney of normal or reduced size. In acute occlusion the kidney may be of decreased echogenicity in the first week, and intrarenal arterial traces may be absent. Duplex Doppler studies may demonstrate the stenosis directly, or infer it by elevated absolute or relative peak velocities in the main renal arteries or by alterations of waveform shape in the intrarenal vessels. A disadvantage is the technically demanding nature and poor specificity of the examination, with false-negatives arising from multiple renal arteries and collateral vessels.
- Scintigraphy is considered elsewhere (p. 93).
- MRA and helical CT angiography can both demonstrate RAS with varying accuracy but variations in technique, repeatability and availability have so far limited their widespread use.
- IVU is now considered non-specific and insensitive for detecting RAS.
- Intravenous digital subtraction angiography is now widely considered inadequate for detecting RAS.

The above investigations have not yet demonstrated the required sensitivity, specificity and repeatability to detect RAS in the routine clinical setting. Their potential use is to screen patients for arteriography, although in patients in whom there is a high index of clinical suspicion arteriography should still be considered even where these screening tests are negative. Arteriography currently remains the most accurate method of diagnosis. A stenosis of greater than 50% diameter (reflecting a 75% area stenosis) is considered significant but where this is difficult to assess, pressure gradients can be confirmatory. Balloon angioplasty or stent insertion may be performed at the same time as a diagnostic examination. Fibromuscular hyperplasia responds well to angioplasty but atherosclerotic stenoses of the renal artery ostium respond less favourably. In this group, and those with more distal short segment occlusions, stenting has proved more effective.

In acute occlusion, US and scintigraphy may be diagnostic. Angiography may be used when necessary to confirm the diagnosis and may allow rapid revascularization in some situations; alternatively surgical revascularization will be necessary. To be successful revascularization must occur within the first hour of the acute event.

Correction of renovascular hypertension by surgery or percutaneous radiological treatment is considered superior to medical therapy as lowering blood pressure medically further decreases renal blood flow, which may lead to ischaemic atrophy or even infarction. Percutaneous techniques have the advantage of a lower complication rate and may be employed in patients considered high risk for surgery.

RENAL A-V MALFORMATIONS AND FISTULAE

These are frequently asymptomatic but may cause audible bruits, haematuria and occasionally increased cardiac output or even renal impairment (due to renal ischaemia). Fistulae may be congenital but are most commonly iatrogenic (e.g. following renal biopsy or percutaneous nephrostomy).

- Colour Doppler US will demonstrate most lesions clearly.
- Angiography confirms the diagnosis and, where appropriate, permits embolization (the treatment of choice), which is usually successful owing to the end-artery nature of intrarenal vessels.

DIALYSIS ACCESS GRAFTS AND FISTULAE

These are prone to occlusion by thrombus with or without stenoses, which commonly occur close to the venous or arterial anastamoses or in more central veins (the mechanism for the latter is not well understood).

- US will usually diagnose graft thrombosis and may demonstrate stenoses.
- Angiography will also demonstrate stenoses and areas of thrombosis, and permits therapeutic manoeuvres such as thrombolysis, mechanical thrombectomy and balloon angioplasty.
- Venography is helpful for surgical planning of dialysis grafts/fistulae, particularly revision procedures.
- MRA has also been utilized to assess fistula patency and to quantify fistula flow volumes.

Renal parenchymal disease

Imaging techniques have proved effective at demonstrating focal abnormalities of the renal parenchyma, but the diffuse changes associated with many causes of acute and chronic renal failure often produce non-specific findings. Ultrasound is the most appropriate investigation for assessing renal size, which is probably the most important imaging parameter.

In acute renal failure from parenchymal causes the kidneys may be of normal or increased size. A unilateral acutely swollen kidney suggests acute pyelonephritis, acute arterial infarction, acute renal vein thrombosis or acute obstruction. In chronic parenchymal diseases the kidneys may be of normal size but are more commonly reduced in size with global parenchymal loss or scarring. Focal defects or scars in the renal contour may result from infarction, previous trauma, reflux nephropathy, tuberculosis (TB) or calculus disease. Chronic renal enlargement of one or both kidneys often indicates an infiltrative process.

GLOMERULONEPHRITIS

Except for documenting reduction in overall renal size, imaging techniques have little to offer in the diagnosis of chronic glomerulonephritis. A spectrum of changes in parenchymal appearances has been described, such as loss of corticomedullary differentiation on ultrasound, but these changes are non-specific. There is no focal cortical loss and the papillae and calyces are usually normal.

ACUTE TUBULAR NECROSIS

Acute tubular necrosis (ATN) presents with acute oliguric renal failure that is usually reversible. It may be caused by drugs (including intravenous X-ray contrast media but not MRI agents) and ischaemia from many causes.

- Scintigraphy is usually diagnostic and demonstrates maintained perfusion with poor excretion (considered in detail on p. 91).
- Plain radiographs are rarely useful but may allow assessment of renal size and exclusion of nephrolithiasis.
- US is often used to exclude obstruction (but see below). In 90% of cases the renal size and texture is normal but oedema may result in renal enlargement with a relatively hypoechoic medulla and pyramids. The arterial trace may show an elevated resistive index (peak systolic velocity minus end diastolic velocity divided by peak systolic velocity), which is uncommon in prerenal failure (where the kidney is not oedematous).

- CT is rarely used but may demonstrate early ATN as an unsuspected finding when intravenous contrast has been employed. The renal parenchyma enhances but the collecting systems fail to opacify. In general, the use of intravenous iodinated contrast media should be avoided in patients with known marked renal impairment so as to avoid any exacerbation.

ACUTE CORTICAL NECROSIS

Many of the causes of ATN may also cause acute cortical necrosis which, unlike ATN, is irreversible. Obstetric hypovolaemic shock is the commonest cause, although unusual causes such as snake venom are more easily remembered. There is partial or total necrosis of the cortex with preservation of the medulla. The peripheral 1–2 mm of cortex is usually preserved due to its supply from separate capsular vessels.

- A calcified rim can be identified on plain radiographs as early as three weeks, but it usually takes longer to develop.
- The kidneys are smoothly enlarged in the early stages on US and may show loss of normal corticomedullary differentiation with hypoechoic outer cortex. Later the kidney shrinks, becomes hyperechoic and may show acoustic shadowing from peripheral calcification.
- CT may show peripheral calcification as early as the first week. The calcification can be patchy or linear (single 'pencil-line' or double 'tram-line'). The preserved rim of subcapsular cortex enhances on contrast-enhanced CT or MRI.

ACUTE PYELONEPHRITIS

Imaging is rarely indicated in uncomplicated pyelonephritis, but when flank pain or fever persist despite antibiotic treatment, then a renal abscess or underlying renal obstruction should be excluded. Radiological investigation can be useful at an earlier stage to help distinguish between renal colic and pyelonephritis, particularly if the patient is immunocompromised. Acute pyelonephritis may be diffuse or focal.

- US is normal in the majority of cases but non-specific renal enlargement may be seen in diffuse involvement. Occasionally focal disease may be apparent as a wedge of reduced echogenicity, or rarely high echogenicity, where there has been secondary haemorrhage.
- CT is often more informative than US as, in addition to renal enlargement, unenhanced CT may show focal or diffuse decreased attenuation (or increased attenuation if there is associated haemorrhage). A perirenal 'cobweb' with thickening of the perirenal fascia can occur. Following

intravenous contrast medium the main renal vein(s) will enhance (unlike in renal vein thrombosis), but wedges of reduced enhancement extending from the papillae to the cortical surface may be demonstrated. Delayed images (three to six hours) may show accumulation of contrast medium in these areas, which may form foci for subsequent abscess formation. The enhancement changes can persist over several weeks and may lead to the development of focal scarring.

- IVU is rarely required but may be performed to exclude obstruction. It is normal in up to 75% of patients and in the remainder there may be diffuse or focal swelling, reduced or delayed pelvicalyceal opacification or, in severe pyelonephritis, a persistent, striated or even absent nephrogram.

Rarely, infection by gas-forming organisms (usually due to facultative anaerobes such as *E. coli* or *Proteus*) results in emphysematous pyelonephritis. Diabetes mellitus or underlying obstruction are common associations. Plain films (or more sensitively CT) will demonstrate perinephric or collecting system gas. US may be difficult to interpret because of the high reflectivity at the gas/tissue interface.

INFILTRATIVE PROCESSES

In early **amyloid** there is deposition of extracellular protein resulting in enlargement of the kidneys and patchy or uniform increased cortex echogenicity, but quite rapidly the kidneys become damaged and scarring occurs, leading to the small contracted kidneys commonly found at the time of presentation. The kidneys are involved in about one-third of the patients with primary amyloidosis and in over 80% of those with secondary disease. The incidence of renal vein thrombosis is increased in these patients. Multiple myeloma may lead to amyloidosis but can also impair function by precipitation of abnormal proteins, reduced blood flow due to its high viscosity, or nephrocalcinosis.

Leukaemia is the commonest malignant cause of bilateral smooth generalized renal enlargement but it may also present as a focal mass prior to the development of more generalized disease.

Lymphoma is shown at post-mortem to have involved the kidneys in about half the patients with non-Hodgkin's lymphoma (NHL), whereas only 10% of Hodgkin's lymphoma patients have autopsy evidence of renal involvement. Imaging tends to underestimate involvement, with renal changes apparent in only about 5% of patients with NHL. US findings include diffusely enlarged hypoechoic kidneys and focal hypoechoic masses.

In focal disease, contrast enhanced CT may reveal homogeneous low attenuation masses, often with ill-defined borders.

DIABETES MELLITUS

The kidneys can be damaged structurally by three mechanisms in diabetes: glomerulosclerosis, ischaemia and ascending infection. In early glomerulo-sclerosis the GFR is increased and the kidneys enlarged. Ischaemia results from both the increased risk of atherosclerosis and afferent and efferent arteriolar lesions due to hypertrophy and hyalinization. Renal impairment and hypertension result and the kidney reduces in size. Ascending infection may result in pyelonephritis or renal papillary necrosis (p. 69 and p. 76, respectively). Administration of iodinated contrast media (X-ray contrast media) to diabetic patients carries an increased risk of ATN, particularly if they are dehydrated. US is the preferred method of assessing renal size. Investigation and treatment of large vessel disease is described above (p. 65–67).

AIDS

HIV nephropathy is considered a poor prognostic indicator, with mortality near to 100% at six months. Focal and segmental glomerulosclerosis leads to rapidly progressive renal impairment with marked proteinuria but only mild hypertension. Imaging is again relatively non-specific: there may be renal enlargement with increased echogenicity on US. Contrast enhanced CT may reveal a striated nephrogram after contrast medium, although in a small number the medulla may be hyperdense precontrast. Renal *Pneumocystis carinii* infection has become more common since the introduction of inhaled prophylaxis for *Pneumocystis carinii* pneumonia (PCP), because of the poor systemic distribution of pentamidine. The infection may result in focal renal cortical calcification (also seen in *Cytomegalovirus* (CMV) and *Mycobacterium avium-intracellulare complex* infections).

CONNECTIVE TISSUE DISEASES

In general the connective tissue diseases produce non-specific imaging changes in the kidneys indistinguishable from most other parenchymal diseases. One exception is polyarteritis nodosa, which involves the kidney in 85% of cases. *Arteriography* demonstrates multiple small intrarenal aneurysms of the interlobar, arcuate and interlobular arteries with or without arterial narrowing or cortical infarcts. Occasionally the aneurysms may be microscopic, preventing detection at arteriography.

NEPHROCALCINOSIS

Nephrocalcinosis is the deposition of calcium salts in the parenchyma whereas nephrolithiasis is the deposition of calculi in the collecting systems.

Medullary nephrocalcinosis describes pyramidal calcification (usually in the distal convoluted tubules). Hyperparathyroidism, medullary sponge kidney (p. 76) and renal tubular acidosis account for over 70%. Less common causes include sarcoidosis, idiopathic hypercalciuria and renal papillary necrosis.

- Plain radiography shows normal or enlarged (medullary sponge) kidneys with granular or linear calcification.
- CT is more sensitive than plain films for detecting renal calcification, but is rarely required for initial diagnosis.
- US can demonstrate early deposition. With absence of the normal hypoechoic renal pyramids and with more established deposition there may be focal or diffuse hyperechogenicity of the pyramids +/− acoustic shadowing (depending on the size of deposits).
- IVU may narrow the differential diagnosis, e.g. by confirming a diagnosis of medullary sponge kidney (see below).

Cortical nephrocalcinosis is rare. The characteristic patchy or continuous peripheral calcification may result from acute cortical necrosis or occasionally from chronic glomerulonephritis or renal transplant rejection.

Focal renal calcification may be caused by trauma (calcified haematoma), vascular problems (atherosclerosis, aneurysms), infections (tuberculosis, hydatid and atypical infections in immunocompromised patients such as CMV and PCP), or complicated cysts and tumours.

CYSTIC DISEASE

Simple (serous) renal cysts

These are considered to be a part of the normal ageing process, occurring in up to 50% of 50-year-olds, increasing with age. They may vary from several millimetres to several centimetres in diameter. They are acquired lesions, probably secondary to tubular obstruction. They are rare in childhood (incidence: 1 in 500) and adolescence. Simple renal cysts may be seen as a component of a number of rare inherited conditions including Turner's syndrome, tuberous sclerosis, von Hippel–Lindau syndrome and neurofibromatosis.

Adult polycystic kidney disease (APKD)

This is an autosomal dominant condition encoded for by more than one gene locus. Polycystic kidney disease 1 (PKD1), localized to chromosome 16, is both the most severe and most common (85%) form of APKD. Until all the gene loci have been identified, imaging is required to identify affected individuals in susceptible families. The presence of at least two cysts (unilateral or bilateral) has been suggested as sufficient to establish a diagnosis in an at risk individual under the age of 30 years. In 30–59-year-olds, at least two bilateral cysts, and in the over 60s, in whom simple cysts are common, at least four cysts on each side are the suggested diagnostic criteria. There is a spectrum of severity of APKD and different criteria may be required in older family members of non-PKD1 families. APKD is progressive and if there is doubt a follow-up examination can be useful. The cysts may be so extensive as to almost completely obscure the functioning renal parenchyma and markedly expand the overall renal size. Additional cysts may occur within the liver (30%) and pancreas (10%). MRA is increasingly being used as a non-invasive screening technique for the associated cerebral aneurysms in these patients.

Acquired cystic kidney disease

Also known as acquired cystic disease of uraemia, this is commonly demonstrated in the native kidneys of patients on chronic dialysis (both peritoneal and haemodialysis) and occasionally predialysis in chronic renal failure. Multiple small cysts (typically < 1 cm) are present. They are thought to arise as part of a proliferative parenchymal response to chronic renal impairment, but oxalate crystal deposition and vascular insufficiency have also been proposed as aetiologies. Renal adenomas and carcinomas are also more common in these patients, and it may prove difficult to distinguish between these and a complicated cyst.

Parapelvic cysts

These are extraparenchymal and intimately related to the renal pelvis but do not communicate with it and therefore typically do not opacify after intravenous contrast medium. It has been suggested that they arise from obstructed lymphatics, but some are probably due to simple cysts close to the renal sinus. They can be mistaken for hydronephrosis on US (particularly by inexperienced operators), and occasionally they may exert sufficient pressure on the adjacent renal pelvis to actually cause true obstruction.

- Ultrasound is diagnostic for the demonstration of most renal cysts that have the characteristic appearances (hypoechoic, homogeneous, well defined with posterior acoustic enhancement). Variations of appearance can occasionally create diagnostic problems: echoes visible within a cyst on ultrasound may be the result of haemorrhage or, rarely, infection, and CT may be required to confirm their cystic nature.

- Cysts can be diagnosed on CT by their well defined shape, homogeneous appearance and 'water' attenuation value (0–15 Hounsfield units). 'Hyperdense' cysts on CT may occur owing to a high protein content in the fluid, and their cystic nature may be confirmed by the absence of enhancement following intravenous contrast administration or by ultrasound; calcification may be present in the wall of an apparently simple cyst and this may reflect previous trauma and evolution of a subcapsular haematoma.

- On MRI, cysts demonstrate marked high signal on T2w images (owing to the long T2 value of water) and fail to enhance on T1w images following intravenous gadolinium administration.

Renal collecting ducts and pelvis

RENAL OBSTRUCTION

Renal obstruction is defined as an increased resistance to urinary flow. Most clinically significant obstruction causes hydronephrosis, but not all dilated collecting systems are obstructed (e.g. chronic vesico-ureteric reflux). The renal pelvis is normally maintained at low pressure despite high pressures in the ureter during peristalsis and in the bladder during micturition. In acute obstruction an elevated pressure develops in the renal pelvis and, as a result, structural and functional changes develop in the kidney (obstructive nephropathy). Dilatation of the renal pelvis is frequently minimal in the first few hours. The glomerular filtration rate (GFR) decreases after several days as the collecting system usually distends, and if the obstruction is prolonged over a period of months the renal pelvis pressure eventually becomes normal or subnormal and the renal pelvis chronically dilates. The degree of renal pelvis dilatation is, however, a notoriously poor indicator of the severity of obstruction, particularly in the acute phase. Non-invasive imaging methods can diagnose obstruction in many cases, but invasive urinary tract studies or a trial of percutaneous or retrograde drainage is occasionally necessary. It is particularly important in the investigation of suspected renal tract obstruction that imaging findings are interpreted in the context of the clinical history and examination and that previous renal imaging is available for comparison.

- A plain radiograph should be undertaken to exclude radio-opaque renal tract calculi, which remain the commonest cause of acute renal obstruction.

- IVU remains widely used for the diagnosis of acute obstruction and will typically demonstrate a delayed and increasingly dense nephrogram with delayed calyceal opacification of the collecting system. Spontaneous partial decompression may occur due to forniceal tears into the pyelo-sinus, leading to urinomas, or into the pyelovenous system, resulting in decompression into the circulation. Although ruptures can appear dramatic at IVU, urine leaks are rarely of clinical significance unless the urine is infected or the urinoma is large and persistent. In chronic obstruction, the findings vary. The kidneys may be markedly enlarged (indicating partial obstruction that is not sufficiently severe to significantly reduce the GFR), or small and atrophic.

- In established acute obstruction US may demonstrate a dilated pelvicalyceal system, usually with an otherwise relatively normal renal appearance. However, US may overlook acute obstruction in the earliest stages, when an IVU is more appropriate. In chronic obstruction US will demonstrate the dilated collecting system and allows an assessment of the renal size and parenchyma, which is often thinned and atrophic.

- Scintigraphy is frequently diagnostic and provides much more functional information than other radiological techniques but suffers from inherently poor spatial resolution. It is therefore often used in combination with other imaging investigations to determine the level and aetiology of obstruction.

- CT is not usually a first line investigation in the diagnosis of renal obstruction. Moderate and severe hydronephrosis may be found serendipitously on CT examinations performed for other reasons. Acute obstruction may result in a very dense nephrogram on one side following intravenous contrast medium with failure to opacify the collecting system. CT is most useful in demonstrating the cause of obstruction (e.g. radiolucent stones, periaortitis and other causes of retroperitoneal 'fibrosis', retroperitoneal malignancy, etc.).

- MR urographic techniques have been described that produce images similar to the IVU, but they have no functional component and therefore suffer the same limitations as US: potentially useful in chronic obstruction but limited in the acute phase.

- Antegrade pyelography may be rarely required in difficult cases where IVU is inconclusive, inadequate owing to renal impairment, or where obstruction is partial. Pressure-flow studies may be undertaken to assess ureteric obstruction directly.

- Retrograde pyelography may also be useful in patients where other investigations have been unhelpful and an intraluminal cause such as tumour is suspected.

RENAL CALCULI

Calculi vary widely in size and related symptoms. Stasis, dietary factors (high purine and protein intake), acquired and inborn errors of metabolism, and infection are important factors in many 'stone formers'. Calcium oxalate and phosphate stones (the most common, accounting for 70% of calculi), magnesium ammonium phosphate (also called triple phosphate or struvite) stones, and cystine stones are usually radiopaque. Triple phosphate stones are caused by infection with urea-splitting organisms (classically *Proteus*, but *E. coli*, *Klebsiella* and *Pseudomonas* also produce urease). Uric acid stones and xanthine stones are usually radiolucent on plain films, but a low kV technique film may detect them. Sloughed renal papillae resulting from papillary necrosis (see below) may calcify. They have a characteristic triangular shape with a rim that is denser than the centre.

RENAL PAPILLARY NECROSIS

This is a relatively uncommon but important cause of renal failure as progression may be halted if the cause is treatable. It may also present with recurrent ureteric colic, infections or sterile pyuria. There are multiple causes including analgesic abuse, diabetes mellitus, sickle cell disease, pyelonephritis (usually with obstruction), transplant rejection and poly-arteritis nodosa. The mechanism of papillary necrosis may lead to varying appearances at imaging. In partial necrosis there is dissection leading to cleft and cavity formation around the base of the papillae. As the papillae become necrotic they may calcify *in situ*, occasionally without cleft forma-tion, or slough off into the collecting system where they may cause obstruction and become foci for calcification. At this stage the affected calyces will appear excavated. Imaging may demonstrate a range of appear-ances relating to the degree of necrosis in adjacent papillae. Early on an important feature is the preservation of renal size and contour, although some scarring may occur late in the disease. This allows differentiation from other conditions such as renal TB and chronic pyelonephritis.

- IVU is usually diagnostic, demonstrating the development of clefts and cavities along with the later stages of papillary destruction, sloughing and calcification. Diagnosis is usually made on IVU. The renal outline and size are usually well preserved.

- Plain radiographs will demonstrate calcified papillae, which typically have angular margins and 'hollow'-appearing calcification.
- US will not detect the earliest stages but may suggest the diagnosis by detecting medullary cavity formation, or the sloughed papillae, particularly if calcified.

MEDULLARY SPONGE KIDNEY

Medullary sponge kidney is a sporadic congenital abnormality in which there is abnormal dilatation of the pyramidal collecting tubules within which stone formation commonly occurs. It may affect both kidneys, one kidney or only a portion of one kidney. An affected kidney is often mildly enlarged. There is an association with Caroli's disease and hemihypertrophy. It can present with urolithiasis, infection, and haematuria, or as an incidental finding.

- Plain radiographic demonstration of clustered multiple small medullary calculi may suggest the diagnosis.
- IVU is frequently diagnostic as contrast will collect around the concretions in the dilated terminal ducts and may demonstrate thick bands of contrast enhancement, which may be beaded, radiating from papillae ('bunch of flowers' appearance). It should be distinguished from a normal papillary blush in which there is no nephrocalcinosis or parenchymal banding.
- US may detect the early medullary calcification as regions of increased echogenicity, and is capable of detecting these changes before plain radiographs or CT.

Renal transplantation

DONOR IMAGING

In living-related donor transplantation imaging is required to establish that the donor will retain a normal functioning kidney post-nephrectomy and that there is no major structural or vascular abnormality of the proposed donor kidney (such as accessory renal arteries, which are associated with a poorer transplant outcome). The left kidney is usually preferred due to its longer vascular pedicle.

- US will detect solitary kidney, horseshoe kidneys, adult polycystic kidney disease, renal tumours and most calculus disease.

- Arteriography is still performed in many transplant centres to assess the renal vasculature. It is sensitive for demonstrating accessory renal arteries and occult vascular disease such as fibromuscular hyperplasia.
- Contrast enhanced helical CT and MRA techniques are evolving and where available may reduce the need for arteriography in the future.

EARLY GRAFT FAILURE

This may result from ATN, acute rejection, vascular thrombosis or ureteric obstruction.

- Scintigraphy in the form of serial ^{99m}Tc-DTPA (diethylenetriamine pentaacetic acid) studies will usually distinguish ATN from acute rejection primarily on the basis of the reduced perfusion that occurs in rejection.
- US provides good views of the transplant kidney and may demonstrate ureteric obstruction, when any surgical tube drainage has been withdrawn or is not employed, although as in the native kidney caliceal dilatation is minimal in early obstruction and serial studies may be required. US in experienced hands can also be diagnostic in the demonstration of renal artery or vein thrombosis.
- Angiography may be required to confirm a diagnosis of vascular occlusion.

PERIOPERATIVE COMPLICATIONS

Perinephric collections and ureteric leaks may occur.

- Antegrade pyelography via a drainage catheter sited in the renal pelvis at surgery is the preferred method, if available, for confirming a urinary leak.
- Scintigraphy is a sensitive alternative when antegrade studies are not possible, as IVU is often unhelpful in the early postoperative period owing to poor opacification.
- US will demonstrate perinephric collections, such as haematomas and urinomas, and guide any required percutaneous intervention such as drainage or aspiration. CT can provide the same information and guidance when US is technically difficult, for example in the obese patient or, rarely, when bowel gas obscures the view.
- Percutaneous stent insertion may be helpful for treating ureteric leaks and reducing the need for surgical repair.

LATE GRAFT COMPLICATIONS

Lymphocoeles may occur as persisting or recurring perirenal collections; they may be septated, and are well demonstrated by US, CT or MRI. Renal artery stenosis relating to the surgical anastamosis or from superimposed atherosclerosis may occur. Doppler US may detect these directly (colour Doppler) or indirectly by relative velocity changes, but in transplant vessels the anastamotic disturbance of blood flow makes interpretation difficult. Arteriography remains the definitive procedure and permits balloon dilatation or stenting where appropriate. Imaging is of little value in the diagnosis of chronic rejection or cyclosporin toxicity but may be helpful to exclude other causes of renal impairment such as obstruction.

Musculoskeletal imaging

RENAL OSTEODYSTROPHY

The musculoskeletal changes related to chronic renal failure are termed renal osteodystrophy and include hyperparathyroidism, rickets and osteomalacia, osteoporosis and soft tissue calcification. With the improved management of renal failure in recent years, the prevalence of severe radiological changes has reduced. Plain radiographs remain the primary method of demonstrating these changes, although scintigraphy is a more sensitive means of detecting the underlying metabolic changes.

HYPERPARATHYROIDISM

The prolonged hypocalcaemic stimulus of chronic renal failure may lead to secondary hyperparathyroidism with hypertrophy of all the glands or occasionally tertiary hyperparathyroidism with autonomous gland overproduction of parathyroid hormone. The skeletal changes observed on serial plain radiographs reflect the long-term activity of the underlying hyperparathyroidism and remain a useful means of monitoring the effectiveness of management.

Bone resorption is common and is manifested in several ways.

- Subperiosteal resorption of cortical bone is characteristic of hyperparathyroidism and is most frequently demonstrated along the radial aspect of the middle phalanges (especially of the middle and index fingers) of the hand. The medial proximal aspect of the long bones and the lamina dura of the teeth are other locations in which similar changes may be detected by plain radiography. More extensive resorption of bone leads to a 'lace-like' trabecular pattern, and eventually to complete cortical resorption. When marked these changes, may lead to resorption of the terminal phalanges (acro-osteolysis).

- Subchondral resorption of bone may occur particularly around the axial skeletal joints, e.g. sacro-iliac joints, where the changes may mimic sacro-ileitis.
- Brown tumours are, now rarely demonstrated, focal bone lesions where bone resorption has led to replacement by fibrous tissue and giant cells. Typically single, they may be centrally or eccentrically placed and involve the facial bones, pelvis, ribs or femora. They are usually well defined and radiolucent. They are more commonly found in primary hyperparathyroidism, and when treated may heal and become sclerotic.

Bone sclerosis is relatively common in secondary hyperparathyroidism and may be patchy or diffuse. When diffuse it may be difficult to detect initially but within vertebral bodies the sclerosis tends to be subchondral, deep to the endplates, leading to characteristic horizontal banding ('rugger jersey' spine). When combined with bone resorption severe changes may lead to fracture and vertebral body collapse.

RICKETS AND OSTEOMALACIA

These changes are now relatively uncommon and, in addition, are difficult to distinguish from other components of renal osteodystrophy. Osteopenia but more specifically Looser's zones may occur in the pubic rami, iliac bones, ribs, femoral necks and scapulae. They are usually narrow radiolucent bands, frequently symmetrical and perpendicular to the bone surface, and may underlie 'insufficiency' fractures. In children there may be irregularity and widening of growth plates, maturation delay and an increased risk of slipped epiphyses (especially of the femur).

SOFT TISSUE AND VASCULAR CALCIFICATIONS

Soft tissue and vascular calcifications are a frequent finding in renal failure. Soft tissue calcification is related to the product of calcium and phosphate concentration and may occur quite rapidly (in weeks) in a wide variety of soft tissues including the cornea, viscera and peri-articular tissues. They are best demonstrated by plain radiographs or CT, which usually underestimate the extent of such deposits when compared with histological examination. They are more frequently seen in patients treated with haemodialysis or transplantation. Vascular calcification, particularly of the media in arteries, occurs and may be both linear and nodular. It results in luminal narrowing and arterial ischaemia.

Haemodialysis and transplantation

The effects of haemodialysis on renal osteodystrophy are complex and improvement occurs in many cases. However, in some cases there is further progression of bone disease, which is thought to be due to aluminium toxicity causing primarily osteomalacia-type changes. Fractures of the ribs and proximal femora are common manifestations. Osteomyelitis and osteonecrosis are both more common in patients undergoing haemodialysis or transplantation.

OSTEOMYELITIS

Infection is more common in the transplant patient and imaging will confirm bony involvement.

- Scintigraphy with early phase views forms the mainstay of diagnosis in many institutions.
- MRI has more recently been of value with fat-suppressed T2w or STIR images employed to detect bone oedema, which although relatively non-specific may be diagnostic in the appropriate clinical context.
- Changes usually take 10–14 days to become apparent on plain radiographs, with subtle bone destruction often being the first manifestation. Later a periosteal response and healing may be demonstrated.

OSTEONECROSIS

Osteonecrosis or avascular necrosis is more common in both transplant and haemodialysis patients. It occurs most commonly in the femoral heads but may occur in almost any other site, including the distal femur, humerus, talus, cuboid and carpal bones.

- MRI has proved the most sensitive and clinically useful method both for detecting the earliest changes and monitoring their progression. Loss of signal on T1 weighted imaging and the so-called 'double line' sign on T2w imaging may be diagnostic.
- Scintigraphy is also sensitive and will detect changes before plain radiographs.
- Plain radiographs demonstrate the late sequelae well with sclerosis and collapse of the affected areas.

Further reading

Grainger, R.G. and Allison, D.J. (eds) (1997) *Diagnostic Radiology: A textbook of medical imaging*, Churchill Livingstone, Edinburgh.

Holley, K.E., Hunt, Brown, A.L. Jnr *et al.* (1964) Renal artery stenosis in normotensive and hypertensive patients. *Am. J. Med.*, **161**, 577–86.

Miller G.A., Ford, K.K., Braun, S.D. *et al.* (1985) Percutaneous transluminal angioplasty vs surgery for renovascular hypertension. *Am. J. Radiol.*, **144**, 447–50.

Ravine, D., Gibson, R.N., Walker, R.G. *et al.* (1994) Evaluation of ultrasonographic diagnostic criteria for autosomal dominant polycystic kidney disease. *Lancet*, **343**, 824–2.

RCR Working Party (1995) *Making the Best Use of a Department of Clinical Radiology: Guidelines for doctors*, The Royal College of Radiologists, London.

Resnick, D. (ed.) (1995) *Diagnosis of Bone and Joint Disorders*, 3rd edn, W.B. Saunders, Philadelphia.

Robidoux, M.A., Dunnick, N.R., Klotman, P.E. *et al.* (1991) Renal vein renins: Inability to predict response to revascularisation in patients with hypertension. *Radiology*, **178**, 819–22.

Sherwood, T., Davidson, A.J. and Talner, L.B. (1980) *Uroradiology*, Blackwell Scientific, Oxford.

Nuclear medicine

Philip Wraight

Radionuclide methods

A wide variety of radionuclide investigations contributes to the management of nephrological patients (Table 6.1).

BODY SPACES

Isotopic measurements of electrolyte distribution and exchange have been of vital importance in much of the physiological research on which nephrology is based. However these tests are rarely useful in clinical management and will not be discussed further here.

Table 6.1
Radionuclide investigations in nephrology

Tests related to renal function	Non-renal imaging

• Body space measurements
  − total body water (^3H_2O)
  − sodium ($^{24}Na^+$) and potassium ($^{42}K^+$ and $^{43}K^+$)
• Clearance measurements
  − Glomerular filtration rate (^{51}Cr-EDTA and ^{99m}Tc-DTPA)
  − Renal plasma flow (^{125}I- or ^{131}I-OIH, ^{99m}Tc-MAG$_3$)
• Dynamic imaging
  − GFR tracer (^{99m}Tc-DTPA)
  − GFR and secretion agents (^{123}I- or ^{131}I-OIH, ^{99m}Tc-MAG$_3$)
    ○ perfusion, secretion and excretion
    ○ pharmacological intervention (frusemide, captopril)
    ○ micturating cystography
• Parenchymal imaging (^{99m}Tc-DMSA)
	• Bone scintigraphy (^{99m}Tc-MDP)
	• Leucocyte imaging (^{111}In- or ^{99m}Tc-HMPAO leucocytes)
	• Gallium scintigraphy (^{67}Ga citrate)

CLEARANCE METHODS

Glomerular filtration rate (GFR)

Substances suitable for measuring this fundamental parameter of renal function must have low protein binding and negligible non-renal excretion, and must be freely filtered, chemically stable and inert (not being metabolized, secreted or reabsorbed in the kidneys). Inulin has been shown to meet these requirements and has been the gold standard in renal physiological research. However, the use of radioactive tracers greatly simplifies sample measurements and allows single injection techniques. No suitable radiotracer of inulin is available for clinical use but [51]chromium ethylenediamine tetraacetic acid (^{51}Cr-EDTA) was introduced many years ago as a suitable alternative, and remains the agent of choice. ^{99m}Tc-diethylenetriamine pentaacetic acid (^{99m}Tc-DTPA) can be used, but it is prepared from kits and there is variability in stability and protein-binding. The short half-life of [99m]Tc (six hours) creates logistic problems for sample counting, but there is the advantage that if ^{99m}Tc-DTPA is used for imaging (see below), a GFR measurement can be performed at the same time.

The most accurate measurement of GFR involves infusing the tracer at a constant rate, after a loading dose, and measuring tracer output in the urine while monitoring blood concentration. This is not convenient for routine clinical use and methods based on blood sample concentration after a single injection are almost universal.

After intravenous injection, ^{51}Cr-EDTA rapidly diffuses throughout the bloodstream and equilibrates more slowly with the extravascular fluid. Exact calculation of clearance from this two compartment system requires at least six blood samples over a four hour period – not convenient for routine use. A simplification, shown to give accurate results in most cases, is to measure the plasma concentration at two, three and four hours after injection. Back extrapolation to the time of injection gives the distribution volume of the extracellular space, and the slope of declining concentration is the fractional clearance of this space, the GFR. This may be expressed directly in ml/min or normalized for body surface area. Alternatively, it may be expressed simply as the fractional clearance of the extracellular space, which may be more useful in some conditions where disturbance of extravascular volume or fluid exchange rates may distort the apparent measured GFR.

A number of attempts have been made to simplify GFR measurements. The tracer concentration in a single sample, taken when equilibrium with the extravascular space has occurred, correlates inversely with the GFR, and a number of algorithms have been published for calculating GFR on this basis (Picciotto *et al.*, 1992). However, there is considerable variation due to age and body dimensions, and the errors may be unacceptably high for some clinical use, especially when renal function is poor. The method may, however, be acceptable for monitoring changes in an individual patient's GFR with regard to progress of disease or for monitoring the response to therapy. Attempts to measure GFR from gamma camera images alone are subject to considerable error, but accuracy is improved when the external counting data are calibrated by a blood sample.

It should be remembered that all single injection methods of measuring GFR assume the patient is in a steady state with respect to haemodynamics and fluid exchange. Measurements are not accurate following, for example, major surgery, transfusion or dialysis.

Renal plasma flow

Tracers that are both filtered and actively secreted by renal tubules are extracted with high efficiency from the plasma perfusing the kidneys, and can be used to measure renal plasma flow (RPF) by similar methods to those used for the GFR. Nearly 90% of ortho-iodohippurate (OIH) is removed by the kidneys on a single pass, so that the effective renal plasma flow (ERPF), which is plasma flow multiplied by extraction efficiency, approaches true plasma flow. However, this tracer is now less widely available since ^{99m}Tc-labelled compounds have largely replaced it for imaging. ^{99m}Tc mercapto acetyl triglycine (MAG$_3$) has higher protein binding than OIH and lower extraction efficiency. Clearance of this compound is generally referred to as the tubular extraction rate (TER). The protein binding and rapid excretion necessitates multiple blood samples for accurate analysis.

Since GFR correlates well with ERPF in most clinical conditions, the greater simplicity and accuracy of GFR measurements have meant that measurements of ERPF have never achieved widespread utility in nephrology. Measurement of TER gives useful additional information about total renal plasma flow when imaging is performed with ^{99m}Tc-MAG$_3$.

DYNAMIC IMAGING

More detailed information about renal function can be obtained by continuous measurements over the kidneys following intravenous injection of clearance agents labelled with radionuclides suitable for external detection. ^{131}I-OIH was introduced for this purpose 40 years ago when measurements were made by non-imaging probes. Following the invention of the gamma camera and development of ^{99m}Tc agents, imaging superseded probe studies and ^{99m}Tc-DTPA became the agent of choice. Not only could sequential images be obtained of tracer within the kidney, but computer-aided analysis of the region of interest produced functional curves of renal activity (renograms). In the past decade agents like MAG$_3$ have been developed. Although providing the same information in most cases as

^{99m}Tc-DTPA, the faster clearance of ^{99m}Tc-MAG$_3$ provides images with greater contrast, and functional curves with better counting statistics, which is particularly helpful when renal function is poor. ^{99m}Tc-MAG$_3$ is now the preferred imaging agent except when acute tubular necrosis is suspected as ^{99m}Tc-DTPA is more specifically diagnostic. A further advantage of ^{99m}Tc-MAG$_3$ is that during the parenchymal phase (the first three minutes of renal tracer uptake), focal defects such as infarcts or pyelonephritic scars may be demonstrated.

The most complete diagnostic information is obtained by analysing the functional renal curve (renogram) in conjunction with inspection of sequential renal images (Figure 6.1(a)). A wide variety of methods of analysis has been published (Britton, Maisey and Hilson, 1991; Taylor and Nally, 1995). Empirical descriptions of 'vascular', 'secretory' and 'excretory' phases are over-simplified since much of the initial vascular bolus is retained in the kidney, extrarenal vascular activity overlies the kidney throughout the study and tracer uptake by the kidney (filtration and secretion) continues in the third phase even when excretion occurs at a faster rate, leading to a falling curve (Figure 6.1(b)). Whichever method of analysis is chosen, it is important that the relative function of the kidneys and the transit time through each is calculated. During the first two and a half minutes, before any tracer has left the kidneys, the relative uptake in each kidney reflects its fractional contribution to GFR or ERPF, depending on the tracer. This information can also be obtained by deconvolution analysis, a mathematical technique that takes a vascular curve as an input function and combines it with the renogram to obtain a retention function (a time/activity curve that would be observed if a bolus of tracer were injected directly into the renal artery (Figure 6.1 6.1(c))). The height of this curve gives the relative function of the kidney, and the shape describes the time course of the passage of tracer, the pattern of prolongation reflecting pathology such as ureteric obstruction or vascular stenosis.

In order to distinguish between retention in a dilated renal pelvis and prolonged transit through the tubules of the renal parenchyma, deconvolution analysis can be performed using a region of interest confined to the parenchyma and excluding the pelvicalyceal system, giving the so-called parenchymal transit time.

If a duplex system is present, region of interest analysis can be applied separately to the upper and lower moieties. This enables the contribution of each to be calculated along with their transit times, which may be very different if, for example, one has been obstructed or subject to reflux.

If there is clinical suspicion of ureteric reflux, an indirect micturating cystogram can be performed at the end of the renographic study. The patient continues to drink, and when the bladder is full micturates with his/

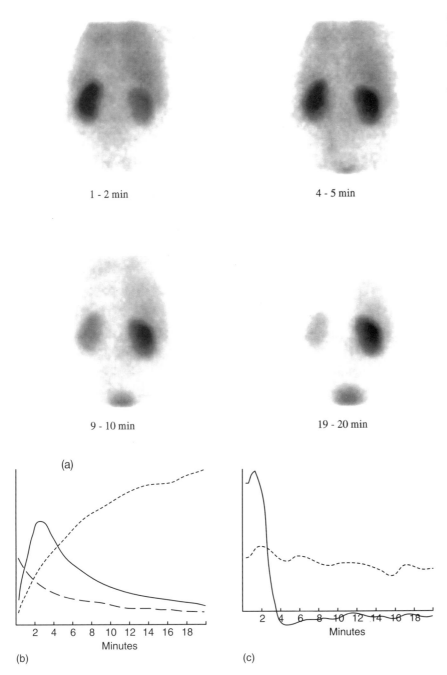

1 - 2 min

4 - 5 min

9 - 10 min

19 - 20 min

(a)

(b)

Minutes

(c)

Minutes

Fig. 6.1
(a) Posterior images of ^{99m}Tc-MAG$_3$ study. The left kidney is normal. The right side shows reduced function (low initial uptake) and markedly prolonged retention of tracer. (b) Region of interest time/ activity curves over kidneys and blood background, quantifying reduced rate of tracer uptake on the right and a continual rising curve showing severe retention. Solid line, left; dotted line, right; dashed line, blood × 10. (c) Retention curves for both kidneys derived by deconvolution analysis, quantifying reduced function (relative height of curves) and prolonged transit time on the right. Solid line, left; dotted line, right.

her back to the gamma camera, when rapid sequence imaging demonstrates any reflux into the upper ureters and renal areas. This has a sensitivity comparable with that of the radiological micturating cystogram (Gordon,

Peters and Morony, 1990), but involves a lower radiation dose and avoids the need for catheterization.

The diagnostic information available from dynamic renal imaging can often be enhanced by pharmacological intervention. Administration of frusemide to increase urine flow during a study is helpful in distinguishing a non-obstructed dilated pelvicalyceal system from an obstructed one where increased outflow pressure impairs renal function. Rapid complete washout excludes obstruction and a continually rising curve confirms obstruction. In some cases the response is equivocal. Numerical analysis of the washout curve can achieve greater definition but it is important to take the kidney function and size of the outflow tract into consideration. There may be relatively slow washout from a very large renal pelvis even in the absence of obstruction, and a poorly functioning kidney may respond inadequately to frusemide, also leading to slow washout without obstruction. Administration of frusemide 15 minutes before injection of the radiopharmaceutical may unmask intermittent obstruction that is only present at high flow rates.

Combining renography with a captopril challenge increases the sensitivity and specificity of the technique in diagnosing renovascular hypertension. Since the main effect of inhibiting the angiotensin-converting enzyme (ACE) is on glomerular filtration, one would expect ^{99m}Tc-DTPA to be the most effective agent for captopril renography, but results with ^{99m}Tc-MAG$_3$ appear to be equally good. When compared with the standard renogram, the captopril study shows reduced relative function, prolonged parenchymal transit time, or both on the side of the renal artery stenosis.

Renography in renal transplant recipients differs from conventional renography in that the relative function analysis of two kidneys is obviously not available. An empirical index of renal perfusion can be obtained by integrating the rate of arrival of the injected bolus in the kidney and in the vessel supplying it. As originally described (Hilson *et al.*, 1978), the perfusion index was the ratio of iliac to renal activity. It seems more logical to use the reciprocal (i.e. renal/iliac activity) so that a low perfusion index is indicative of poor perfusion. Region of interest analysis of the functional curves is similar to two-kidney renography, but inspection of the serial images and time of arrival of activity in the bladder are important in diagnostic interpretation.

RENAL PARENCHYMAL IMAGING

^{99m}Tc dimercaptosuccinic acid (DMSA) is slowly cleared from the circulation and, although there is some urinary excretion, the majority accumulates in the tubular cells of the renal cortex. There is disagreement over the exact mechanism, but it is probably a combination of tubular reabsorption from the glomerular filtrate and direct uptake into the tubules from the bloodstream. Imaging is normally performed between two and four hours after injection. High resolution posterior and posterior oblique views are obtained (Figure 6.2(a)). Region of interest analysis gives the relative renal function, which generally correlates very well with that calculated from dynamic imaging, although in obstruction, sufficient excreted activity may be retained in the renal area to overestimate relative function by 10%. In a small percentage of cases when there is nephroptosis or one kidney is displaced anteriorly (usually obvious from visual inspection), the posterior view alone gives significant error, which can be avoided by also obtaining an anterior view and calculating the relative function from the geometric mean of each kidney's counts in the two views.

Fig. 6.2
(a) Posterior ^{99m}Tc-DMSA images. Right kidney is normal. Left is small with irregularly reduced cortical uptake due to scarring from reflux. (b) Region of interest analysis to give relative function.

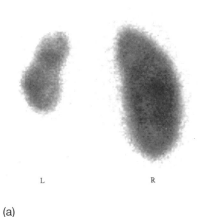

L   R

(a)

RELATIVE UPTAKE
LEFT   RIGHT
21%   79%

L   R

(b)

The main value of DMSA scintigraphy is in the sensitive depiction of functioning renal parenchyma and both diffuse and focal reductions indicate pathology such as reflux nephropathy and infarcts with greater sensitivity than anatomical imaging procedures such as ultrasound or computed tomography (CT) (Figure 6.2). In some cases of trauma or reflux there may be focal reduction in tracer uptake due to reduced blood flow. This may not be associated with permanent tissue damage and improvement can be seen on serial scans performed at a later date.

NON-RENAL IMAGING

A number of other radionuclide investigations (Table 6.1) not directly related to renal function can be important in the management of nephrological patients. Reference will be made below to clinical indications. Technical details of these tests are given in textbooks of nuclear medicine (e.g. Murray and Ell, 1994).

Clinical applications

ACUTE RENAL FAILURE

Radionuclide techniques have no part in the initial assessment of acute renal failure. When initial biochemical and haematological investigations and the response to the initial treatment have failed to establish a clear clinical picture, isotope methods can help in diagnosis, guiding management and indicating prognosis. In the selected cases where radionuclide imaging is necessary, this should not be delayed too long, since after about two weeks the secondary effects of many causes of failure may result in similar renograms with non-specific appearances reflecting poor perfusion and poor function.

Vascular patency

Renal perfusion can be demonstrated by the early phase of either a DTPA or MAG_3 study. Whether vascular impairment is the direct result of vascular occlusion (e.g. embolism or aortic dissection) or secondary to other renal pathology of drugs such as ACE inhibitors, early renal uptake can indicate how much blood flow is preserved and which kidney is better perfused if intervention is planned.

Acute tubular necrosis (ATN)

^{99m}Tc-DTPA is the preferred agent to confirm this diagnosis, as the appearances with MAG$_3$ are non-specific. Perfusion is generally well preserved and the kidneys are clearly visualized as the initial tracer bolus passes into the tubules by glomerular filtration. However, as circulating concentration falls with redistribution to the extravascular fluid, tracer leaks out through the damaged tubules and is removed in the blood, so that total renal activity falls steeply instead of rising to the normal peak at about three minutes. There is little excretion of activity in the urine. At a later stage, increasing excretion of radionuclide in the urine is a sign of resolution of the ATN.

Ureteric obstruction

Ureteric obstruction leading to acute renal failure is normally demonstrated by ultrasound, and the cause by antegrade or retrograde pyelography. However, when the obstruction has been relieved, residual function is well demonstrated by MAG$_3$, giving prognostic information and in some cases indicating which kidney merits interventional treatment.

Acute interstitial nephritis

This leads to high renal uptake of ^{67}gallium, which can help to confirm the diagnosis in doubtful cases.

Rhabdomyolysis

When rhabdomyolysis is the cause of acute renal failure the clinical picture is usually clearcut, but in cases where this is not so, bone scintigraphy with ^{99m}Tc-methylene diphosphonate (^{99m}Tc-MDP) can be helpful in confirming the diagnosis. There is high tracer uptake in the muscle groups affected and irregular increased uptake in the kidneys themselves.

CHRONIC RENAL FAILURE

Renal function

While radionuclide techniques are valuable in the diagnosis of some of the conditions leading to renal failure (see below), nuclear medicine has little to contribute to diagnosis in most cases of established chronic renal failure. The GFR may fall to about 50% of normal while circulating levels of urea and creatinine remain within the normal range, and abnormal concentrations correlate poorly with actual renal functional reserve. GFR measurements can therefore be helpful in monitoring renal function in treatable conditions such as diabetes and hypertension, where demonstration of falling renal function can have prognostic significance and influence management. Occasionally GFR measurements can be helpful in severe chronic renal failure in demonstrating any residual function or recovery of function following supportive dialysis.

Complications

Radionuclide methods can be helpful in the diagnosis of a number of complications in patients with renal failure. ^{111}In-labelled leucocytes can demonstrate the site of occult infection; for example, tunnel infection or peritonitis in peritoneal dialysis, shunt infection in haemodialysis, cyst infection in polycystic kidney disease and occult sepsis after renal transplantation. ^{99m}Tc-MDP bone scintigraphy detects renal osteodystrophy with much greater sensitivity than radiology and is also useful in demonstrating fractures and avascular necrosis in patients receiving steroids.

Renal transplants

Radionuclide techniques provide a useful non-invasive method for monitoring renal transplant function and diagnosing complications. Since comparison of serial studies is important for some diagnoses, particularly rejection, a baseline study should be performed within one to two days of operation and thereafter when there is concern because of deteriorating renal function. ^{99m}Tc-DTPA is the tracer of choice in the early stages after surgery. Later studies can be performed with DTPA or MAG_3.

The initial concern is about the perfusion of the transplant kidney, monitored both by inspection of serial images and a perfusion index (see above). Complete vascular occlusion is usually obvious, the transplant being a photon deficient region with no tracer uptake on early or delayed images. (The only differential diagnosis here is hyperacute rejection, which is now very rare.) Renal artery stenosis tends to develop later and can be diagnosed by comparing the perfusion index in studies with and without captopril. Serial measurements of the perfusion index provide the best non-invasive method of diagnosing acute rejection, suggested by falling perfusion and no specific evidence of other complications.

The other common early cause of oliguria is ATN, which can be diagnosed by preserved perfusion followed by the immediately falling renal region of interest curve described above. At a later stage, cyclosporin toxity can present a similar picture, although there is usually an accompanying fall in blood flow.

Unless renal function is very poor, ureteric leaks can be detected with high sensitivity, usually as perirenal photon deficient regions that accumulate tracer later in the study. In contrast, a lymphocoele will remain photon deficient. (Both appear as fluid on ultrasound.) Ureteric obstruction can develop at a variable period after transplantation. It is characterized by a 'negative pyelogram' during the early parenchymal phase of the study, build up of activity within the pelvis and ureter, and delay in tracer reaching the bladder. If the cause of obstruction is external compression by haematoma, lymphocoele or urinoma this may also be visualized as described above.

OTHER CONDITIONS LEADING TO OR COMPLICATING RENAL FAILURE

Renovascular hypertension
Uncontrolled hypertension of any type can lead to renal failure, but only about 1% of cases originate as renal artery stenosis. Non-invasive detection of these cases is attractive because of the possibility of cure by percutaneous angioplasty and, as described above, captopril renography is the investigation of choice. Hypertension is so common that it is not cost-effective to screen all cases. Factors increasing the probability that hypertension is due to renal artery stenosis include rapid onset, young patients, difficulty in medical control, abdominal bruit, evidence of atherosclerosis elsewhere, deterioration of renal function with ACE inhibitor medication and development of renal failure in hypertensive patients. In cases selected by these criteria, captopril renography is useful not only in diagnosing renal artery stenosis but in predicting which cases are likely to achieve a satisfactory reduction in blood pressure with angioplasty. Renography is unlikely to be helpful in chronic renal failure with long-standing hypertension as the findings will be non-specific due to secondary hypertensive renal impairment.

^{99m}Tc-DMSA imaging can be of value in investigating hypertension in younger patients, demonstrating not only pyelonephritic scarring (see below), but also focal ischaemic areas due to segmental arterial stenosis or previous trauma. In older patients it is the non-invasive investigation of choice to confirm suspected renal infarcts.

Pyelonephritis
^{99m}Tc-DMSA scintigraphy has been shown to be far more sensitive than ultrasound or intravenous urography in detecting pyelonephritis and is the investigation of choice in establishing this diagnosis and in distinguishing between upper and lower urinary tract infections. Abnormalities include focal areas of reduced uptake (both scars and areas of acute inflammation which may progress to scars), and diffusely reduced renal cortical uptake, reflecting global reflux. The main application of DMSA is in the investigation of paediatric urinary tract infection, where early diagnosis and treatment can prevent later progression to chronic renal failure.

In adults, the DMSA scintigram will demonstrate the extent of renal damage due to pyelonephritis. In some patients with chronic pyelonephritis the diagnosis may not be clear-cut, and in these cases ^{111}In-labelled leucocyte scans can be helpful in demonstrating active renal infection.

References

Britton, K.E., Maisey, M.N. and Hilson, A.J.W. (1991) Renal radionuclide studies in *Clinical Nuclear Medicine*, 2nd edn (eds M.N. Maisey, K.E. Britton and D.L. Gilday), Chapman and Hall, London.

Gordon, I., Peters, A.M. and Morony, S. (1990) Indirect radionuclide cystography: a sensitive technique for the detection of vesico-ureteral reflux. *Pediat. Nephrol.,* **4** 604–6.

Hilson, A.J.W., Maisey, M.N., Brown, C.B. *et al.* (1978) Dynamic renal transplant imaging with Tc-99m DTPA (Sn) supplemented by a transplant perfusion index in the management of renal transplants. *J. Nucl. Med.,* **19**, 994–1000.

Murray, I.P.C. and Ell, P.J. (eds) (1994) *Nuclear Medicine in Clinical Diagnosis and Treatment*, Churchill Livingstone, Edinburgh.

Picciotto, G., Cacace, G., Cesana, P. *et al.* (1992) Estimation of chromium-51 ethylene diamine tetra-acetic acid plasma clearance: a comparative assessment of simplified techniques. *Eur. J. Nucl. Med.,* **19**, 30–5.

Taylor, A. and Nally, J.V. (1995) Clinical applications of renal scintigraphy. *Am. J. Radiol.,* **164**, 31–41.

Further reading

Dubovsky, E.V., Russell, C.D. and Erbas, B. (1995) Radionuclide evaluation of renal transplants. *Semin. Nucl. Med.,* **25**, 49–59.

Renal biopsy

Sathia Thiru

Clinical and biochemical investigations seldom provide a precise nephrological diagnosis or indicate a prognosis. A biopsy, on the other hand, provides information regarding the diagnosis, extent and state of evolution of the disease and therefore, to some extent, a prognosis, thus helping in the management of the patient. Indications for biopsy are relative rather than absolute and it is essential to have full clinical details when examining biopsy material. The biopsy procedure is invasive and the tissue obtained is small; it is therefore imperative that the specimen is studied systematically and in detail by light microscopy in addition to immunohistochemistry and, ideally, electronmicroscopy as well.

Types of biopsy material

NEEDLE BIOPSY

A specimen consists of a core of 1–1.5 cm long and 0.1 cm wide containing cortex and medulla, including interlobular and arcuate arteries. An adequate biopsy is one that contains a minimum of five glomeruli, though most contain 10–20 on average. The greater the number of glomeruli, the better the accuracy of diagnosis, particularly when the disease process involves only scattered glomeruli. There are some conditions where even a single glomerulus is sufficient for a definite diagnosis, e.g. membranous glomerulonephritis or amyloidosis. However, small samples will not give a true picture of the severity and extent of the disease process; this applies to glomerular diseases as well as to tubulointerstitial nephritis and, in particular, to vascular sclerosis, where the lesions can be focal.

SURGICAL BIOSPY

An open subcapsular wedge biopsy contains an adequate number of glomeruli but suffers from the lack of inner cortex, medulla, interlobular and arcuate arteries. Moreover, in older patients, incidental, age-related, subcapsular nephrosclerotic scarring may complicate the diagnosis and assessment of disease severity.

Renal histology

The peripheral cortex consists of glomeruli with closely packed proximal and distal convoluted tubules. Within the medulla are the loops of Henle, which are composed of the straight portion of the proximal tubule and the thin and the thick ascending limbs of the distal tubule, and the collecting ducts. Nephrons arising in the superficial cortex have short loops of Henle that extend up to the outer medulla, whereas the juxtamedullary glomeruli have long loops that enter the deep inner medulla. The renal artery at the hilum divides into five or six segmented arteries that are virtually end-arteries. At the corticomedullary junction, they give rise to arcuate branches, from which a series of perpendicular interlobular arteries traverse the cortex. Afferent arterioles from these supply individual glomeruli from which smaller efferent arterioles emerge. These break into peritubular capillaries that form a network around the tubules and eventually drain into arcuate veins via interlobular veins. The efferent arterioles emerging from the juxtamedullary glomeruli are large and extend into the deep medulla, divide into the descending vasa recta and subsequently into the capillary plexus that supply the inner medulla. Within the cortex the interstitium is sparse, containing the peritubular capillaries between the closely packed tubules. It is more prominent in the medulla.

NORMAL GLOMERULUS

The glomerular tuft is composed of a bundle of capillaries invaginated into the modified and dilated end of the proximal tubule, the **urinary Bowman's space**. The capillaries are held together and supported by a slender branching stalk of specialized connective tissue called the **mesangium**, which also contains a few **mesangial cells**. The glomerular capillaries arise by subdivision of the afferent arteriole and reunite into the efferent arteriole, which leaves the glomerulus at the hilus.

The capillary wall consists of a basement membrane covered by a thin sheet of **endothelial cell cytoplasm** on its inner aspect and by **epithelial cells** on the outer aspect facing the urinary space. The epithelial cells are attached to the basement membrane by projections known as foot-processes or podocytes. The mesangial and endothelial cells are also known as **endocapillary cells** and the epithelial cells as **extracapillary cells**.

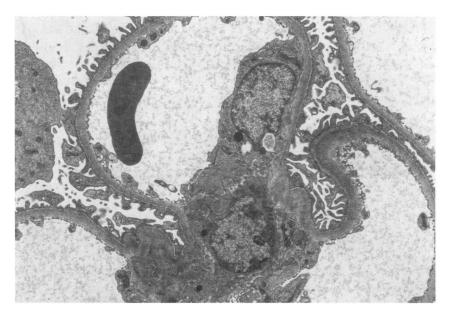

Fig. 7.1
Normal electronmicrograph illustrating segment of a glomerulus demonstrating the relationship between endothelial cells, mesangial cells and visceral epithelial cells.

The appearance of the normal glomerulus is shown in Plates 6 and 7 and Figure 7.1.

Handling the biopsy

Ideally, a histology technician should attend the biopsy procedure with a renal biopsy kit containing:

- sharp blade
- dental wax
- wooden sticks to handle the tissue
- hand lens to recognize glomeruli
- fixative for paraffin sections (10% neutral buffered formalin, Bouin's solution, Carnoy's solution)
- flask of liquid nitrogen
- 3% phosphate-buffered glutaraldehyde.

The biopsy specimen should be handled with care to avoid crushing; forceps should never be used. It is essential that the specimen is transferred rapidly into the fixatives to prevent drying. The specimen is laid on the dental wax and examined with the hand lens to identify the glomeruli, which are seen as tiny red pinhead structures. Ideally, two cores should be obtained. One is then transferred into the fixative for light microscopy, and the second core should be bisected longitudinally, with one half being snap-frozen in liquid nitrogen and the second immersed in the electronmicroscopy fixative. If only one core of tissue is available it should be divided for all three procedures, with the largest fragment being used for light microscopy; it is important to ensure that glomeruli are present in all the fragments.

PROCESSING AND SECTIONING

Light microscopy

A needle biopsy specimen or small subcapsular biopsy requires fixation for a minimum of one to two hours. The tissue is then processed overnight by a method standard to the individual laboratory. Urgent biopsies can be processed rapidly within three hours. The processed specimen is transferred to an embedding medium, paraffin or glycol methacrylate. Serial thin sections of 2–3 µm depth are cut and the slides are numbered, each slide containing three sections. Slides 1, 5 and 10 are stained with haematoxylin and eosin (H&E), and the intervening slides with special tinctorial stains. Periodic acid–Schiff (PAS) stain accentuates basement membranes, the mesangial matrix and the brushborder of the proximal tubules, sclerotic lesions, hyalinosis and cryoglobulin deposits. Methanamine silver (MethAg) with H&E counter stain is an exquisite combination that shows up similar structures to the PAS stain and is also extremely photogenic. A trichrome stain shows up fibrin and immune deposits as well as foci of fibrosis. The unstained slides can be held in reserve and where necessary used for other stains, such as elastin, or for immunohistochemistry. If the initial sections are insufficient to evaluate the disease process, further serials can be cut. When amyloid is suspected, a section of 7 µm is required to demonstrate Congo red staining; only a thick section will bind sufficient dye for visualization by polarizing microscopy.

Immunohistochemistry

The snap-frozen tissue is cut on a cryostat, the sections approximately 5 µm in thickness, one to two sections on each slide. Sections are fixed for 5–10 minutes in acetone, dried at room temperature, washed in buffered saline and incubated for 30 minutes with fluorescein-labelled antiserum in a covered moist chamber. After three washes with buffer the sections are mounted using buffered glycerol. The slides are viewed under a fluorescence microscope equipped with appropriate excitation and barrier filters. As the fluorescent stains fade on exposure to ultraviolet and incident light, the sections should be photographed if a permanent record is required. We have developed the technique of immunofluorescent stains on paraffin sections and this technique is used when the frozen sections do not contain glomeruli. The method requires dewaxing paraffin sections, treating them with trypsin to break the protein bonds created by formalin fixation, and then staining the sections with fluorescein-labelled antiserum.

Immunoperoxidase staining techniques for identification of cell surface markers produce excellent results with a clean background. However, identification of proteins in extracellular deposits has not been successful in most laboratories because of the presence of high background. The advantages of this method are that frozen tissue is not required and the slides are available as a permanent record.

Electronmicroscopy

The fragments used for electronmicroscopy should be no larger than 1 mm cubed to ensure penetration of the fixative. The fixative used in most laboratories is 3% phosphate-buffered glutaraldehyde, which must be refrigerated to prevent deterioration. After fixation for a minimum of four hours, the tissue is rinsed in buffer, post-fixed in 1% osmium tetroxide, dehydrated and embedded in resin. Glass knives are used for sectioning and thick 1 µm sections are stained with toluidine blue to select the areas for thin sectioning. Thin sections are then cut and stained with uranyl acetate and lead citrate.

If no glomeruli are present in the electronmicroscopy material, the tissue remaining in the paraffin block can be used. A small area containing glomeruli is identified and cut from the block and reprocessed for electronmicroscopy.

MATERIAL AVAILABLE FROM RENAL BIOPSY

Using light microscopy:

- serial thin sections 2–3 µm thick; three sections per slide
- routine H&E stains
- routine PAS, MethAg and trichrome stains
- Congo red stain for amyloid
- other stains as required.

Using immunohistochemistry.

- frozen or paraffin sections stained with fluorescein isothiocyanate conjugated antisera to IgG, IgA, IgM, light-chains, complement components C_1, C_3, C_4 and fibrinogen; viewed under ultraviolet light and photographed.
- Immunoperoxidase stains for Ig, complement, light-chains, amyloid, cytomegalovirus (CMV), Epstein–Barr virus (EBV), lymphocytes and subsets, monocytes.

Using electronmicroscopy.

- Electronmicrographs of relevant lesions.

Interpretation of renal biopsy

The nephron is a single unit and therefore, although the primary site of injury may be a particular component, e.g. the glomerulus, in time the entire nephron will be affected, resulting in secondary tubular atrophy and associated interstitial fibrosis. In the acute or early phase of the disease the primary injury is therefore quite clear, e.g. acute glomerulonephritis or acute interstitial nephritis. With progressive disease and secondary involvement of the rest of the nephron there is a lack of predominance of lesions in a particular compartment, and with the superadded effects of hypertensive vascular sclerosis, it can be impossible to be certain of the primary disease process. Biopsy of an end-stage kidney is, in most cases, an unrewarding exercise.

Interpretation of a renal biopsy must always be done in the context of the clinical history, blood and urinary abnormalities. This is particularly the case when the initial biopsy is performed in the later phase of the disease process. Interpretation must be systematic, detailed and semiquantitative.

LIGHT MICROSCOPY

- Adequacy of biopsy → cortex, medulla, vessels, number of glomeruli.
- Site of lesion → glomeruli, tubules, interstitium or vessels.
- Distribution → focal or diffuse; global or segmental.
- Type of lesion → Glomeruli: cellularity, capillary wall abnormality, necrosis, sclerosis
  Tubules: necrosis, inflammation, atrophy
  Interstitium: oedema, inflammation, fibrosis
  Vessels: necrosis, sclerosis, occlusion.
- Severity → mild, moderate, severe
- Proportion of tissue involved
- Indicators of prognosis → reparable or irreparable injury; onset of secondary changes.

IMMUNOHISTOCHEMISTRY

- Adequacy of sample → number of glomeruli.
- Specificity → positive immune stain or non-immunological trapping, e.g. necrotic sites, hyalin in glomerular sclerotic segments or arterioles; tubular protein reabsorption droplets.

- Site and distribution → glomerular mesangium or capillary wall; tubular basement membrane; focal, segmental or diffuse.
- Pattern → granular, coarse, linear.
- Components → Ig heavy-chains, light-chains, complement fractions, fibrinogen.

ELECTRONMICROSCOPY

Results should be interpreted in the context of the findings from light microscopy.

- Adequacy → number of glomeruli, tubules, vessels.
- Structure of glomerular basement membrane → integrity and contour, width, inclusions, immune and non-immune deposits.
- Structure and location of immune deposits → mesangial, glomerular capillary wall: subepithelial, intramembranous, subendothelial; tubular basement membrane; vessels.
- Cellular changes → podocytes, cell swelling, cell proliferation, cell infiltration; inclusions.

Aspects of renal biopsy

INDICATIONS FOR RENAL BIOPSY

Indications are often relative and depend on the entire clinical picture as well as the personal preference of the nephrologist:

- acute renal failure
- persistent proteinuria
- nephrotic syndrome in adults
- steroid-resistant nephrotic syndrome in children
- recurrent haematuria with or without proteinuria
- acute nephritic syndrome
- rapidly progressive glomerulonephritis
- acute renal failure
- renal involvement in systemic disorders
- transplant management
- chronic renal insufficiency?

CONTRAINDICATIONS TO RENAL BIOPSY

Absolute contraindications are:

- bleeding diathesis

- Hypertension.

Relative contraindications are:

- single functioning kidney
- small kidneys < 9.0 cm
- infection → acute pyelonephritis, abscess
- renal mass or cysts.

COMPLICATIONS OF RENAL BIOPSY

The complications of renal biopsy are:

- inadequate tissue → 5–10%
- adjacent organ trauma → 1%
- bleeding → microscopic haematuria 100%; gross haematuria 5–10%
- arteriovenous fistula → 15–18%; 1% require intervention
- nephrectomy
- death.

Glomerular disorders

Glomeruli have a limited repertoire of responses to injury and histologically there can be similarity between immune and non-immune injury. Moreover, presence of immunoglobulin and complement components in damaged tissues does not invariably indicate immune injury; C_3, Clq and IgM are 'sticky' molecules. Conversely, the absence of immune deposits or circulating immune complexes does not automatically exclude an immunopathogenic mechanism.

The various glomerular disorders are characterized by one or more basic tissue reactions.

- Cellular proliferation: increase in mesangial and endothelial cells.
- Leucocyte infiltration: neutrophils, lymphocytes and monocytes.
- Mesangial matrical increase: a by-product of mesangial cell hypercellularity.
- Capillary wall thickening: due to deposits, new basement membrane material, swelling of endothelial cells.
- Adhesions: cellular attachment between capillary wall and Bowman's capsule.
- Crescents: epithelial cell proliferation and infiltration of macrophages within urinary space secondary to glomerular basement membrane rupture and escape of fibrin.

- Hyalinosis/hyaline change: eosinophilic, glassy, acellular accumulation of glycoproteins and lipids within capillary walls.
- Necrosis: loss of structure with disruption of capillary loops and matrix, associated with fibrin and nuclear debris (karyorhexis).
- Sclerosis: increased, extracellular, fibrillar material within mesangium or collapse and condensation of glomerular capillary loops.

These manifestations can be:

- diffuse: 50% or more glomeruli involved
- focal: 50% or fewer glomeruli involved
- global: entire glomerulus involved
- segmental: part of the glomerular tuft involved.

PATHOGENESIS OF GLOMERULONEPHRITIS

There is strong evidence that most glomerulonephritides are due to injury caused by immunopathogenic mechanisms. The following mechanisms are responsible for the initiation of glomerulonephritis (GN) and are not necessarily mutually exclusive.

- Circulating antibodies react with non-basement membrane glomerular antigens or with antigens from the plasma that have become trapped within the glomerular basement membrane. Immune complexes are formed *in situ*, e.g. membranous GN. Granular deposition of Ig and C occurs.
- Circulating immune complexes may be filtered out in the glomerular basement membrane; e.g. acute serum sickness, post-streptococcal GN. Granular deposition of Ig and C occurs.
- Antibodies may form to constituents of the glomerular basement membrane; immune complexes form *in situ*, e.g. Goodpasture's syndrome. Continuous linear staining of IgG along capillary walls.
- Non-antibody substances within the glomeruli may activate the alternative complement pathway and cause damage. Deposition of C_3, but usually no Ig.
- Cell-mediated immune injury may occur via action of cytokines.

The formation and site of deposition of immune complexes depends on: haemodynamic factors; the size, shape and charge of molecules; the availability of receptors; and vascular permeability.

Once deposited, immune complexes cause glomerular injury by:

- activation of the complement cascade: chemotaxis, platelet aggregation, anaphylatoxin effects, immune adherence, membrane damage, cell lysis and release of enzymes;

- local activation of the coagulation cascade secondary to complement activation and/or by the release of enzymes and protein breakdown products from damaged cells;
- release of vasoactive amines from platelets.

FUNCTIONAL EFFECTS OF GLOMERULAR DISORDERS

Glomerular diseases produce symptoms that differ from one condition to another more in quantity than in quality. Secondary hypertension complicates many renal diseases, especially in the later stages. Individual disease processes can produce diverse clinical manifestations and, conversely, a particular syndrome may have multiple causes: e.g. mesangiocapillary GN type I may present with nephrotic syndrome, nephritic syndrome, proteinuria or haematuria; nephrotic syndrome may be due to minimal change disease, focal segmental glomerulosclerosis, membranous GN, lupus nephritis, diabetic nephropathy, renal amyloid, and so on. Characteristic symptoms of some common glomerular disorders are shown in Table 7.1.

Table 7.1

Characteristic symptoms of some common glomerular disorders

Nephritic syndrome	Nephrotic syndrome	Rapidly progressive glomerulonephritis (RPGN)	Recurrent/ persistent haematuria	Acute renal failure	Chronic renal insufficiency
Abrupt onset of: • Haematuria • Proteinuria • Hypertension • Fall in glomerular filtration rate • Retention of Na and H_2O • Oliguria	• Heavy proteinuria • Hypoalbuminaemia • Oedema • Hyperlipidaemia • Lipiduria	Abrupt or insidious onset of: • Haematuria • Proteinuria • Oliguria • Anaemia • Rapid renal failure	Insidious or abrupt onset of: • Haematuria (gross or microscopic) • With or without proteinuria	Abrupt onset of: • Oliguria • Fall in glomerular filtration • Increase in plasma creatinine and urea	Slowly developing renal failure: • Proteinuria • Haematuria • Oliguria • Hypertension

CLASSIFICATION OF GLOMERULONEPHRITIS

There are innumerable classifications of GN, all quite complex and none ideal. Classification can be based on clinical, aetiological, pathogenetic or morphological criteria. As aetiology and pathogenesis are as yet poorly understood, the most acceptable classification is currently based on morphology. The patterns themselves do not represent disease entities, but when

Category	Description and type
I	Minor glomerular abnormalities or normal • Minimal change disease

II	Diffuse glomerulonephritis
	(a) Proliferative glomerulonephritis
	  • Endocapillary proliferative glomerulonephritis
	  • Mesangial proliferative glomerulonephritis
	  • Mesangiocapillary glomerulonephritis types I and II
	  • Extracapillary proliferative glomerulonephritis (crescentic glomerulonephritis)
	(b) Membranous glomerulonephritis
	(c) Sclerosing glomerulonephritis (end-stage disease)

III	Focal and/or segmental glomerular abnormalities
	  • Focal segmental glomerular necrosis
	  • Focal proliferative glomerulonephritis with or without necrosis (often associated with systemic diseases such as Wegener's granulomatosis, microscopic polyangiitis or SLE)

Table 7.2
Morphological classification of glomerulonephritis

used with clinical, immunological and other laboratory data do appear to be consistent entities. Table 7.2 gives the most widely accepted classification.

Minimal change disease

Minimal change disease is a clinicopathological entity composed of the nephrotic syndrome in association with normal glomeruli by light microscopy and immunohistochemistry, and non-specific electronmicroscopic changes of obliteration of the epithelial cell foot processes.

Minimal change disease is predominantly a disease of young children but it can also be seen in adults of all ages. The onset is rapid, the proteinuria is selective, especially in children, and the syndrome is characterized by multiple remissions and exacerbations over a period of years. It accounts for almost 80% of all cases of nephrotic syndrome in the paediatric age group and 20–30% in adults. The response to steroids is excellent, particularly in children. A therapeutic trial of steroids is therefore instituted in most children presenting with the nephrotic syndrome and a biopsy is performed only if there is no response to therapy. Adults with the nephrotic syndrome, on the other hand, are routinely biopsied.

By light microscopy the glomeruli appear entirely normal or may show mild segmental or global mesangial hypercellularity. Minimal change disease is a diagnosis of exclusion and it is imperative that a careful examination be made of multiple sections and a thorough search be made for the presence of even the smallest adhesion to Bowman's capsule, peripheral capillary foam cells or sclerosis of even a single loop. If any of these lesions is present the diagnosis is more likely to be the sinister condition of focal segmental glomerulosclerosis (see below).

Tubules are unremarkable except for protein reabsorption droplets and lipid vacoules secondary to lipoprotein reabsorption. If even a single focus of atrophic tubules is present, especially in children, great caution is necessary in the interpretation of the biopsy as this may indicate early focal segmental glomerulosclerosis in which the glomerular lesions have been missed by the pathologist or were not included in the biopsy.

With immunohistochemistry there is usually a total absence of staining for immunoglobulins and complement components. In some cases there is mesangial staining for IgM, occasionally accompanied by C_3. The clinical behaviour and prognosis in these patients is no different.

By electronmicroscopy there is diffuse obliteration or effacement of the epithelial cell foot processes. The epithelial cells often show villous hyperplasia and the cytoplasm contains clear and lipid-filled vacuoles. Electron deposits are not identified.

Diffuse endocapillary proliferative GN

This is the classic example of immune complex-mediated GN associated with streptococcal and other bacterial infections and also with systemic lupus erythematosus (SLE). The onset is two or three weeks after the episode of infection and the patient presents with an acute nephritic syndrome accompanied by immune complexes in serum and transient hypocomplimentaemia. An elevated and rising titre to streptococcal antigens establishes streptococcal infection as the most likely cause. The majority of patients make a complete recovery, although 1% go into rapidly progressive renal failure. Fewer than 5% have persistent or latent disease progressing to renal failure months to years later.

By light microscopy the glomeruli are enlarged, hypercellular with mesangial and endothelial cell proliferation, and are often infiltrated by neutrophils and monocytes. The increased cellularity together with marked endothelial swelling leads to occlusion of the capillary lumina. In some cases, large fuschinophilic dome-like deposits can be identified with the trichrome stain on the epithelial aspect of the capillary wall (Plate 8).

A few weeks after the onset of the disease there is a reduction in glomerular cellularity with loss of inflammatory cells, endothelial cell proliferation, and restoration of capillary patency. Mesangial cell proliferation persists, often with an accompanying increase in matrix that is reminiscent of a diffuse mesangial proliferative GN. There is generally very little epithelial cell proliferation, but rarely there can be necrosis of tufts with

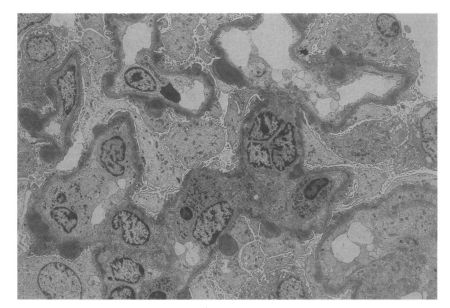

Fig. 7.2
Poststreptococcal glomerulonephritis. Large dome-shaped deposits can be seen on the epithelial aspect of the glomerular basement membrane. There is narrowing of the capillary lumina secondary to endothelial cell swelling.

marked epithelial cell proliferation and crescent formation. The prognosis in such cases is similar to that for other forms of crescentic GN.

Tubules contain red cells and red cell casts, occasionally intermixed with neutrophils. There is interstitial oedema with a mild to moderate in-flammatory cell infiltrate. On immunohistochemistry, there is diffuse bright, granular, staining of glomerular capillary walls for IgG and C_3 (Plate 9). With electronmicroscopy, the pathognomonic feature is the presence of large dome-shaped deposits irregularly studded along the epithelial aspect of the glomerular basement membrane. Mesangial deposits are also often present. The marked hypercellularity together with the swelling of the endothelial cells can make it very difficult to identify landmarks within the glomerulus (Figure 7.2).

Diffuse mesangial proliferative GN
Mesangial proliferation can be seen in a number of conditions, including some cases of lupus nephritis, Henoch–Schönlein purpura, postinfectious GN and, of course, IgA nephropathy.

IgA nephropathy is the commonest GN seen by nephrologists. Patients present with micro- and macroscopic haematuria, with or without protein-uria. There is often a history of respiratory tract infection at the time or immediately preceding the renal symptoms. It can be associated with chronic liver disease or gastrointestinal disorders such as coeliac disease, or be part of the spectrum of Henoch–Schönlein purpura. Some 20–30% of patients progress to renal failure, and IgA nephropathy is the most common cause of chronic, progressive GN in the developed world.

IgA nephropathy can show a spectrum of histological abnormalities ranging from mild focal and segmental mesangial proliferation to diffuse mesangial proliferation with significant matrical increase (Plate 10). In the early phase of the disease, occasional small foci of necrosis with accompanying epithelial cell proliferation may be present. With progressive disease, sclerotic segments with synechiae to Bowman's capsule and global sclerosis become prominent features. The PAS stain is ideal for highlighting the abnormalities seen in IgA nephropathy.

In the early phase of the disease, tubules contain red cells and red cell casts, which, on occasion, can be quite abundant even with mild glomerular abnormalities. With progression, the tubulointerstitial changes correspond to the severity of the glomerular damage, and the degree of renal functional impairment and the foci of tubular atrophy with accompanying interstitial fibrosis are present in the vicinity of sclerosed glomeruli. Vessels are normal in the early phase, but with progressive nephron injury vascular sclerosis becomes significant and gets much worse if there is superadded hypertension.

Immunohistochemistry is crucial in the diagnosis of IgA nephropathy. There is diffuse brilliant granular staining of the mesangium for IgA and C_3, with similar but less intense staining for IgG and IgM in at least half the cases. Clq and C_4 are generally absent. The diffuse staining for IgA is evident even when the light microscopic abnormalities are mild and focal. In a few cases there can be additional scattered granular staining of glomerular capillary walls for IgA (Plate 11).

On electronmicroscopy there is a prominent increase of mesangial cells and matrix with small to large aggregates of electron-dense deposits within the mesangium and paramesangial subendothelium. Unlike the diffuse IgA positivity on immunohistochemistry, electronmicroscopic deposits can be focal and segmental with some mesangial regions totally lacking in deposits (Figure 7.3).

Diffuse mesangiocapillary GN

Mesangiocapillary glomerulonephritis (MCGN) (membranoproliferative GN) is a chronic, progressive GN that occurs predominantly in children and young adults. Most patients need renal replacement therapy within 20 years of onset. Histologically it is characterized by proliferation of mesangial cells accompanied by thickening of peripheral glomerular capillary walls. There are two distinct types of MCGN.

MCGN Type I The nephrotic syndrome is the most common presentation in the adult, often with an active urine sediment containing red cells and casts. Occasional patients may have symptomless proteinuria, macroscopic haematuria or the nephritic syndrome. Complement abnormalities

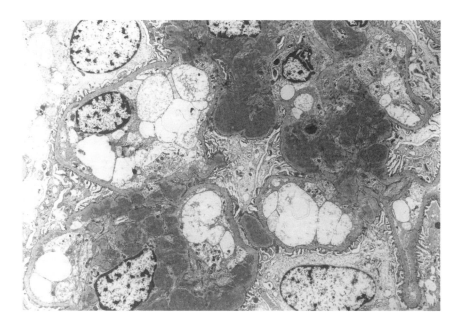

Fig. 7.3
IgA nephropathy. Deposits of varying size can be seen in the mesangium and paramesangial subendothelium. There is associated expansion of the mesangial matrix.

are frequent and about 50% of patients have low plasma CH_{50} and C_3 levels and, less frequently, low Clq and C_4 as well. The majority of cases of MCGN type I are idiopathic, but some can be associated with chronic infections (infective endocarditis, infected ventriculoatrial shunts, hepatitis B, malaria), SLE, macroglobulinaemia, cryoglobulinaemia, or lymphoid malignancies.

By light microscopy the glomeruli are enlarged, hypercellular with increased mesangial matrix, and have a lobular appearance. The hypercellularity can be accentuated by an infiltration of neutrophils. The expanded mesangium encroaches on the capillary lumina, which are further compromised by diffuse thickening of the capillary wall. The thickening is due to a characteristic, circumferential double-contoured tram track appearance of the glomerular basement membrane, with interpositioning of mesangial cell cytoplasm between the two layers (Plate 12). Large, ovoid deposits are also present within the double contours. As the disease progresses, the cellularity decreases but the mesangial matrix increases, causing further narrowing of the capillary lumina and eventually solidification of the tuft. Rarely, in the acute phase there can be epithelial cell proliferation forming crescents.

Tubular changes are secondary and consist of red cells within the lumina, protein reabsorption droplets and hyalin casts, and eventually tubular atrophy with interstitial fibrosis.

With immunohistochemistry there is a coarse, bright, garland-type granular positivity of all peripheral glomerular capillaries for C_3, IgG and

Fig. 7.4
MCGN type I. Multiple small to large, subendothelial and mesangial deposits (lower right); mesangial cell extensions into capillary walls (upper left).

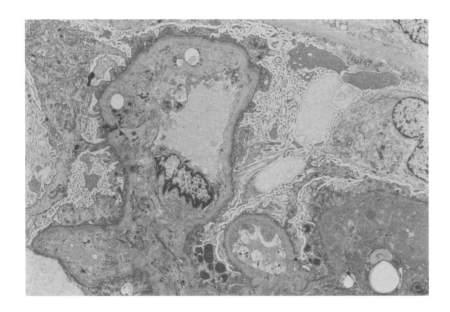

IgM, and less often for Clq and C_4. Mesangial C_3 is frequent. IgA deposits are unusual (Plate 13). By electronmicroscopy the double contoured appearance is seen to be due to native basement membrane on the epithelial aspect with new discontinuous basement membrane on the subendothelial aspect, the intervening space contains mesangial cell cytoplasm and matrix together with electron-dense deposits. These subendothelial deposits vary in size and are usually accompanied by aggregates of mesangial deposits (Figure 7.4). Subepithelial deposits are present in approximately 20% of cases and can be small and numerous or scattered, large and dome-shaped. In patients with cryoglobulinaemic nephropathy the subendothelial deposits often have a distinct structure composed of straight or curved parallel fibrils.

MCGN Type II   Also known as dense-deposit disease, this disorder presents with the nephrotic syndrome, the nephritic syndrome or haematuria with proteinuria. Serologically there is persistent severe depletion of serum C_3 with normal values for early complement components. In the majority of patients the serum contains a circulating IgG autoantibody termed C_3 nephritic factor (NeF), which is responsible for the persistent activation of C_3.

The majority of cases are idiopathic, but in approximately 10% there is an association with partial lipodystrophy, suggesting that the renal disorder is part of a systemic disease. MCGN type II is slowly progressive, with at least half the patients being in renal failure 10 years after clinical onset.

There is a characteristic histological appearance: the glomeruli are enlarged, often lobular, and have a striking eosinophilic ribbon-like thickening of the capillary walls. In the early phase, the thickening can be discontinuous, rather like a string of sausages (Plate 14). Similar lesions can be seen within the mesangium and also in Bowman's capsule. These lesions are intensely PAS-positive, and stain brown rather than black with methanamine silver. Glomerular hypercellularity is only moderate, unlike in MCGN type I. With progressive disease there is increasing mesangial sclerosis. Glomerular crescents may be present in a minority of cases.

Tubular basement membranes, peritubular capillary membranes and even arterioles may have PAS-positive lesions similar to the glomeruli. Tubulointerstitial abnormalities are otherwise non-specific and simply reflect the consequences of glomerular damage.

With immunohistochemistry there is faint to bright pseudolinear staining of the deposits in the glomerular capillary walls and other basement membranes for C_3. Mesangial deposits stain in a ring pattern. Occasionally there may be some IgM staining and rarely IgG staining. On electronmicroscopy the lamina densa of the glomerular basement membrane is replaced by linear-ribbon-like, homogeneous, intensely electron-dense material (Figure 7.5). Similar material in nodular form may be present in the mesangial regions. As with light microscopy, changes similar to those in the glomerular basement membrane can be identified in Bowman's capsule, and in the tubular basement membranes and capillaries.

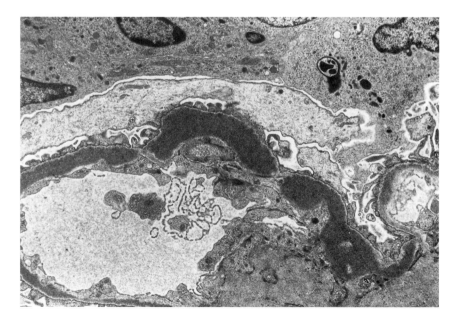

Fig. 7.5
MCGN type II. Dark, electron-dense, ribbon-like material within the thickened glomerular basement membrane.

Diffuse extracapillary proliferative glomerulonephritis

Also known as crescentic glomerulonephritis or rapidly progressive glomerulonephritis, this condition is characterized by the presence of large collections of proliferating epithelial cells and infiltrating monocytes within Bowman's space. The cells cover 50% or more of the circumference of the glomeruli. Crescentic GN includes a number of conditions that have the common features of crescents in at least 50%, and usually 80%, of the glomeruli and a clinical course characterized by abrupt onset and rapid progression to renal failure. Crescents probably form in response to breaks in the glomerular basement membrane, which allow fibrin and its precursors into Bowman's space; there is subsequent influx of monocytes and also proliferation of glomerular epithelial cells.

On the basis of immunofluorescence staining, three pathogenic forms of crescentic glomerulonephritis can be identified: antiglomerular basement membrane antibody-mediated (anti-GBM). GN with linear IgG; immune complex-mediated GN with granular immunoglobulins and complement components; and pauci (scanty) immune GN with no significant immune staining. Renal biopsy is essential to distinguish between the various causes of crescentic glomerulonephritis.

Pulmonary haemorrhage is a complication in approximately 30% of patients with anti-GBM nephritis, almost all of whom have a history of smoking or other pulmonary injury.

Patients with immune complex-mediated crescentic GN often have an underlying disorder, e.g. systemic or visceral bacterial infection, SLE, mesangiocapillary GN, Henoch–Schönlein purpura or, less commonly, cryoglobulinaemic nephropathy. Pauci immune crescentic GN is associated with vasculitic disorders, e.g. Wegener's granulomatosis, microscopic polyangiitis and, less commonly, severe hypertension.

Patients with crescentic GN are adults with vague prodromal symptoms of lethargy, fever and joint pains followed by acute nephritic syndrome with or without macroscopic haematuria. Screening for antiglomerular basement membrane (anti-GBM) antibodies, complement levels, antinuclear factor, antibodies to neutrophil cytoplasmic antigen and antistreptolysin antibodies is essential.

Renal biopsy is essential in the diagnosis and management of crescentic GN. As crescent formation is rapid and leads to permanent scarring, it is crucial that pathologists report the light and immunofluorescence microscopy findings with the least delay possible.

On light microscopy, the most striking feature is the presence of proliferating epithelial cells and macrophages, two to three layers thick, within Bowman's space of the majority of glomeruli. Mitotic figures are frequent and fibrin, neutrophils and red cells are present within the crescents. The crescents can be circumferational and may almost totally

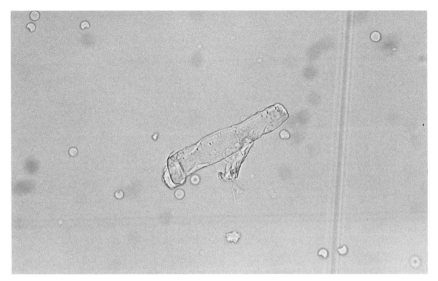

Plate 1
Hyaline cast. The field also contains numerous red cells, some with normal morphology (e.g. those adjacent to the left hand end of the cast), others dysmorphic (e.g. those in the top left hand and bottom right hand corners).

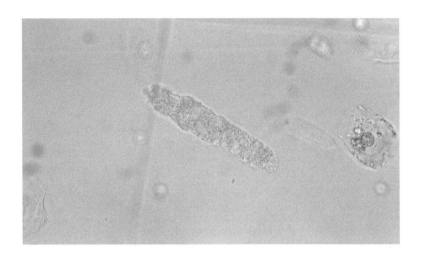

Plate 2
Fine granular cast. The field also contains a large nucleated epithelial cell, probably a renal tubular cell.

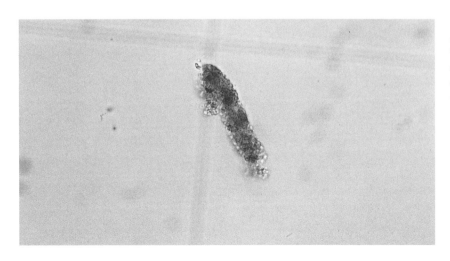

Plate 3
Coarse granular cast. Typically (as in this case) darker in colour and containing larger fragments of debris.

Plate 4 Red cell cast. Brownish-red in colour, with intact red cells visible, especially at the edges: it is difficult to get the whole cast in focus, and the structure is best visualized by moving the plane of focus of the microscope up and down. The field also contains a fragment of a granular cast (top right).

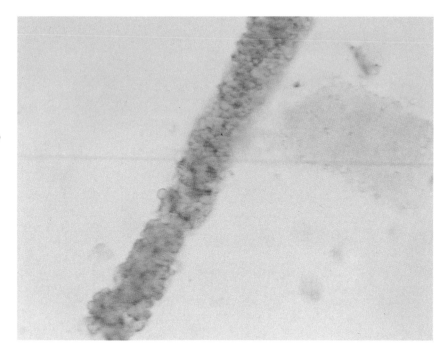

Plate 5
White cell cast. Intact nucleated cells, each larger than a red cell, again best visualized by moving the focus up and down.

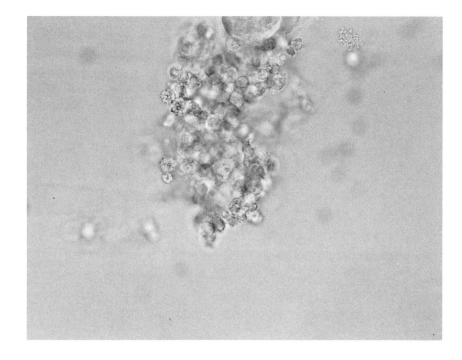

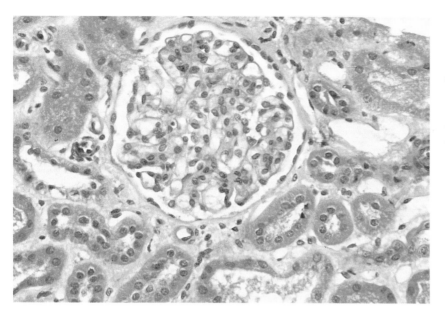

Plate 6
Normal glomerulus. Widely patent capillary loops, sparse mesangium and a few nuclei within mesangial regions can be seen. Surrounding tubules are arranged compactly with sparse interstitium. (H&E low power.)

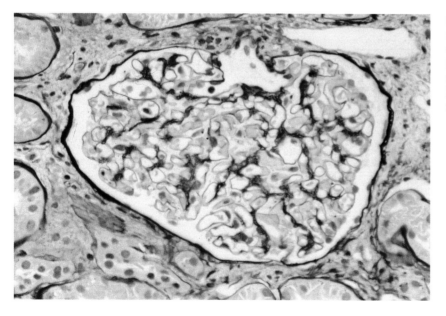

Plate 7
Normal glomerulus. Glomerular capillary walls, Bowman's membrane and mesangium stain dark brown/black. (MethAg, medium power.)

Plate 8
Poststreptococcal glomerulonephritis. The glomerulus is enlarged, hypercellular and infiltrated by neutrophils. The capillary lumina are occluded secondary to endothelial cell swelling and proliferation of mesangial cells. (H&E, medium power.)

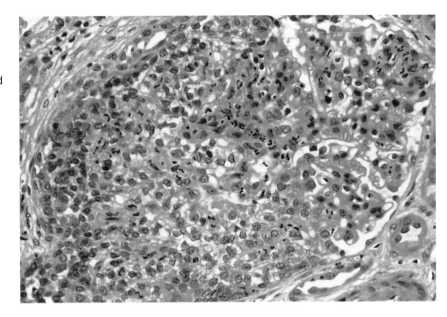

Plate 9
Poststreptococcal glomerulonephritis. Diffuse, brilliant, granular staining of capillary walls for IgG. (IF stain, medium power.)

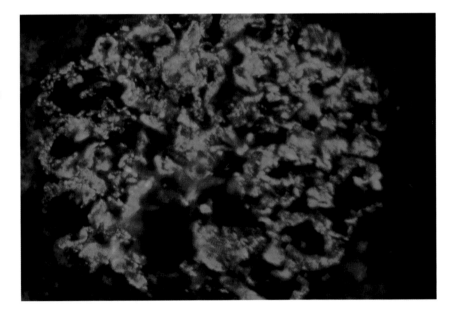

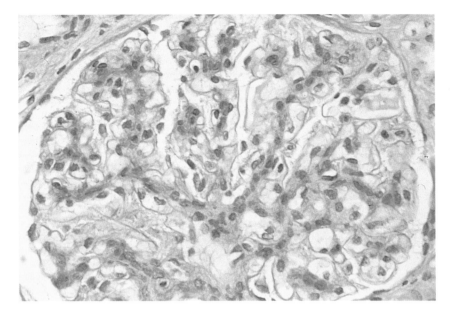

Plate 10
IgA nephropathy. Diffuse mesangial matrical and cellular increase; capillary loops patent. (PAS, medium power.)

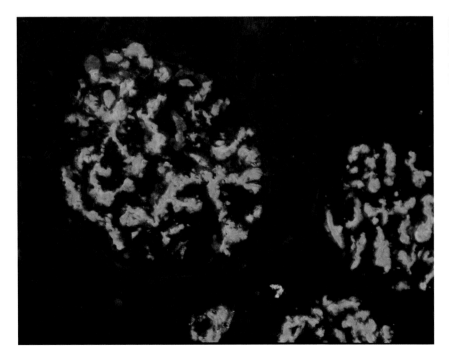

Plate 11
IgA nephropathy. Brilliant, coarsely granular positivity of mesangium for IgA. (IF, low power.)

Plate 12
MCGN type I. The glomerulus is enlarged, has a lobular appearance secondary to mesangial matrical and cellular increase, and many of the capillary lumina are narrowed. Glomerular capillary walls have mesangial interposition and duplication of the glomerular basement membrane. (MethAg, medium power.)

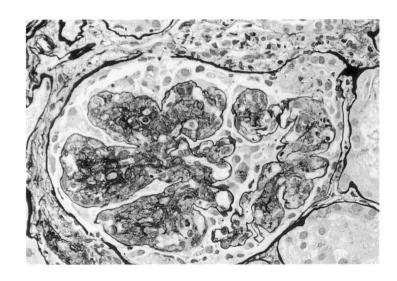

Plate 13
MCGN type I. Coarse, granular positivity of peripheral capillary loops (garland pattern) for IgG. (IF, medium power.)

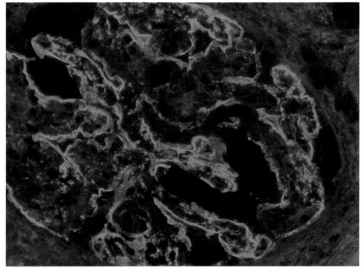

Plate 14
MCGN type II. Enlarged hypercellular glomerulus with the capillary walls outlined by thick, diffuse, almost continuous refractile material. (PAS, medium power.)

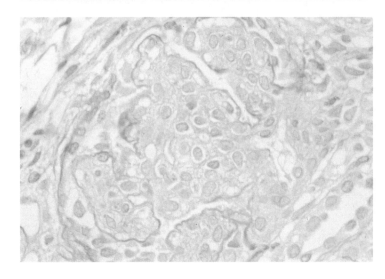

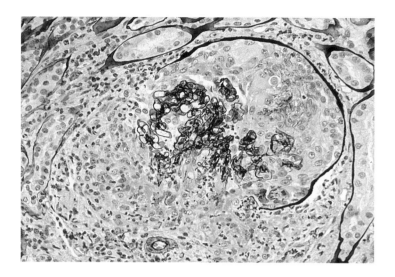

Plate 15
Crescentic glomerulonephritis. Segmental necrosis of glomerular tuft with fibrin deposition; Bowman's membrane is ruptured and the space is obliterated by a cellular crescent composed of macrophages and proliferating epithelial cells. (MethAg, medium power.)

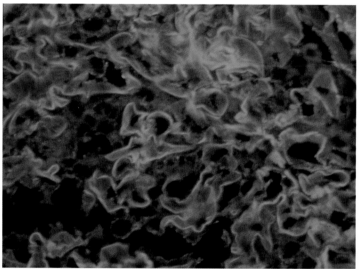

Plate 16
Anti glomerular basement membrane nephritis. Diffuse, brilliant, linear flourescence for IgG. (IF, high power.)

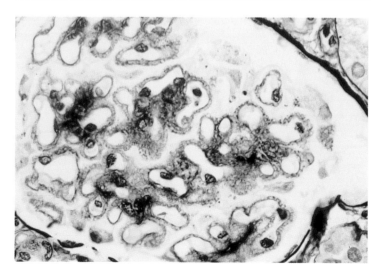

Plate 17
Membranous glomerulonephritis. The glomerulus is enlarged, has rigid capillary walls, and is only marginally hypercellular. Small evenly distributed spikes are present on the subepithelial aspect of the capillary wall. (MethAg, medium power.)

Plate 18
FSGS. Segmental sclerosis of capillary loops (3 o'clock) with some containing eosinophilic insudative 'deposits' within capillary walls (7 o'clock). (MethAg, medium power.)

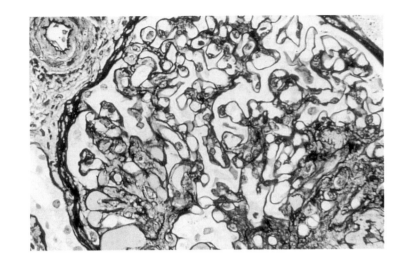

Plate 19
Lupus nephritis class III. Focal, segmental necrosis with fibrin deposition, endocapillary proliferation and neutrophil infiltration. (H&E, medium power.)

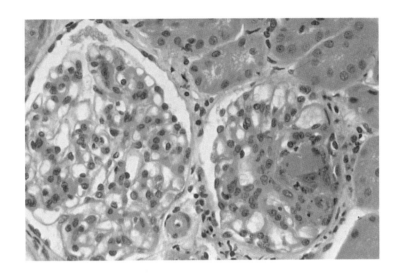

Plate 20
Lupus nephritis class IV. Enlarged hypercellular glomerulus; large subendothelial deposits almost occluding the capillary lumina, so-called 'hyalin thrombi'. (MethAg, medium power.)

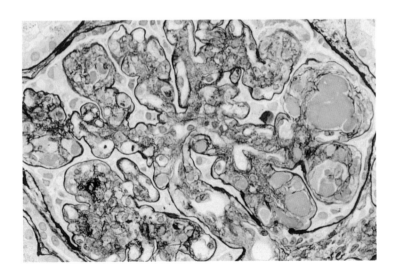

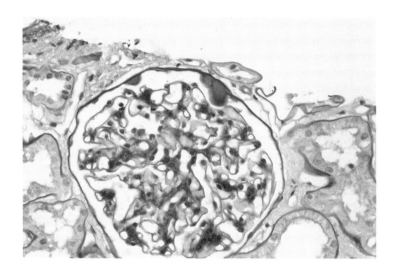

Plate 21
Diabetic nephropathy.
Diffuse increase in
mesangial matrix with only
modest hypercellularity.
The capillary loops are
widely patent. Two
PAS-positive capsular
drop lesions on Bowman's
membrane (around 12
o'clock). (PAS, low power.)

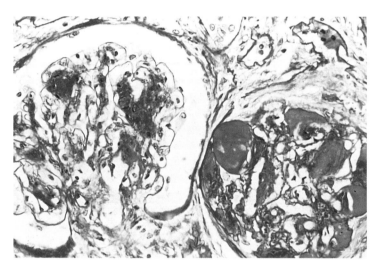

Plate 22
Diabetic nephropathy.
Segmental fibrillar nodular
mesangial matrical
increase (11o'clock in tuft
on left) on a background of
diffuse increase in the rest
of the glomerulus. The tuft
on the right looks similar at
first glance but shows
multiple homogeneous,
insudative lesions within
the capillary walls. With
silver stains the expanded
matrix will be black and
insudative lesions pink.
(H&E, medium power.)

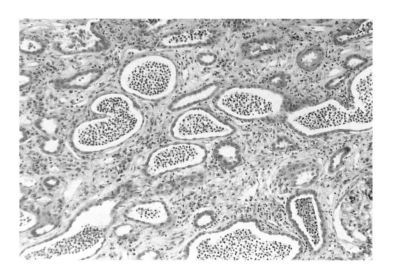

Plate 23
Acute pyelonephritis.
Abundant neutrophils
within tubular lumina,
tubular epithelial cell
damage, oedema and
cellular infiltration in
surrounding interstitium.
(H&E, medium power.)

Plate 24
Allergic TIN. Diffuse
infiltrate of predominantly
mononuclear inflammatory
cells within the interstitium
and tubular epithelium: a
modest number of
eosinophils is also present.
Significant tubular epithelial
damage. (H&E, medium
power.)

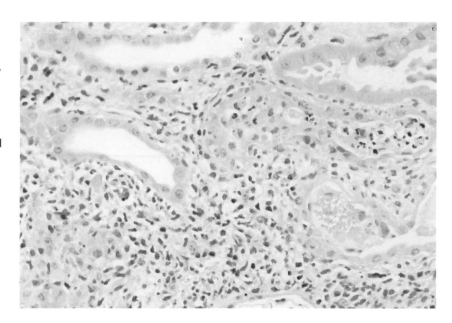

Plate 25
Allergic TIN. The majority
of the infiltrating cells are
of T-cell phenotype; note
'tubulitis' with lymphocytes
within the tubular epithelium.
(Immoperoxidase stain,
CD3, medium power.)

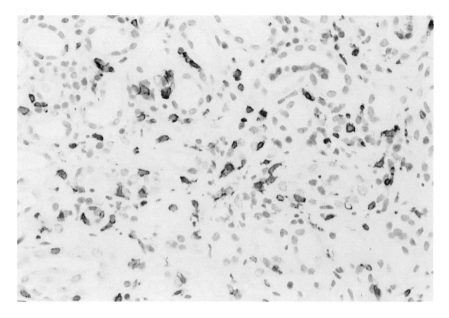

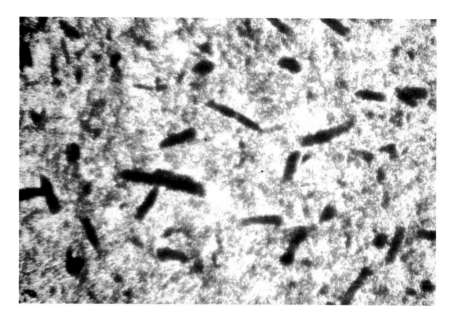

Plate 26
'Muddy brown' granular pigmented casts seen in ATN.

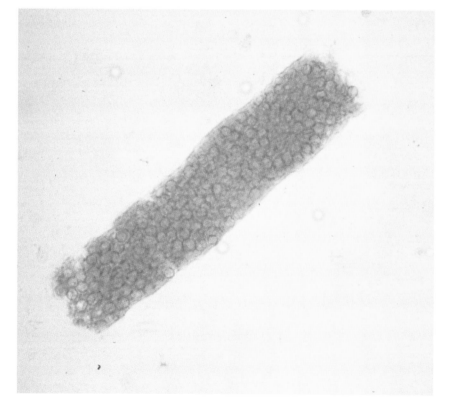

Plate 27
Red blood cell cast seen in glomerulonephritis.

Plate 28
White blood cell cast seen in pyelonephritis or allergic interstitial nephritis.

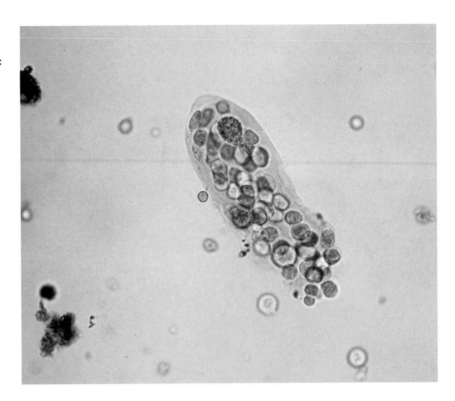

Plate 29
Calcium oxalate crystals seen in ethylene glycol poisoning.

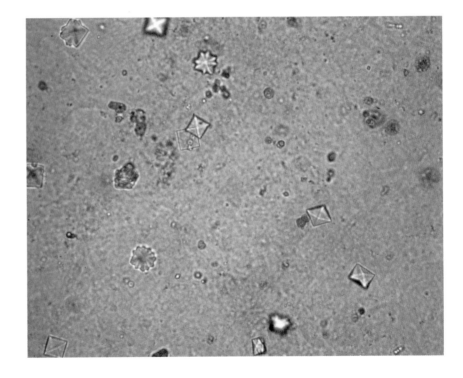

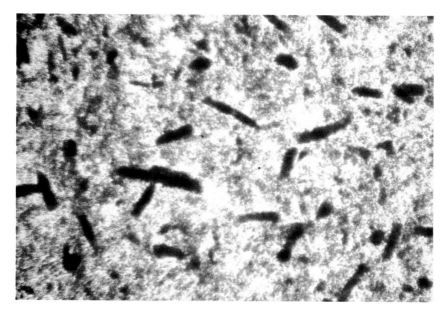

Plate 26
'Muddy brown' granular pigmented casts seen in ATN.

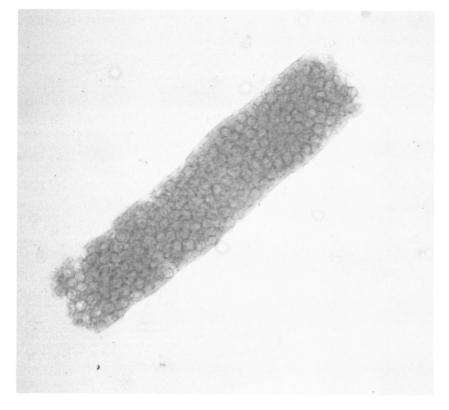

Plate 27
Red blood cell cast seen in glomerulonephritis.

Plate 28
White blood cell cast seen
in pyelonephritis or allergic
interstitial nephritis.

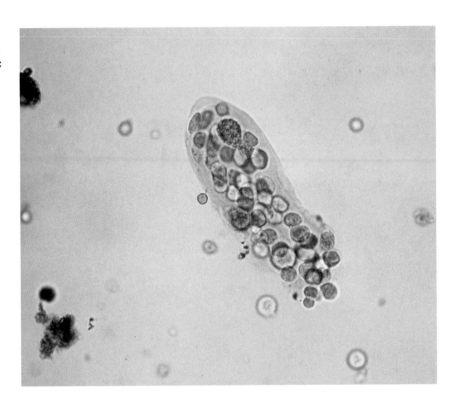

Plate 29
Calcium oxalate crystals
seen in ethylene glycol
poisoning.

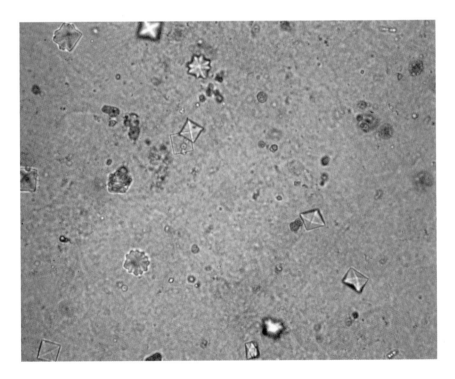

replace the glomerular space. The glomerular tufts show a spectrum of changes from segmental to global necrosis with or without endocapillary proliferation and neutrophil infiltration. Sometimes the glomerular destruction can be so extensive that only a few remnants of capillary walls can be identified with silver stains (Plate 15). Cellular crescents start to undergo fibrosis and progress to fibrocellular crescents and then fibrotic crescents. This progression can be rapid, occurring in the course of four to five weeks, and at the same time the injured glomerular segments become sclerotic.

In anti-GBM nephritis the glomerular lesions tend to be of the same age, whereas in immune complex and pauci immune crescentic GN the lesions tend to be in different stages of resolution, indicating that the injury is ongoing or recurrent. The tubules and interstitium reflect the severity of the process with red cells within tubules, acute tubular necrosis, tubulitis, interstitial oedema and inflammation. In patients with Wegener's granulomatosis or microscopic polyangiitis, focal necrosis of arteries and capillaries may be present.

In anti-GBM nephritis, immunohistochemistry shows brilliant diffuse linear fluorescence of all glomerular capillary walls for IgG (Plate 16). On occasion, C_3 can be positive, but IgA and IgM are usually absent. The appearance and distribution of immune reactants in immune complex crescentic GN depends on the associated disease. In patients with infections it is granular staining of capillary walls for IgG and C_3; in IgA nephropathy and Henoch–Schönlein purpura there is predominant mesangial staining for IgA and C_3; in lupus nephritis diffuse granular staining of capillary walls and mesangium for IgG, IgA, IgM, C_3, C_4 and Clq. In pauci immune crescentic GN there are scattered flecks of staining with 'sticky' molecules IgM and C_3 in the necrotic foci.

Electronmicroscopy can be difficult to interpret because of the glomerular destruction and disorganization. Surviving capillary loops may show perforation in the glomerular basement membrane, with extravasation of fibrin into Bowman's space. In immune complex crescentic GN, electron-dense deposits may be identified. Bowman's space is filled with epithelial cells, macrophages, and fibrin in different stages of polymerization, and there are time-dense bands of organizing matrix between the cells.

Diffuse membranous GN

Membranous GN is the most frequent cause of nephrotic syndrome in adults. Patients usually present with persistent proteinuria, with or without the nephrotic syndrome. Microscopic haematuria and hypertension are also common. Serum complement levels are normal and immune complexes are not elevated. The majority of the cases with membranous GN are idiopathic, but a significant number can be associated with chronic infections (e.g. hepatitis B, malaria, syphilis), autoimmune disorders (e.g. SLE, rheumatoid arthritis), drugs (e.g. captopril, penicillamine, gold) and malignant neoplasms (e.g. carcinomas of the bronchus or breast and non-Hodgkin's lymphoma). Recovery is usual in most secondary cases when the primary cause is removed. In the idiopathic cases the disease is stationary or slowly progressive, with periods of remission and relapse.

On renal biopsy there is generally no material difference between idiopathic and secondary membranous glomerulonephritis. With light microscopy, the glomeruli are large with stiff capillary loops but no significant cellular proliferation. Silver stains are essential to demonstrate short regular subepithelial spike-like projections of the glomerular basement membrane (Plate 17). In the early phase, the spikes are delicate and slender and not present in all loops, but with progression the spikes become extensive, thicker, longer and fuse with each other to give a chain-link, double-contoured, thickened basement membrane. With further deterioration there is segmental sclerosis and hyalinosis, and eventually the glomeruli become globally sclerotic and obsolescent but still maintain their size and outlines of the thickened capillary walls.

In the early phase, the proximal tubules contain lipid and proteinaceous casts and the cells contain prominent reabsorption droplets. Later, there is tubular atrophy, with accompanying interstitial fibrosis and accumulations of small lymphocytes. In patients with heavy lipidaemia, interstitial collections of foam cells are a frequent finding. Vascular lesions, when present, are either age-related or secondary to progressive scarring and the development of hypertension.

With immunohistochemistry there is brilliant diffuse granular staining of capillary loops for IgG in all cases. Similar staining for C_3 is seen in 20–50%, and more variable staining for IgA and IgM. Mesangial deposits are unusual, and C_4 and Clq are generally absent; if they are present, it is highly probable that the patient has membranous GN secondary to SLE.

The main abnormality on electronmicroscopy is the presence of subepithelial deposits in glomerular capillary walls. With the aid of electronmicroscopy the evolution of the disease has been divided into four stages which parallel the light microscopic abnormalities.

Stage I Small scattered subepithelial deposits are present in the glomerular basement membrane. The capillary walls appear normal on H&E sections, but with silver stains there are short spikes in scattered capillary loops.

Stage II More extensive, almost diffuse, subepithelial deposits are shown by electronmicroscopy, with the intervening space of basement membrane seen as silver-positive spikes on light microscopy (Figure 7.6).

Stage III The basement membrane between the deposits extends over to enclose the deposits, thereby causing thickening of the glomerular basement

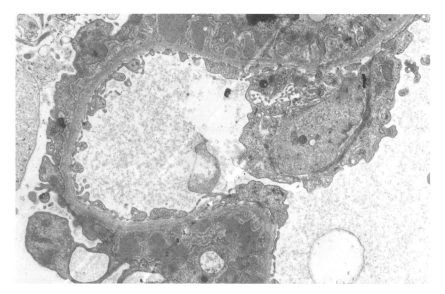

Fig. 7.6
MGN stage II. Irregularly shaped deposits on the epithelial aspect of the glomerular basement membrane with extensions of the lamina densa between the deposits (the spikes seen by light microscopy). There is diffuse obliteration of the epithelial cell foot processes.

membrane and a double-contoured chain-link appearance on light microscopy. Some of the deposits resolve producing electronlucent foci. In patients with relapsing diseases, the glomerular basement membrane shows marked thickening, with 'waves' of recent subepithelial deposits overlying older, partly resolved, deposits incorporated within the glomerular basement membrane (Figure 7.7).

Stage IV The glomerular basement membrane is grossly thickened and distorted, with obliteration of the capillary lumina, and shows a spectrum of

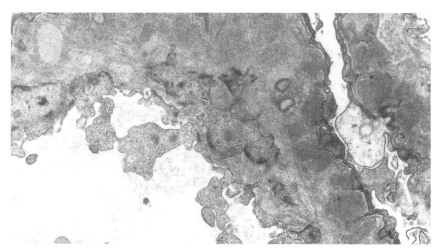

Fig. 7.7
MGN stage III. The glomerular basement membrane is thickened, the deposits are surrounded by lamina densa (chain-link appearance on light microscopy); some of the deposits are showing resolution, leaving electronlucent areas.

changes including residual deposits, intramembranous lucencies and endothelial invaginations.

The deposits resolve in patients with prolonged remission, leaving electronlucent areas that gradually disappear to leave an essentially unremarkable glomerular basement membrane.

Focal segmental glomerulosclerosis

Focal segmental glomerulosclerosis (FSGS) is a clinicopathological entity in which the presentation is heavy proteinuria with or without the nephritic syndrome, and renal biopsy is characterized by focal and segmental glomerular lesions consisting of intracapillary foam cells, synechiae, sclerosis of capillary loops, and hyalinosis. Although distinctive, the lesions are not exclusive to FSGS and can be seen in a number of renal diseases in which there has been previous glomerular damage, e.g. postinfectious GN, diabetic glomerulosclerosis, Alport's syndrome, reflux nephropathy, or any end-stage glomerular disease. It is therefore clear that a diagnosis of FSGS should not be made on histological grounds alone. It should be made only when the lesions are present at the time of initial presentation with heavy proteinuria.

Patients with long-term minimal change disease may, in later biopsies, demonstrate segmental synechiae or sclerosis. This has led to the as yet unresolved debate about whether minimal change disease and FSGS are separate disorders or are at the two ends of a spectrum with a common pathogenesis.

Focal segmental glomerulosclerosis is characterized by heavy proteinuria and the rapid development of oedema. It is common in children and young adults, and slightly more frequent in males. The proteinuria may exceed 10 g in 24 hours, is non-selective, even in children, and in the majority is accompanied by microscopic haematuria. At least one-third of patients are hypertensive at the time of presentation. A severe and relentless form of FSGS is seen in AIDS nephropathy and heroin-associated nephropathy.

FSGS is a progressive disease, but the rate of deterioration is variable. Approximately 50% of patients will develop chronic renal failure within 10 years. There are no specific criteria that indicate a poor prognosis, although mesangial hypercellularity, mesangial IgM, the proportion of glomeruli with global sclerosis, tubular atrophy at the time of presentation, and the degree of heavy proteinuria have all been suspected. FSGS recurs in approximately 30% of renal allografts, occasionally with amazing rapidity. The condition in some cases can be familial, and it is therefore prudent to avoid live-related donor transplants in patients with end-stage FSGS.

The initial lesions of FSGS can be very subtle and are easily missed, thereby leading to the mistaken diagnosis of minimal change disease. Moreover, the initial lesions are sparse and characteristically found in the deep juxtamedullary glomeruli; if this region is not included in the biopsy the diagnosis can again be missed.

In the early lesions, a few glomerular capillaries contain lipid-laden foam cells, often with swelling of the overlying epithelial cells containing PAS-positive droplets and adherence to Bowman's capsule. With progression, segmental capillary loops become sclerotic and contain hyaline, intensely PAS-positive silver-negative insudative lesions within the capillary walls (Plate 18). In the early phase there may be mild mesangial matrical and cellular increase. With time, the sclerotic segments increase in distribution, and within individual glomeruli the segmental lesions spread to involve the whole tuft, leading to global sclerosis. Even in end-stage FSGS with obsolescent glomeruli, there is persistence of the segments of hyalinosis, indicating the underlying initial pathology.

Well established FSGS is invariably associated with tubular atrophy and interstitial fibrosis. As the glomerular lesions are few and far between, and therefore easily missed, in early cases, the presence of even a few atrophic tubules in the biopsy sample should alert the pathologist to a diagnosis of FSGS rather than minimal change disease. This is particularly so in the case of biopsies from children and young adults. Arteriolar hyaline sclerosis, even in the absence of hypertension, is present in about half of cases.

With immunohistochemistry, the most characteristic appearance is the presence of coarse aggregates of IgM and C_3 within the sclerotic segments and often in arteriolar walls.

On electronmicroscopy, the sclerotic segments show irregular collapse of capillary loops, mesangial matrical increase, obliteration of epithelial cell foot processes and villous hyperplasia of epithelial cells containing numerous vacuoles, some filled with lipid. Fibrillar material, representing synechiae, may be present bridging the sclerotic segment to Bowman's capsule. The hyaline insudative lesions of light microscopy appear as large electron-dense subendothelial 'deposits', often containing lipid vacuoles, and should not be mistaken for immune deposits.

Focal proliferative glomerulonephritis

Focal proliferative glomerulonephritis is invariably associated with a systemic disease, e.g. SLE, Henoch–Schönlein purpura, Wegener's granulomatosis, microscopic polyangiitis, anti-GBM nephritis, subacute bacterial endocarditis, or hypertension. The clinical presentation can be variable and includes haematuria, proteinuria, nephrotic syndrome, nephritic syndrome and acute renal failure.

The characteristic appearance is the presence of segmental lesions in some glomeruli with the rest being normal. The segmental lesions include mild endocapillary proliferation with or without necrosis, foci of epithelial cell proliferation and scarring. On occasion, the proliferation and necrosis may be severe and global and be accompanied by cellular crescents.

In mild cases, fewer than 10% of the glomeruli examined may be abnormal; when severe, 50% or more of the glomeruli are involved and there is associated acute tubular necrosis, interstitial oedema and inflammation. Arterial and arteriolar inflammation and necrosis may be present in Wegener's or microscopic polyangiitis.

Immunohistochemical findings depend on the underlying systemic disease: linear IgG in anti-GBM nephritis, mesangial IgA in Henoch–Schönlein purpura and IgA nephropathy, 'full house' IgG, IgM, IgA, C_3 and Clq in lupus nephritis, granular IgG and C_3 in subacute endocarditis and pauci immune in Wegener's granulomatosis and microscopic polyangiitis.

Electronmicroscopic abnormalities will again reflect the underlying condition. These have been described elsewhere.

Diffuse global sclerosis

Biopsy of patients in end-stage renal failure, with or without previous history of renal problems, is generally unproductive. Diffuse glomerular scarring is the final common pathway of many of the glomerulonephritides and in most cases it is not possible to make any assessment of the initial pathology. The majority of these patients are hypertensive and the secondary parenchymal damage it causes adds further to the problems of interpreting the biopsy.

The kidney in systemic diseases

Renal involvement complicates many systemic diseases, the majority of which have an immunological, infectious, metabolic or hereditary basis. There is often a significant relationship between the degree of renal involvement and the patient's clinical course. The glomerular abnormalities form a spectrum that is essentially similar to that seen in primary glomerulonephritis.

SYSTEMIC DISEASES WITH RENAL INVOLVEMENT

Immune diseases

The main systemic diseases with renal involvement that have an immunological basis are:

- systemic lupus erythematosus
- rheumatoid arthritis
- mixed connective tissue disease

- Sjögren's syndrome
- Henoch–Schönlein purpura
- sarcoidosis
- systemic sclerosis
- anti-GBM disease with pulmonary haemorrhage (Goodpasture's syndrome)
- allograft rejection.

Infectious diseases

There is often an immunopathogenetic mechanism to the infectious diseases that have renal involvement. These include:

- bacterial endocarditis
- hepatitis B and C
- malaria
- HIV.

Vascular diseases

The main vascular diseases with renal involvement are:

- microscopic polyangiitis
- classic polyarteritis nodosa
- Wegener's granulomatosis
- Churg–Strauss syndrome
- haemolytic uraemic syndrome
- thrombotic thrombocytopenic purpura
- hypertension.

Metabolic diseases

The main metabolic diseases that have renal involvement are:

- diabetes mellitus
- amyloidosis
- multiple myeloma
- cryoglobulinaemia and paraproteinaemias
- gout.

Hereditary nephropathies

Renal involvement is present in the following hereditary nephropathies:

- Alport's syndrome
- thin membrane nephropathy
- hereditary metabolic disorders.

It is beyond the scope of this chapter to discuss all of these conditions and many have been alluded to in the previous sections. Alport's syndrome is discussed in Chapter 8. Lupus nephritis and diabetic nephropathy are discussed below.

SYSTEMIC LUPUS ERYTHEMATOSUS

SLE is a multisystem disorder in which there is production of autoantibodies against a spectrum of self-antigens. The immunological abnormalities are discussed elsewhere (p. 57). The pathogenesis of the glomerular involvement is thought to be due to the following mechanisms:

- circulating DNA is localized to the glomerular basement membrane and anti-DNA antibodies are fixed to it to form immune complexes *in situ*
- circulating immune complexes are filtered through the glomerulus and deposited within the mesangium and capillary wall.

Subsequently there is complement fixation, which leads to inflammation and tissue injury. Patients with renal involvement present with a spectrum of urinary abnormalities ranging from asymptomatic proteinuria and haematuria to nephrotic syndrome or the nephritic syndrome. There can be poor correlation between the laboratory findings, urinary sediment and the degree of renal involvement. Renal biopsy is therefore mandatory in patients suspected of having lupus nephritis, not only for diagnosis but also for management and assessment of prognosis.

As with the clinical presentation, lupus nephritis can have a number of morphological patterns with marked irregularity in the distribution of lesions. The World Health Organization (WHO) has proposed a classification that correlates morphology with clinical symptoms and prognosis (Churg, Bernstein and Glassock, 1995). However, the predictive value of the WHO classification is not entirely satisfactory and a semiquantitative histological scoring system with activity and chronicity index has been introduced. These indices also help to compare different patients and assess the progress of the disease in an individual patient (Table 7.3).

Classification of lupus nephritis (WHO)
The biopsy must be evaluated by light microscopy, immunohistochemistry and electronmicroscopy.

Class I – normal or minor lesions Patients have no urinary sediment abnormalities and are biopsied as part of the work-up of patients in a prospective study of SLE.

Class II A and B – mesangial proliferative GN Patients have mild proteinuria with or without microscopic haematuria but the renal function

Index	Maximum score
Activity index	
Fibrinoid necrosis and karryorrhexis	6
Cellular crescents	6
Wire loops and hyaline thrombi (subendothelial deposits)	3
Neutrophil infiltration	3
Monocyte infiltration	3
Interstitial inflammation	3
Chronicity index	
Glomerular sclerosis	3
Fibrous crescents	3
Tubular atrophy	3
Interstitial fibrosis	3

Source: Austin *et al.*, 1993.

Table 7.3
Activity and chronicity index in lupus nephritis

is normal. The glomerular abnormality consists of mesangial hypercellularity and matrical increase; the change is mild in IIA and more advanced in IIB. By immunohistochemistry there is mesangial IgG, C_3, Clq, and perhaps IgA and IgM. On electronmicroscopy mesangial hypercellularity and matrical increase are more apparent and immune deposits are identified within the mesangium and paramesangium, few in IIA but more abundant in IIB.

Class III – focal segmental proliferative GN Patients present with proteinuria, haematuria and an active urinary sediment. The lesions are focal and segmental and consist of endocapillary proliferation, neutrophil infiltration and karryorrhexis, which may or may not be accompanied by necrosis. Epithelial proliferation and cellular adhesions overlie the necrotic foci. All these changes tend to occur on a background of mild mesangial hypercellularity. The mesangium and peripheral capillary loops contain large deposits that are eosinophilic by H&E stain and magenta with PAS. Circumferential subendothelial deposits in capillary walls cause a thickened wire-loop appearance, and large nodular deposits appear as intraluminal masses known as 'hyalin thrombi'. Along with such active lesions there can be foci of glomerular sclerosis (Plate 19).

Tubulointerstitial inflammation and atrophy correlate with the severity of the glomerular changes. Arteries and arterioles may show vascular sclerosis.

There is diffuse granular mesangial positivity together with large subendothelial and fine subepithelial positivity of segmental capillary walls for IgG, IgM, C_3 and Clq; IgA is occasionally present. There may also be deposits of IgG and complement in tubular and capillary basement membranes.

On electronmicroscopy, abundant deposits of varying sizes are present within the mesangium, and there are scattered subepithelial and subendothelial deposits.

Class IV – diffuse proliferative GN   This is essentially a continuum of class III in that the lesions are no longer focal and segmental but tend to be diffuse and global. With progressive disease, class III can become class IV, or with therapy and improvement class IV may revert to class III, with active proliferation co-existing with healed focal segmental sclerosis.

Patients with class IV lupus nephritis present with proteinuria and haematuria, and nephrotic syndrome or nephritic syndrome, renal function is usually compromised.

Histologically class IV can have three predominant patterns, which are not mutually exclusive:

- diffuse proliferative, necrotizing and sclerosing GN
- diffuse endocapillary proliferative GN
- diffuse mesangiocapillary type I proliferative GN (Plate 20).

Any of these types can have superimposed cellular crescents. Wire-loop lesions and capillary hyaline thrombi are frequent. Interstitial inflammation is common and tubilitis is frequent. Vessels may have intimal proliferation with medial thickening, and rarely there may be necrosis. Patients with anticardiolipin antibody can have vascular thrombi with glomerular and parenchymal necrosis.

Immunofluorescence microscopy presents a 'full house' picture, with large coarse, granular deposits along capillary walls and mesangium for IgG, IgM, IgA, C_3, C_4 and Clq. Large occlusive deposits of IgG are quite characteristic. Tubular membranes and arteriolar walls are often positive for IgG.

Electronmicroscopic appearances correspond to the immunohistochemical findings. Numerous and often large deposits are seen in the mesangial, intramembranous, endothelial and subepithelial regions. Large occlusive subendothelial deposits are frequent and if circulating cryoglobulins are present some of the deposits may have a parallel fibrillar structure (Figure 7.8).

Patients with class IV nephritis tend to have a poor prognosis, particularly when subendothelial deposits are extensive.

Class V – membranous GN   Patients with class V lupus nephritis present with heavy proteinuria with or without the nephritic syndrome. Criteria for

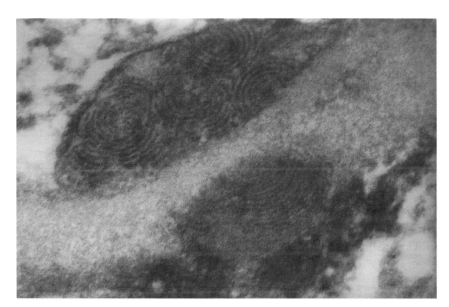

Fig. 7.8
Lupus nephritis class IV, Cryoglobulins. Subendothelial and subepithelial deposits with characteristic fibrillar structure.

the diagnosis of membranous lupus nephritis have to be strict as sub-epithelial deposits can be seen in the diffuse lesions of class IV. Class V should be reserved for biopsies with almost pure membranous change in which mesangial proliferation is minimal and mesangial and subendothelial deposits are sparse. By light microscopy the abnormalities are essentially similar to those seen in primary membranous GN. However, on immunohistochemistry there can be 'full house' positivity for IgG, IgM, IgA, C_3, C_4 and Clq.

Class transformation in lupus nephritis
The most striking feature of lupus nephritis is the histological variability between and within biopsies, as a result of which it can be difficult to assign a biopsy to a particular class. Moreover, repeat biopsies in patients have shown that transformation in either direction may occur between classes.

The factors involved in transformation are ill understood, but effective therapy must certainly play a part in transferring a severe class of disease to a milder form.

DIABETES MELLITUS

Renal disease is a major cause of morbidity and mortality in diabetes mellitus. Approximately 40–50% of patients with type I insulin-dependent diabetes mellitus (IDDM) develop renal insufficiency that becomes clinically evident 15–20 years after the onset of the disease. The frequency of diabetic nephropathy in type II non-insulin dependent diabetes mellitus

(NIDDM) is uncertain, but the average time of onset is about a decade earlier than in type I. In both types the susceptibility to diabetic nephropathy is determined by a number of factors including control of blood sugar, systemic hypertension and heredity. Once clinically manifest, the progression of nephropathy is irreversible, and it is often accompanied by diabetic retinopathy, neuropathy and hypertension. Proteinuria is the commonest manifestation. Initially mild and intermittent, over a period of time the proteinuria becomes heavy and continuous and there is progressive deterioration of renal function.

The classic features of diabetic nephropathy consist of glomerular and vascular abnormalities together with accompanying tubular atrophy. However, papillary necrosis and acute pyelonephritis are also frequent complications of diabetes.

Renal biopsy in the early phase reveals enlarged and hypertrophied glomeruli with varying degrees of mesangial matrical increase. With time there is marked PAS-positive mesangial accentuation producing a diffuse glomerulosclerosis that is accompanied by thickening of the capillary walls (Plate 21). In 1936 Kimmelsteil and Wilson described nodular glomerulosclerosis, which is considered to be diagnostic of diabetic glomerulopathy. It is present in the kidney of approximately 25% of diabetic patients and is invariably accompanied by diffuse glomerulosclerosis. The nodules are composed of homogeneous, eosinophilic, PAS- and silver-positive acellular masses of mesangial matrix that often have concentric lamination. They vary in size and distribution both within a glomerulus and between glomeruli (Plate 22). The capillaries at the periphery of the nodules are potent and may be dilated, even aneurysmal. With progressive disease, localized accumulations of eosinophilic deposits within the substance of the basement membrane of Bowman's capsule are known as 'capsular drop lesions' and are considered specific for diabetic glomerulopathy.

The glomerular abnormalities are accompanied by vascular changes of hyaline arteriosclerosis, which is of course not specific for diabetes being seen in hypertension and as a part of the 'normal ageing process'. However, arteriolar sclerosis is seen in diabetic patients at a much younger age, is much more extensive and, pathognomonic of this condition, involves both afferent and efferent arterioles. Accompanying the glomerular and vascular changes there is tubular atrophy characterized by thickening of the basement membranes and interstitial fibrosis.

Diabetic patients with significant small vessel disease are prone to renal papillary necrosis, especially when there is an accompanying urinary tract infection.

Immunofluorescent staining has no specific features, but there is often diffuse linear staining of glomerular and tubular basement membranes for

IgG and albumin and, in advanced disease, IgM and C_3 within sclerotic glomeruli and hyaline vessels.

By electronmicroscopy the earliest abnormality to be seen is significant thickening of the glomerular basement membrane; normally 300–380 nm, it can reach 1600 nm. With progressive diseases there is mesangial matrical increase, diffuse and nodular, with compression of the capillary lumina. In late disease electron dense subendothelial accumulations, many containing lipid droplets, are present within arterioles and glomerular capillaries.

Tubulointerstitial nephritis

Disorders of the tubules or interstitium lead to abnormalities in both compartments because of their anatomical proximity and functional interdependence. The emphasis can vary, however. In acute tubular necrosis the abnormalities are predominantly in the proximal tubules with very little, if any, interstitial pathology, whereas in acute drug-induced allergic-type tubulointerstitial nephritis the abnormalities are primarily in the interstitium together with mild to severe involvement of tubules.

In the initial phase of tubulointerstitial nephritis (TIN), glomerular and vascular pathology is mild, but with advanced disease there can be glomerular scarring and secondary hypertensive vascular disease.

CLINICAL PRESENTATION

Clinically tubulointerstitial nephritides can be distinguished from glomerular diseases by the absence of symptoms of glomerular injury, i.e. persistent proteinuria, nephrotic syndrome, significant haematuria or nephritic syndrome. The most common presentation is oliguria, anuria or non-oliguric renal failure. Patients with drug-related interstitial nephritis may have accompanying fever, rash and eosinophilia. Similarly, patients with acute infectious tubulointerstitial nephritis may have fever, loin pain, leucocytosis, and urgency of micturition; examination of the urine sediment will reveal white cell casts. In patients with advanced and chronic tubulointerstitial nephritis, defects in tubular function (inability to concentrate urine, salt wasting and diminished ability to excrete acids) may be present.

CLASSIFICATION OF TUBULOINTERSTITIAL NEPHRITIS

Tubulointerstitial nephritis has diverse aetiologies and pathogenic mechanisms, and in a signficant minority a causative factor is never identified. The

WHO classification of tubulointerstitial nephritis is quite extensive and there is considerable overlap between the various categories (Table 7.4). Only some of the commoner entities are discussed here.

Table 7.4

Classification of tubulo-interstitial nephritis (modified by WHO classification)

1. Infections
   (a) Ascending urinary tract infection – pyelonephritis
   (b) Associated with systemic infection
   (c) Xanthogranulomatous pyelonephritis
   (d) Malakoplakia
2. Acute tubular injury/necrosis
   (a) Ischaemic
   (b) Toxic
   (c) Septicaemia
   (d) Crush injury
3. Drug-induced nephritis
   (a) Allergic-type tubulointerstitial nephritis
   (b) Acute tubulotoxic injury
   (c) Chronic tubulointerstitial nephritis
4. Vesicoureteric reflux nephropathy
5. Obstructive uropathy
6. TIN associated with papillary necrosis
   (a) Diabetes mellitus
   (b) Analgesic nephropathy
   (c) Obstructive nephropathy
7. Heavy metal-induced nephritis
8. TIN associated with metabolic disorders
   (a) Hypercalcaemic nephropathy
   (b) Urate nephropathy
   (c) Oxalate nephropathy
9. Hereditary tubulointerstitial disorders
10. TIN associated with neoplastic disorders
    (a) Plasma cell dyscrasias
    (b) Leukaemia and lymphomatous infiltration
11. TIN associated with immune disorders
    (a) Allograft rejection
    (b) Anti-GBM disease
    (c) Systemic lupus erythematosus
    (d) Sjögren's syndrome
12. Tubulointerstitial lesions in end-stage renal disease
13. Miscellaneous disorders
    (a) Sarcoid granulomatous nephropathy
    (b) Idiopathic TIN – acute, granulomatous or chronic

Acute infectious TIN (acute pyelonephritis)

In most cases this is accompanied by cystitis and is due to ascending infection of the urinary tract by *E. coli* or other faecal bacteria. Oedema and inflammation of the bladder wall impairs competence of the ureterovesical valvular effect resulting in reflux of infected urine into the ureter and pelvis and then, via intrarenal tubular reflux, into the renal parenchyma.

It is unusual to biopsy patients with obvious clinical symptoms of acute pyelonephritis as the diagnosis can be confirmed by microbiological examination of the urine. The biopsy findings are quite characteristic, with linear streaks of suppuration; aggregates of neutrophils are present not only within the tubules but also in the surrounding interstitium. There is interstitial congestion and oedema, and in severe cases considerable tubular epithelial destruction (Plate 23). Bacteria are only very rarely demonstrated. Glomeruli are remarkably well preserved.

Acute tubular necrosis

The cause of acute tubular necrosis is either ischaemia (hypotension, shock, septicaemia, burns, rhabdomyolysis, haemolysis, incompatible blood transfusion) or toxins (antibiotics (gentamicin, cephalosporins, rifampicin), sulphonamides, chemotherapeutic agents, heavy metals, carbontetrachloride, ethylene glycol and abnormal light-chains as in multiple myeloma). The pathogenesis of ischaemic acute tubular necrosis is not clearly understood and a number of theories, including prolonged renal vasoconstriction, tubular obstruction by casts, leakage of tubular fluid and tubuloglomerular feedback, have been proposed. The most likely scenario is that all of these mechanisms may be playing a part.

Clinical presentation is usually oliguria or non-oliguric renal failure. The urine is loaded with granular and cellular casts, including epithelial cells. There is mild proteinuria, the osmolarity of the urine is close to that of plasma, and urinary sodium is high, indicating poor reabsorption of sodium.

Biopsy findings vary depending on the time of biopsy in relation to the initial insult, and it is important to remember that histological findings may not always correlate with functional status, i.e. profound anuria may be accompanied by a relatively normal appearing renal biopsy.

The tubules, particularly the proximal tubules, are dilated and lined by cuboidal or flattened cells that have lost the surface microvilli and their specialized appearance. Focal collections of tubules show sloughing with gaps in the lining of the epithelium where clusters of cells have been shed. It is unusual to see necrotic epithelial cells attached to the tubular basement membrane. In a minority of cases there is rupture of the tubular basement membrane, with a cellular reaction in the interstitium. The distal tubules and collecting ducts contain an admixture of hyaline, granular or pigmented casts. The pigmented casts are orange–brown on H&E stain and are composed of Tamm–Horsfall protein with haemoglobin or myoglobin. The presence of large fractured casts with a surrounding epithelial cell reaction is highly suspicious of myeloma. In ethylene glycol toxicity oxalate crystals are found in the lumen and tubular epithelial cells.

The interstitium is oedematous with wide separation of tubules. There is only a very scant infiltration of mononuclear inflammatory cells; if these are present in larger numbers they are clustered around ruptured tubules. This paucity of interstitial inflammation is a helpful feature in differentiating acute tubular necrosis due to ischaemia or direct toxicity from acute tubular necrosis seen as part of a predominantly interstitial nephritis such as allograft rejection and allergic TIN.

The glomeruli are essentially normal and may appear bloodless. Blood vessels are normal or have pre-existing lesions of arteriosclerosis. A careful search for cholesterol/atherosclerotic emboli should be made as this may be the cause of sudden clinically unexplained ischaemic acute tubular necrosis. The vasa recta may show evidence of haemopoiesis, particularly myelopoiesis, with immature precursors filling the vascular spaces. The pathogenesis of this phenomenon has not been worked out.

In the recovery phase there is evidence of regeneration, with tubules lined by cells with basophilic cytoplasm and scattered mitotic figures. If the patient is treated with hypertonic solutions the proximal tubular epithelial cells have a finely vacuolated appearance. The interstitial oedema gradually subsides, but in severe long-standing cases it may progress to interstitial fibrosis with consequent tubular atrophy. Prognosis in acute tubular necrosis is discussed elsewhere.

Drug-induced allergic-type TIN

Many drugs can cause acute hypersensitivity injury. Those most often implicated are: antibiotics (penicillin and derivatives, cephalosporins, rifampicin); sulphonamides; thiazides and non-thiazide diuretics (frusemide); anticonvulsive agents (phenytoin, carbamazepine); non-steroidal anti-inflammatory agents (indomethacin, ibuprofen).

Patients usually have fever, skin rash, mild proteinuria, microscopic haematuria, eosinophilia and, in severe cases, acute renal insufficiency. Serum levels of IgE may be increased. In most cases there is dramatic clinical improvement when the drug is withdrawn.

On biopsy, there is marked interstitial oedema with a focal to diffuse infiltrate of lymphocytes, including many activated forms, prominent numbers of eosinophils, macrophages and some plasma cells. The macrophages may sometimes be in aggregates forming granulomas. Neutrophils are unusual unless there is much acute tubular necrosis. Characteristically, the tubules are invaded by lymphocytes (tubulitis) and there may be small collections of lymphocytes within tubular lumina (Plate 24). In some cases there can be prominent necrosis of tubular epithelial cells. Glomeruli and blood vessels are usually normal.

With immunohistochemical stains the majority of infiltrating lymphocytes are CD4-positive T lymphocytes with fewer CD8-positive cells (Plate 25).

Drug-induced toxic TIN

The kidney is especially susceptible to toxic injury because the tubules concentrate a number of drugs locally to high levels. It is usually dose-related and results in direct tubular toxicity causing acute renal insufficiency. The drugs most often implicated are: *antibiotics* (penicillins, aminoglycosides, cephalosporins, amphotericin); *non-steroidal anti-inflammatory agents* (indomethacin, aspirin); *mercuric chloride; heavy metals* (lithium, gold); *cyclosporin.* Tubular toxicity can also be caused by subtle, cumulative injury to tubules and vasculature causing renal insufficiency after a silent latent period, e.g. injury from analgesic mixtures containing phenacetin, paracetamol and aspirin; and cyclosporin (discussed elsewhere).

In biopsies of patients with acute drug-induced toxic TIN there is acute tubular necrosis, predominantly involving the proximal tubules, together with interstitial oedema and a mild to moderate infiltrate of mononuclear cells. In aminoglycoside nephrotoxicity characteristic myeloid bodies can be seen within proximal tubular cells by electronmicroscopy.

Chronic cumulative drug-induced nephrotoxicity is exemplified by analgesic nephropathy. The mechanism of this toxicity is not well understood but the following mechanisms, which are not mutually exclusive, are thought to play a part:

- The metabolite acetaminophen (paracetamol), a known oxidant, is concentrated in the medulla and causes oxidative damage to the tubules and vasa recta.
- Aspirin inhibits prostaglandin synthesis thereby inhibiting vasodilatation and further predisposing to ischaemia of the medulla and papilla.
- Normal papilla has a borderline blood supply and the tubular damage and ischaemia caused by analgesics makes it very vulnerable to necrosis.

A renal biopsy can only rarely pick up diagnostic evidence of papillary necrosis. More commonly the abnormalities seen are of diffuse interstitial fibrosis with atrophic tubules showing markedly thickened basement membranes. Collecting ducts are often spared. There is very little, if any, cellular infiltrate. The capillary basement membranes and vasa recta are thickened with considerable luminal narrowing. As the medullary damage intensifies there are secondary cortical abnormalities of oedema and fibrosis around medullary rays progressing to tubular atrophy with crowding of glomeruli, which appear remarkably normal. Eventually there is periglomerular fibrosis, glomerular sclerosis, and arteriolar and arterial sclerosis.

References

Austin, H.A., Muenz, L.R., Joyce, K.M. *et al.* (1993) Prognostic factors in lupus nephritis. Contribution of renal histologic data, *Am J Med*, 75, 382–91.

Churg, J., Bernstein, J. and Glassock, R.J. (1995) *Renal Disease: Classification and Atlas of Glomerular Diseases*, 2nd edn, Igaku Shoin, New York.

Kimmelsteil, P. and Wilson, C. (1936) Intercapillary lesions in the glomeruli of the kidney, *Am. J. Pathol.*, **12**, 83–98.

Further reading

Neilson, E.G. and Conser, W.G. (eds) (1996) *Immunologic Renal Diseases*, Lippincott-Raven, Philadelphia.

Tisher, C.G. and Brenner, B.M. (eds) (1994) *Renal Pathology with Clinical and Functional Correlations*, J.B. Lippincott, Philadelphia.

Inherited renal diseases and genetic counselling

Richard Sandford

Introduction

Inherited renal diseases form a major part of both paediatric and adult nephrology practice. Up to 20% of patients with end-stage renal failure and those entering renal transplant programmes will have a primary renal genetic disease. Two of the commonest inherited disorders in humans are primarily renal diseases. Autosomal dominant polycystic kidney disease (ADPKD) has an incidence greater than 1 per 1000 of the population, and vesico-ureteric reflux (VUR) is estimated to occur in 1 in 100 to 1 in 1000 of the population. ADPKD is responsible for up to 10% of cases of adult end-stage renal failure, while VUR may be responsible for a similar number of adults with end-stage renal failure but is a common cause in children. Our understanding of the genetic nature of VUR and the establishment of screening protocols for at-risk individuals is likely to have great benefit in the future as prophylactic antibiotics will almost certainly prevent the serious complication of renal scarring in this condition (VUR is more fully discussed on pp. 269–271). At present no disease-specific treatments exist for ADPKD, so management is principally concerned with the early treatment of known complications that may adversely affect renal function, such as hypertension and urinary tract infection (UTI).

The interface between the nephrologist and the geneticist will therefore become more important as the molecular basis of these conditions is defined. Direct molecular diagnosis may become available, replacing or complementing existing investigations; the relationship between the underlying gene mutation and the clinical phenotype may allow more precise predictions of disease progression to be made; and individuals may request presymptomatic genetic testing in the presence of a significant family history.

The first manifestation of this new genetic information is likely to be a greater demand for better information, and clearer more detailed explanations of the disease that will allow individuals to be more involved in making decisions about their own management. This brief account of the role of genetic counselling in inherited renal disease, and recent molecular and clinical advances in their management will illustrate the current use of diagnostic and screening tests and the current and potential future applications of molecular testing.

A chapter on renal genetic disease in a book called *Diagnostic Tests in Nephrology* suggests that many new molecular genetic tests are available for the specific diagnosis of these conditions. While the identification of the genes responsible for this clinically very diverse range of conditions is rapidly increasing (Table 8.1), direct mutation analysis and other molecular genetic tests that may be routinely employed in diagnosis and management are still at the research stage in most cases. The potential of automation and 'chip' technology in genetic testing, which offers great hope for 'routine' testing, still remains to be realized. The current reality is that standard investigations such as blood and urine biochemistry (Chapter 1), renal imaging (Chapter 5) and renal biopsy (Chapter 7) are still the principal methods used in the diagnosis and screening of inherited renal disease. Nephronophthisis provides a possible exception where the demonstration of large homozygous deletions at 2q13, diagnostic of the condition in most affected individuals, removes the requirement to consider renal biopsy. The ultimate benefits of the molecular investigation of inherited renal disease will be in therapeutic and preventive interventions and in developing appropriate screening protocols for affected individuals and those at high risk of inheriting these diseases. For example, the suggestion that the molecular defect in ADPKD may be in an ion channel raises the possibility of disease-specific pharmacological therapy. In addition, the suggestion that ADPKD families with a mutation at the PKD2 locus on chromosome 4 have a slower rate of decline in renal function may make genotyping in this condition routine, with clear implications for the screening and follow-up of other family members.

Disease classification

There is no single classification of inherited renal diseases in common use that reflects the broad nature of the pathological findings and the uncertainty about molecular pathophysiology in most cases. Some individual diseases can be classified on the basis of the underlying gene mutation (e.g. ADPKD and Alport's syndrome), but this has yet to have widespread clinical relevance. The conditions described in this chapter will broadly fall in to one or more of the following categories:

Table 8.1

Inherited renal diseases for which genes have been identified

Disease	Gene	Location	Inheritance	Function
Primary Structural Disorders				
ADPKD	PKD1	16p13.3	AD	Unknown
	PDK2	4q21–q23	AD	?Ion channel
	PDK3	Unknown	AD	
TSC	TSC1	9q34	AD	Unknown
	TSC2	16p13.3	AD	Tumour suppressor gene
VHL	VHL	3p	AD	Tumour suppressor gene
Wilms' tumour	WT1	11p13	AD	Unknown
Alport's syndrome	COL4α5	Xq22	XR	Collagen
	COL4α4	2	AD, AR	Collagen
	COL4α3	2	AD, AR	Collagen
Thin basement membrane disease	COL4α3	2	AD	Collagen
Branchio-otorenal syndrome	EYA1	8q13.3	AD	Unknown
Renal Transport Disorders				
Liddle's syndrome	ENaC	16	AD	β, γ subunit, epithelial sodium channel (activating mutations)
Type 1 pseudohypoaldosteronism	ENaC	16	AR	Epithelial sodium channel subunits (loss of function mutations)
Bartter's syndrome	NKCC2		AR	Bumetanide-sensitive co-transporter
	ROMK	11	AR	K+ channel
Gitelman's syndrome	NCCT		AR	Thiazide-sensitive co-transporter
Nephrogenic DI	AVPR2	Xq28	XR	ADH receptor
	AQP2	12q13	AD, AR	Water channel
Hypercalciuric nephrolithiasis	CLCN5	X	XR	Chloride channel
VUR with eye abnormalities	PAX2	10q24–q25	AD	Transcriptional regulator
X-linked hypophosphataemic rickets	PEX	Xp22.1	XD	Endopeptidase

ADPKD, autosomal dominant polycystic kidney disease; TSC, tuberous sclerosis complex; VHL, von Hippel–Lindau syndrome; VUR, vesico-ureteric reflux; AD, autosomal dominant; AR, autosomal recessive; XR, X-linked recessive; XD, X-linked dominant; ADH, antidiuretic hormone.

- congenital abnormalities (p. 281)
- abnormalities as part of chromosomal/dysmorphic syndromes
- primary renal structural disorders
- renal tubular transport disorders (p. 16)
- mitochondrial diseases
- renal tumour syndromes
- secondary renal involvement in other inherited disorders.

The diagnosis of inherited renal disease is often made both by considering the clinical features, and specifically asking for a full family history. The detailed description of a pedigree will often suggest a diagnosis by identifying other features of the disease in family members and by indicating the likely mode of inheritance. For example, the commonest X-linked nephritis is Alport's syndrome and the identification of a distinctive type of brain tumour in a relative of an early onset case of renal carcinoma will suggest a diagnosis of von Hippel–Lindau syndrome. This chapter will therefore concentrate on updating the reader on some of the recent advances in renal genetics and their relevance to our current understanding of the commoner conditions, rather than providing an exhaustive clinical description of the numerous genetic conditions characterized or complicated by renal involvement. The essential discussion points will be the molecular genetics of the condition, the use of screening and diagnostic tests in affected and at-risk individuals, and the role of genetic counselling. Chapter 14 deals with congenital disorders, ARPKD and VUR, while the biochemical tests necessary for the investigation of the renal tubular transport disorders are discussed in Chapter 1. The reader is referred to the Further Reading list to obtain descriptions of the many syndromic and systemic conditions that have renal involvement.

Genetic counselling in renal disease

The role of the clinical geneticist in the management and investigation of renal disease can be broadly summarized as follows:

- provision of genetic counselling
- molecular and cytogenetic testing
- family studies
- predictive gene testing.

The process of genetic counselling involves establishing the correct diagnosis if appropriate (referrals to clinical genetics usually comprise individuals or families in which the primary renal diagnosis has been made), estimation of genetic risk, explanation of these risks and the means of altering them, help with understanding all the available facts and how to make decisions based on them. It is an important part of the management of all inherited renal diseases and is mandatory for some conditions, such as those associated with a high risk of renal malignancy or where issues such as prenatal testing are being considered. It should be offered to all affected and at-risk individuals and other family members where the diagnosis of an inherited renal disease is being contemplated or has been made.

A general counselling strategy in the renal genetics clinic will involve all or some of the following areas:

- documentation of individual and family details
- discussion of clinical aspects of the disease
- provision of disease-specific information (if available) for reinforcement
- explanation of patterns of inheritance and identification of at-risk individuals
- the benefits and disadvantages of diagnostic/screening investigations
- follow-up session if screening tests are performed
- collection of clinical data on disease-specific databases.

In some specific conditions such as inherited cancer syndromes, the format may be different; the planning of predictive testing is discussed on p. 154.

Individuals are entitled to be given information in a non-directive and non-judgemental fashion. This information will form the basis of often difficult ethical and social decisions and so the manner in which it is given is important. This is especially so at the time of diagnosis, as little further information will be retained. Discussions about inheritance or screening other family members are best avoided when the results of diagnostic investigations such as biopsy or imaging are being given.

Attitudes to screening or presymptomatic testing have dramatically changed in recent years, especially with respect to children. Early diagnosis has to afford an advantage to the individual such as treatment of early complications. 'Just knowing' is not sufficient to warrant the use of screening tests that vary from routine renal functions tests such as urea and creatinine, even urinalysis, to renal imaging, biopsy and genetic analysis. It must always be borne in mind that a positive test in an individual who is unprepared or unsupported can have devastating effects. Common fears include:

- lack of a cure
- insurance consequences
- fear of the future and ill health

- career difficulties
- loss of self-worth/esteem
- burdening of family and partner.

The issue of prenatal testing may also be discussed, and although it is rarely taken up in conditions such as ADPKD, there is increasing experience with its use in conditions such as autosomal recessive polycystic kidney disease (ARPKD), von Hippel–Lindau syndrome and Alport's syndrome.

Current understanding of renal genetic diseases

PRIMARY RENAL STRUCTURAL ABNORMALITIES

This group of conditions can be broadly split in to cystic and non-cystic disease (Table 8.2).

Autosomal dominant polycystic kidney disease
ADPKD is one of the commonest inherited renal diseases and serves as a paradigm for the management of other conditions. Genetic heterogeneity and extreme phenotypic variability make the process of genetic counselling very important in this condition.

Molecular genetics   This condition demonstrates genetic heterogeneity, with mutations at up to three loci (PKD1, PKD2, PKD3) being clinically indistinguishable. PKD1 maps to 16p13.3 and accounts for 85% of cases, and PKD2 maps to 4q21–q23 and accounts for the remaining 15% of cases. Mutations at the unidentified PKD3 locus appear to be extremely rare. PKD1 and PKD2 have recently been cloned and the spectrum of pathological mutations is being identified. So far no common mutations have been defined. The PKD1 gene encodes a large 460 kDa novel membrane associated glycoprotein that may be involved in cell–cell or cell–matrix interactions. Multiple highly homologous partial copies of the gene are also present on chromosome 16 and have made mutation screening in most of the PKD1 gene extremely difficult. PKD2 is thought to encode an ion channel subunit that undergoes homophilic and heterophilic interactions with the C-terminal domain of PKD1. Both proteins are expressed in a variety of epithelial cell types including normal and cystic renal tubular epithelium. Evidence also suggests that cyst formation may result from a second somatic mutation in the PKD1 gene in the tubular epithelium in

- ARPKD
- ADPKD
  PKD1
  PKD2
  PKD3
- Cystic dysplasia
    sporadic
    ?autosomal dominant
    ?autosomal recessive
    ?X-linked inheritance
    renal-hepatopancreatic dysplasia as part of a syndrome
- Glomerulocystic disease
    sporadic
    autosomal dominant
    early manifestation of ADPKD secondary to obstruction
    as part of a syndrome, e.g. orofaciodigital syndrome type 1,
      tuberous sclerosis complex
- Simple cysts
- Acquired cysts
- Juvenile nephronophthisis/medullary cystic disease
    juvenile nephronophthisis (autosomal recessive)
    renal retinal dysplasia (autosomal recessive)
    medullary cystic disease
- Medullary sponge kidney
    sporadic
    autosomal dominant
    with congenital hemihypertrophy
    early stages of polycystic diseases
- Extraparenchymal cysts

Source: Zerses, 1996.

Table 8.2
Classification of cystic diseases*

addition to the inherited germline mutation, the so-called 'two-hit hypothesis'. The process of cyst formation may therefore be analogous to tumour formation.

Linkage analysis for both the PKD1 and PKD2 loci is available, but mutation analysis is currently performed in only a few research laboratories. Great technical obstacles need to be overcome before PKD1 mutation analysis is available for the whole gene.

Clinical features   ADPKD is a common systemic condition with renal and extrarenal manifestations that occurs in more than 1 per 1000 of the population. Cyst formation is seen in several organ systems and non-cystic features include cardiovascular and connective tissue abnormalities. Cysts are seen in the following organs:

- kidneys
- liver
- pancreas
- spleen.

Cardiovascular abnormalities include:

- hypertension
- mitral valve prolapse (MVP)
- intracranial aneurysm (ICA)
- left ventricular hypertrophy (LVH)
  (aortic aneurysms, aortic root dilatation/dissection, coronary artery aneurysms).

Connective tissue abnormalities include:

- herniae
- diverticular disease.

Patients may present with a wide range of problems. These are commonly hypertension, loin pain, haematuria or UTI, or as a chance finding of renal cysts or renal enlargement during other investigations.

While the rate of decline in renal function is suggested to be slower in PKD2 families, on average 50% of individuals with ADPKD will reach end-stage renal failure in their sixth decade. Accurate genotyping may therefore become important in discussing prognosis with patients.

In childhood ADPKD, the extrarenal manifestations are much rarer, but up to 30% of children have symptoms and signs of the disease, usually pain and frequency. The rare *in utero* form of ADPKD carries a poor prognosis; up to one-third die in the first month and survivors have more aggressive disease than that seen in older children or adults.

Rupture or the presence of an asymptomatic ICA are important extra-renal manifestations of ADPKD. They are present in 4–8% of affected individuals (1.2% of the general population), which rises to about 16% if there is a family history of this condition. They may also be multiple and rupture at a younger age than non-ADPKD ICAs. However, the incidence of rupture in ADPKD patients is not known, but appears to be increased if there is a positive family history. An annual rupture rate of 1–2% is likely based on studies of non-ADPKD ICAs, and as the prognosis is poorer in ADPKD, screening for those at high risk has been advocated.

Age	Minimum number of cysts
< 30	Two cysts, either uni- or bilateral
30–59	Two cysts in each kidney
> 60	Four cysts in each kidney

ADPKD, autosomal dominant polycystic kidney disease.

Table 8.3
Age and number of cysts criteria in the diagnosis of ADPKD

Diagnosis   Diagnosis of ADPKD is usually made by renal imaging and, more rarely, by presymptomatic genetic testing. The presence of other features of the disease should be sought, e.g. liver cysts, and features of other conditions should be excluded. In an ADPKD family the diagnosis is made by the presence of bilateral cysts totalling three or more. However, with the known age-related increase in the number of simple cysts the criteria shown in Table 8.3 are now used in an individual at 50% risk of the condition.

Differential diagnosis   A classification of renal cystic diseases is given in Table 8.2. Conditions that may mimic ADPKD include:

- tuberous sclerosis complex (p. 140); features include facial angiofibromas, fibrous forehead plaque, ungal fibromas, renal angiomyolipomas and visceral hamartomas
- Von Hippel–Lindau disease (p. 151); features include haemangioblastomas, visceral cysts, renal cancer, phaeochromocytoma
- ARPKD
- orofaciodigital syndrome type 1 (OFD1) (p. 144); features include oral frenulae, clefting, polydactyly, syndactyly, renal cysts
- branchio-otorenal syndrome (p. 144); features include deafness, ear pits, branchial fistulae, renal dysplasia/cysts
- renal-hepatopancreatic dysplasia.

Many other conditions may give rise to polycystic kidneys, but other distinguishing features are invariably present. Confusion should be rare following thorough clinical and radiological evaluation.

Genetic counselling and screening   Genetic counselling in ADPKD will generally follow the format described on p. 134. Specific issues that need to be considered are the marked phenotypic variation even within a family, the screening and presymptomatic testing of at-risk relatives including children, and the identification of individuals at high risk of ICA.

Renal ultrasound screening for at-risk individuals is generally deferred until early adulthood. At this age the majority of affected individuals will be detected by ultrasound, but negative scans will need to be repeated and the disease can only be excluded after a negative scan at the age of over 30 years. Computed tomography (CT) or magnetic resonance imaging (MRI) scanning are more sensitive in detecting early cystic changes and can be used to detect early changes of ADPKD following a normal ultrasound. Linkage studies are generally reserved for individuals under the age of 30 years in whom renal imaging is negative but who are considering living-related kidney donation or who would alter family planning based on the result.

Screening for an asymptomatic ICA is generally reserved for individuals aged 18–40 years with a confirmed family history. This is only performed following referral to a neurosurgical unit for a full explanation of the investigation, possible results and available therapeutic options. The diagnosis of ICA has a profound effect on an individual and the choice of treatment may be complicated by the finding of unresectable or multiple ICAs. The frequency of follow-up scans is unresolved; every five years has been suggested, or sooner if a small ICA is discovered that does not warrant intervention.

Prenatal testing   Despite the paucity of mutations in PKD1 and PKD2 at present, the use of PKD1 and PKD2 flanking markers make linkage studies feasible in many families. It is therefore possible to offer prenatal diagnosis for ADPKD, although uptake is very low. It is more likely to be used when a previous case of the *in utero* form of ADPKD has been diagnosed as the risks of further pregnancies being similarly affected is increased.

Tuberous sclerosis complex (TSC)

TSC is an autosomal dominant (AD) trait characterized by the development of hamartomas in multiple organs including brain, skin, heart and kidneys. It may therefore present with a diverse range of symptoms and signs often without a family history. There is considerable phenotypic variation even within families, the diagnosis sometimes being made in a parent only when a child presents with typical features. However, it can be a devastating disease, with a significant proportion of individuals having seizures and mental retardation. Genetic counselling is therefore very important in the management of this condition, especially as 60–70% of cases represent new mutations and will not have a previous family history.

Molecular genetics   TSC is a genetically heterogeneous disorder with mutations at two loci, TSC1 (9q32) and TSC2 (16p13.3), which are equally responsible for the condition. Both genes have now been cloned and their predicted protein products termed hamartin and tuberin, respectively. Germline and somatic mutations have been identified in TSC in both genes, demonstrating that two hits are likely to be required for tumorigenesis and that they function as tumour-suppressor genes. The chromosome 16 gene and its predicted protein product tuberin has a region of homology to the GTPase activating protein GAP3. These proteins bind to Ras proteins and by regulating their activity control cell proliferation and differentiation. The role of TSC2 in tumorigenesis has also been demonstrated by the Eker rat model in which germline and somatic mutations in TSC2 are associated with renal carcinoma and a variety of other tumours. The function of hamartin, however, is not yet known.

TSC2 is adjacent to PKD1 and a contiguous gene syndrome in infants consisting of TSC and severe PKD due to deletions involving both genes and possibly others in the region as well has been described.

The renal manifestations of TSC are second only to the neurological manifestations as a cause of death in this condition. They consist of angiomyolipomas, cysts and renal cell carcinoma (RCC). Focal segmental sclerosis and interstitial fibrosis, lymphangiomatous cysts and vascular dysplasia have also rarely been described.

Clinical features

Renal angiomyolipomas   These are rarely seen in the normal population and are characteristically multifocal and bilateral in TSC. They are present in about 50% of individuals. They are benign non-encapsulated tumours comprising elements containing fat, smooth muscle and arterial tissues. The major risk is haemorrhage, which is related to their size. End-stage renal failure in TSC is more usually related to cystic disease or, bilateral nephrectomies for haemorrhage or tumour rather than to extensive involvement with angiomyolipomas.

Renal cysts   These frequently occur with angiomyolipomas and are multiple and bilateral, occurring in 30% of cases. They also complicate cases of the TSC2-PKD1 contiguous gene syndrome. The possible role of PKD1 in the majority of cases of TSC cystic disease remains to be determined.

Renal cell carcinoma   This is a rare complication but may occur earlier than sporadic disease and be bilateral. Its presence is suspected either by the development of new symptoms or by enlarging non-fatty lesions with or without microcalcifications on imaging.

Diagnostic criteria   These are shown in Table 8.4.

Genetic counselling and screening   The discovery of TSC1 and TSC2 and the ability to detect mutations in both genes is likely to have a significant impact on the diagnosis, screening and prenatal detection of TSC. The great phenotypic variation in the disease makes it impossible to reassure affected parents that any child may be only mildly affected like themselves and that asymptomatic siblings are not gene carriers. At-risk asymptomatic individuals will need to undergo careful clinical evaluation, especially examination of the skin under a Wood's lamp; consider imaging the brain and abdomen to determine disease status.

Juvenile nephronophthisis/medullary cystic disease

This refers to a group of conditions in which medullary cyst formation is regarded as a hallmark accompanied by progressive tubulo-interstitial nephritis with secondary glomerulosclerosis leading to small scarred kidneys and end-stage renal failure. The childhood form is autosomal recessive (AR) and is an important cause of renal failure in children. It may be associated with a variety of extrarenal manifestations including hepatic fibrosis, retinitis pigmentosa and skeletal malformations. The adult form is purely a renal disease and is inherited as an AD trait.

Table 8.4

Diagnostic criteria for tubular sclerosis complex*

Neurological (definite diagnosis: single with histological confirmation or multiple by imaging)
- cortical tuber
- subependymal glial nodule/giant cell astrocytoma
- retinal hamartoma

Dermatological (definite diagnosis)
- facial angiogfibromas
- fibrous forehead plaque
- ungal fibromas
- shagreen patch (histological confirmation)

Visceral (presumptive diagnosis)
- multiple renal angiomyolipomas
- multiple cardiac rhabdomyomas
- multiple renal cysts and an angiomyolipoma
- pulmonary lymphangioleiomyomatosis and a renal angiomyolipoma

Suggestive
- hypomelanotic skin patches
- enamel pits
- angiomyolipoma of kidney, liver, adrenal or gonads
- thyroid adenoma
- infantile spasms
- sclerotic bone patches and cysts

*Source: Torres, 1996.

Some 85% of cases of juvenile nephronophthisis map to 2q13, and in 80% of familial cases large homozygous deletions can be detected by molecular analysis, providing a diagnostic test for the condition. The same deletion is seen in 60% of sporadic cases.

Diagnosis and screening Renal imaging with high resolution ultrasound typically demonstrates hyperechogenic kidneys with loss of corticomedullary differentiation, but medullary cysts may be absent until the disease is advanced. Thin section CT or MRI imaging, which are more sensitive at detecting cysts, may also be indicated when the diagnosis is suspected. This also differentiates it from other cystic diseases which are present in the cortex as well. Renal biopsy may also be indicated, but molecular analysis is likely to play a more important role in the diagnosis of this condition.

Autosomal recessive polycystic kidney disease
This condition is described in Chapter 14.

Simple cysts
These are not inherited and increase in number with increasing age. They are rarely seen below the age of 30 years but are present in 22% of those over 70 (in one-half of these cases they are bilateral). This is important when considering the diagnosis of other cystic diseases (p. 137).

Acquired cystic disease
This describes the development of bilateral renal cysts in individuals with end-stage renal failure that is not cyst-related. It occurs in up to 50% of haemodialysis patients and those with chronic renal failure (CRF), and may resolve following renal transplantation. It is not inherited and not related to age, treatment or primary renal diagnosis. It may cause diagnostic confusion and difficulties during genetic counselling with regard to carrier status, but ADPKD kidneys are frequently massively enlarged unlike those in autosomal recessive cystic disease, which are often small.

Cystic dysplasia
See Chapter 14.

Renal cysts in other syndromes
There are numerous inherited and sporadic conditions in which renal abnormalities including cysts have been described. These are fully described in several texts, one of the best being *The London Dysmorphology Database* (Winter and Baraitser, 1990).

Branchio-otorenal syndrome (BOR)

Molecular genetics   Mutations in the EYA1 gene have been found to be the cause of this rare autosomal dominant syndrome. This gene is a homologue of the *Drosophila* 'eyes absent' gene (eya). Expression is found in all components of the middle ear and in the developing kidney, explaining the phenotype of ear and renal abnormalities in this syndrome. Deletions involving the BOR locus have been described in which it forms part of a contiguous gene syndrome with features of Duane syndrome (congenital strabismus), hydrocephalus and aplasia of the trapezius muscle.

Clinical features   These include:

- mixed hearing loss
- cochlear malformations/abnormal pinnae
- pre-auricular pits
- branchial cleft fistulas
- renal dysplasia/aplasia
- polycystic kidneys.

Diagnosis and screening   Diagnosis is made by the recognition of the clinical features. The association of deafness with renal abnormalities is highly suggestive and the presence of pre-auricular pits and branchial fistula will confirm the diagnosis. Imaging of the ear will demonstrate the typical cochlear hypoplasia, and renal imaging will be required to define accurately the underlying renal abnormality. Mutation analysis is available at only a few research centres. Because of the possibility of renal dysplasia/aplasia genetic counselling is advisable as consideration of prenatal diagnosis may be required. A known mutation may be used to screen a pregnancy, but in its absence linkage studies and detailed ultrasound scanning may be employed.

Orofaciodigital syndrome type 1

Molecular genetics   The OFD1 gene has been mapped to Xp22.2–22.3. This rare X-linked dominant disorder is exclusively seen in females, as males with the condition die *in utero*. The majority of cases are sporadic.

Clinical features   The clinical features are varied but need to be recognized so as not to confuse the diagnosis with ADPKD. The features include:

- Renal: polycystic kidneys.
- Oral: cleft tongue and oral frenulae
            cleft palate
            abnormal dentition.

- Facial: facial asymmetry
            frontal bossing
            hypertelorism
            broad nasal bridge.
- Hands: syndactyly, polydactyly and brachydactyly.
- Other: learning difficulties.

Diagnosis and screening   Renal cystic disease has been reported in only about 20% of cases of OFD1 and not at all in the other OFD syndromes. If the presence of cysts is determined in an affected female, then screening should be offered to other female at-risk members of the family. End-stage renal failure may occur at any age in this condition, and unlike in ADPKD, the screening of children is appropriate.

ABNORMALITIES OF BASEMENT MEMBRANE AND GLOMERULAR DISORDERS

Alport's syndrome

Molecular genetics   Alport's syndrome can now be classified as an abnormality of basement membranes expressing type IV collagen. Each type IV collagen molecule is a trimer of three α-chains, and six different α-chain genes have been identified (COL4α1–6). Alport's syndrome is now proven to be genetically heterogeneous, with mutations in three of these genes being responsible for the same condition. The six α-chain genes are arranged in pairs on three separate chromosomes and this observation explains some of the clinical variation in the condition. COL4α1 and COL4α2 are located on chromosome 13, COL4α3 and COL4α4 on chromosome 2, and COL4α5 and COL4α6 on the X chromosome.

An X-linked inheritance pattern is seen in most Alport's families and this is due to mutations in the COL4α5 gene. Mutations in COL4α6 alone have not been shown to cause Alport's syndrome, but when chromosomal deletions involve both COL4α5 and COL4α6, then the Alport's phenotype is associated with smooth muscle tumours of the oesophagus, tracheobronchial tree and female genital tract (diffuse leiomyomatosis). This represents a further example of a contiguous gene syndrome. Mutations in COL4α3 and COL4α4 are responsible for the rare AD and AR forms of the disease. Table 8.5 summarizes the inheritance pattern. The pattern of distribution of COL4α3–5 predicts the phenotype of Alport's syndrome as they are expressed in the specialized basement membranes of the eye, ear and kidney.

X-linked Alport's syndrome is the commonest form of the disease seen. Mutations in COL4α5 are found in only 50% of families studied,

Table 8.5

Inheritance pattern of Alport's syndrome

Inheritance	Gene
X-linked	COL4α5
X-linked including leiomyomatosis	COL4α5 and COL4α6
Autosomal recessive	COL4α3
	COL4α4
Autosomal dominant	?COL4α3
	?COL4α4

suggesting that mutations in another gene close to COL4α5 may be responsible or more likely that non-coding regions and regulatory elements harbour as yet undetected sequence alterations. Almost all COL4α5 mutations are unique with no common mutation being present. This makes mutation screening in families a large task as the COL4α5 gene spans up to 310 kb of genomic DNA, comprising 51 exons producing a 6.5 kb transcript. Major rearrangements or deletions are seen in up to 15% of X-linked cases and predict a more severe clinical course with early renal failure and deafness (before the age of 30 years). Other mutations such as small deletions, mis-sense and splice site mutations may be associated with a slower onset of end-stage renal failure and deafness (over the age of 30 years). Only a few mutations have been identified in COL4α3 and generally the clinical course is severe.

Clinical features   Gender differences in Alport's syndrome are marked in the X-linked form of the disease but not present in the recessive or dominant forms, which show features of equal severity in males and females.

Males affected with the X-linked disease have persistent microscopic haematuria, probably from birth. Gross haematuria may accompany intercurrent infections. Absence by the age of 10 years indicates an unaffected male. Almost all carrier females will develop haematuria by adulthood. Proteinuria develops eventually in all affected males and may lead to nephrotic syndrome. This is very uncommon in carrier females but many indicate a poorer prognosis.

End-stage renal failure usually occurs in the second or third decades. Families are often divided into those in which end-stage renal failure occurs before the age of 30, and those in which it occurs after that age. In women, childhood nephrotic syndrome, gross haematuria and the presence of deafness and eye signs predict a poor outcome. In women with progressive disease, end-stage renal failure may occur in the sixth decade onwards.

Approximately 30% will develop hypertension; the lifetime risk of CRF in this group is 15%.

Hearing loss occurs in 55% of males and 45% of females. The pattern is of a progressive high tone sensorineural loss.

Ocular signs occur in up to 30% of patients. Anterior lenticonus, which occurs in the second and third decades, is virtually pathognomonic of Alport's syndrome and is associated with a more rapid progression to end-stage renal failure.

Other rarer manifestations include diffuse leiomyomatosis and megathrombocytopenia.

Diagnostic criteria and investigations   The diagnosis of Alport's syndrome can often be made if three of the following four criteria are met:

- family history of haematuria with or without CRF in the absence of evidence of other renal disease
- classic ultrastructural changes on renal biopsy
- high tone sensorineural deafness
- characteristic eye signs.

However, advances in our understanding of the disease phenotype and molecular pathophysiology have broadened the criteria to include the following:

- mutation in COL4α3, COL4α4 or COL4α5
- immunohistochemical evidence of complete or partial loss of Alport's epitopes in kidney or skin
- macrothrombocytopenia or granulocytic inclusions
- diffuse leiomyomatosis of the oesophagus or the female genital tract
- widespread glomerular basement membrane ultrastructural abnormalities
- gradual progression to end-stage renal failure in the index case and at least two family members.

At least four of all of these criteria should be met. Thus the investigations of individuals suspected of having the disease and at-risk family members will include the following in addition to full audiolgical and ophthalmological assessment:

- Renal biopsy – demonstration of classic electronmicroscopy glomerular basement membrane changes of variable thickening, thinning, basket weaving and lamellation.
- Immunohistochemistry – X-linked = absence of COL4α5 in skin, absence of COL4α3, COL4α4, and COL4α5 in glomerular basement membrane, tubular basement membrane and Bowman's capsule

–autosomal recessive = absence of COL4α3 and COL4α4 in glomerular basement membrane, tubular basement membrane and Bowman's capsule, absence of COL4α5 from glomerular basement membrane, COL4α5 present in tubular basement membrane, Bowman's capsule and skin.

It should be noted that skin biopsy has an important role in the diagnosis of Alport's syndrome, especially in those in whom renal biopsy is contra-indicated and in female carriers in whom patchy staining is seen.

Molecular genetics   This may be required for detection of carrier status, prenatal diagnosis and, rarely, for diagnostic purposes. Linkage analysis is possible for most families and mutation screening, although time-consuming and expensive, may be obtained via a few research laboratories. There is a detection rate of 50%.

Genetic counselling   The main practical issues that need to be addressed when counselling an individual or a family about Alport's syndrome are a full discussion of the clinical features and prognosis in both those affected and carriers, and the likely mode of inheritance, which is X-linked, in most cases. The clinical features have been described and the risks for family members of those affected or carriers are shown in Table 8.6.

Individuals identified as being at risk should therefore be offered screening tests. These should include urinalysis and renal function tests, audiometry and full visual assessment. Renal and skin biopsy may also be required to meet the diagnostic criteria in a male. If a female at 50% risk of being a carrier has no clinical features of the disease her risk can be reduced to 2%, giving her a 1% risk of having a son with Alport's syndrome.

Precise carrier status can be offered by molecular testing if the gene mutation is known in the family. Similarly, linkage analysis may be offered. Prenatal testing for Alport's syndrome has also been requested in a small

Table 8.6

Risks for family members of those affected by or carriers of X-linked Alport's syndrome

Family member	Male affected	Female carrier
Father	Unaffected	Affected/unaffected
Mother	Obligate carrier	Unaffected/carrier
Brother	50% affected	50% affected
Sister	50% carrier risk	50% carrier risk
Son	Unaffected	50% affected
Daughter	Obligate carrier	50% carrier risk

number of cases. It must be remembered that mutation screening is lengthy and not widely available and mutations are only found in 50% of cases.

Differential diagnosis   The association between familial renal disease and deafness has been seen in:

- branchio-otorenal syndrome
- renal tubular acidosis
- Barakat syndrome (steroid-resistant nephrotic syndrome, sensorineural deafness, hypoparathyroidism).

These should all be readily distinguishable from each other.

Familial benign haematuria

The condition of benign familial haematuria or thin basement membrane disease is characterized by glomerular basement membrane thinning on electron microscopy and normal renal function. Mutations in COL4α3 have been shown to underlie some cases of this disease. Affected individuals may therefore represent manifesting heterozygous carriers of AR Alport's syndrome.

Nail–patella syndrome

This AD condition maps to 9q34.1 and is characterized by dysplastic nails, absent or hypoplastic patellae, iliac horns, joint problems and occasional proteinuria which may be severe enough to cause nephrotic syndrome. Many collagen fibrils are seen in the thickened basement membranes and mesangial matrix on renal biopsy.

RENAL TUMOURS

Primary renal cancers are rare, with only a small proportion having a major genetic predisposition. Whereas Wilms' tumour is the commonest childhood renal malignancy, renal cell carcinoma predominates in adults. The definition of the molecular events underlying familial cases of these two tumour types has contributed greatly to our understanding of renal development and the development of sporadic tumours. The recent identification of several genes involved in renal malignancy has provided an opportunity to understand the molecular basis of this condition and to identify individuals at high risk of developing it. The ultimate benefits of these discoveries will be in therapeutic and preventive interventions and in developing appropriate screening protocols.

Wilms' tumour

Wilms' tumour, or nephroblastoma, accounts for about 90% of childhood renal tumours, although fewer than 1% are inherited, 1–2% forming part of a syndrome producing an increased risk and the remainder being sporadic. It affects 1 per 10 000 children, with most affected before the age of 6 years. Five per cent are bilateral, and these present at a younger age than those with unilateral tumours (26 v. 36 months). Five per cent of individuals also have urogenital abnormalities, and many tumours arise in kidneys with persistant foci of renal stem cells (nephrogenic rests), illustrating the relationship of these tumours with normal renal development. Syndromes associated with an increased risk of Wilms' tumour are listed in Table 8.7.

Molecular genetics   One out of four possible genes responsible for Wilms' tumour has been identified on the short arm of chromosome 11 (11p13) following the demonstration of chromosomal deletions in patients with WAGR. This region contains the genes for aniridia (Pax6) and Wilms' tumour (WT1). Other genes that produce the other features of this condition may also be present in this region which is therefore a contiguous gene deletion syndrome. Wilms' tumour does not complicate familial aniridia but up to one-third of sporadic cases will develop it. The WT1 gene is principally expressed in the developing genitourinary tract and mesothelium and is essential for formation of the metanephric kidney and gonad. It contains four zinc finger motifs and an effector domain and is involved in DNA binding. The effector domain may act as a repressor or activator of transcription but the genes regulated by WT1 have not been identified.

Table 8.7
Syndromes associated with an increased risk of Wilms' tumour

Syndrome	Features
WAGR	Wilms' tumour, aniridia, genitourinary malformation, mental retardation
Denys–Drash	Glomerulonephropathy, genital anomalies, Wilms' tumour
Beckwith–Wiedemann	Features include macroglossia, congenital overgrowth, abdominal wall defects, earlobe creases, visceromegaly, hemihypertrophy
Hemihypertrophy	
Familial Wilms'	
Perlman	
Simpson–Golabi–Behmel	

Mutations in WT1 have been described in familial and sporadic Wilms' tumour and generally inactivate the protein product. Only 10% of Wilms' tumours have mutations, and a further gene, WT2, is present at 11p15.

Clinical features   Abdominal distension is usually the presenting feature, although pain, haematuria, fever and hypertension may occur. Tumours grow rapidly and invade locally as well as metastasizing via the bloodstream. Five per cent are bilateral and may be solid, undergo necrosis, haemorrhage or cystic change.

Screening   Ninety per cent of tumours have presented by the time the patient has reached age of 7 years, and this defines the period of maximum risk. The screening of children at risk of Wilms' tumour can be performed by ultrasound at regular review. This has not led to an improved prognosis for children with a genetic susceptibility and so regular physical examination by parents has also been advocated, although this is an area of continuing controversy. Early onset, multifocal or bilateral tumours, a positive family history, abnormalities of the genital tract, aniridia and features of the above syndromes suggest a genetic predisposition, and continued screening should be offered. The risk to siblings in cases of unilateral sporadic disease is low and does not warrant screening. If there are two affected siblings the risk rises to 33% and screening is indicated. Children of Wilms' tumour survivors have a risk of up to 10% for unilateral tumours and 33% for bilateral or familial disease and should therefore be screened. Table 8.8 summarizes the risks.

There is no clear pattern or significant risk of secondary primary tumours in individuals with Wilms' tumour and so additional screening is not indicated.

Affected member	Risk for subsequent children
Parent with bilateral tumours	30%
Parent with unilateral tumour + affected relative	30%
Parent unaffected; two affected children	30%
Parent with unilateral tumour	10%
Sibling with bilateral tumours	10%
Sibling with unilateral tumour and no other malformations	< 1%

Table 8.8
Risks for relatives of people with Wilms' tumour

Renal cell carcinoma

This tumour is relatively rare but comprises the majority of primary renal tumours in adults. Only about 1–2% are familial, and they form part of two distinct clinical syndromes: von Hippel–Lindau syndrome and familial renal cell carcinoma. Renal cell carcinoma also complicates TSC in about 2.5% of cases (p. 141). Several features also distinguish TSC from these other familial tumour syndromes. Firstly TSC tumours are very rare in the general population and by themselves may be diagnostic of the condition, and secondly they rarely progress to malignancy.

As predicted by their genetic aetiology, familial RCC occur at a younger age than sporadic forms, may be multifocal and bilateral and are transmitted as autosomal dominant with high age-dependent penetrance.

Molecular Genetics Genes located on chromosome 3 are important in the pathogenesis of familial and sporadic RCC. The von Hippel–Lindau gene has been identified at 3p25 and encodes a small novel predicted protein that functions to down-regulate transcriptional elongation of target genes by binding to the elongin complex. Mutations in the von Hippel–Lindau gene have also been identified in sporadic tumours of the non-papillary type. Cases of familial RCC have been associated with chromosomal transloca-tions involving regions of chromosome 3 distinct from the von Hippel–Lindau locus. In sporadic RCC up to 90% demonstrate allele loss on 3p, defining two further regions that are important in the molecular pathogenesis of this condition. A region on 17p may also be important. Genes at these loci remain to be identified. Of the two types of RCC, papillary and non-papillary, clear genetic differences occur. Non-papillary tumours comprise 80% and are the type seen in von Hippel–Lindau syndrome and familial cases; 3p loss is common in these, whereas it is not seen in papillary tumours.

Clinical Von Hippel–Lindau syndrome manifestations include:

- haemangioblastoma
    - retinal   60%
    - cerebellar   60%
    - spinal   13–44%
    - brain-stem   18%
- renal cell carcinoma   28%
- phaeochromocytoma   10%
- renal cystic disease   76%
- pancreatic cysts/tumours   5%.

Penetrance is almost complete by the age of 60 years, with up to 70% of affected individuals developing RCC by this age. Retinal haemangioblastomas are often the earliest manifestation of von Hippel–Lindau syndrome; RCC is the presenting feature in only 10% of cases.

Diagnostic criteria

If there is a positive family history of haemangioblastoma, a single haemangioblastoma or visceral complication, e.g. RCC, would be diagnostic. If there is no family history, two or more haemangioblastomas or a single haemangioblastoma with a visceral complication is diagnostic.

Screening   Early detection and treatment improves the prognosis of von Hippel–Lindau syndrome, and all affected individuals and at-risk family members should be offered the opportunity to enter a screening protocol and be offered molecular genetic testing. Such a screening protocol for individuals affected by von Hippel–Lindau syndrome comprises:

- Annually:
  - Symptoms and physical examination including blood pressure
  - Direct and indirect ophthalmoscopy
  - Renal ultrasound (CT or MRI depending on local experience and CT every three years especially if multiple renal cysts present)
  - 24-hour urine collection for VMAs
- Three-yearly
  Consider MRI brain scan: definitely if symptomatic otherwise only for those patients who are particularly anxious to have the investigation as treatment is usually only considered for symptomatic lesions.

In at-risk relatives ophthalmological assessment can be started at the age of 5 years, with renal imaging starting at the age of 15 years.

The right to know	The right not to know
• To make reproductive decisions • To have certainty • To plan appropriate action, e.g. prophylactic surgery • To inform other family members • To make provision for the future	• Unable to cope with result • Does not predict disease onset • Fear of increasing risk to children • Insurance/career problems • Burden of positive result on family

Table 8.9
Some reasons to accept or refuse predictive testing

Predictive testing   With the definition of von Hippel–Lindau syndrome mutations it has become possible to offer diagnostic and predictive testing to individuals (including children from the age of 5 years) with features of the condition and to any asymptomatic family members at risk of inheriting it. Mutations can be found in 75% of individuals and linkage analysis can be used in the remainder.

Many difficult issues arise during consideration of predictive testing (issues that are also important when considering any form of screening). A person offered testing may accept or refuse it. Some reasons for the decision made are shown in Table 8.9. Strict protocols for predictive testing must therefore be adhered to. These will have been agreed by local ethical committees and usually follow a basic common scheme (Table 8.10). This protocol is carried out by clinical genetic departments, usually with the back-up and support of medical and surgical services which may become

Table 8.10
Predictive testing protocol

- Initial visit to discuss predictive testing
  - Clinical aspects and screening tests
  - Genetics aspects
  - Personal knowledge/perception of own risk
  - How predictive test works
  - Motivation for the test
  - Effects of the test
    - ○ emotional difference between risk and certainty
    - ○ psychological adjustment to high and low risk results
    - ○ impact on personal life
    - ○ impact on family members
    - ○ financial implications
  - Support during and after test
  - Options
    - ○ test now
    - ○ test later
    - ○ no test
    - ○ prenatal testing
  - Details of test protocol
- Follow-up (clinic or telephone)
  - Further questions
  - ?Proceed
- Consent and blood sampling
  - If proceeding, consent form signed and blood sample taken
  - Arrangements made for results to be given
- Results
- Follow-up
- Arrange screening investigations if appropriate

involved with patient management or may have been involved with other family members. This is important for the planning of regular screening in affected individuals.

References

Torres, V.E. (1996) Tuberous Sclerosis Complex, in *Polycystic Kidney Disease* (eds M.L. Watson and V.E. Torres), Oxford Clinical Nephrology Series, Oxford University Press, Oxford, pp. 283–308.

Winter, R.M. and Baraitser, M. (1990) *The London Dysmorphology Database*, Oxford Medical Databases, Oxford University Press, Oxford.

Zerres, K. (1996) Classification of Cystic Kidneys, in *Polycystic Kidney Disease* (eds M.L. Watson and V.E. Torres), Oxford Clinical Nephrology Series, Oxford University Press, Oxford, pp. 167–88.

Further reading

Davison, A.M.., Cameron, J.S.., Grünfeld, J-P. *et al.* (eds) 1998 *Oxford Textbook of Clinical Nephrology*, Oxford University Press, Oxford.

Eeles, R.A., Ponder, B.A.J., Easton, D.F. and Horwich, A. (eds) (1996) *Genetic Predisposition to Cancer*, Chapman & Hall, London.

Harper, P.S. (1994) *Practical Genetic Counselling*, 4th edn, Butterworth Heinemann, Oxford.

International Study of Genetic Renal Disease (ISGRD) (1998) http://pru6.umds.ac.uk/isgrd/

On line Mendelian Inheritance in Man (1998) http://www.ncbi.nlm.nih.gov/omim/

Rimoin, D.L., Connor, J.M. and Pyeritz, R.E. (eds) (1996) *Emery and Rimoin's Principles and Practice of Medical Genetics*, 3rd edn, Churchill Livingstone, New York.

Scriver, C.R., Beaudet, A.L., Sly, W.S. and Valle, D. (eds) (1995) *The Metabolic and Molecular Basis of Inherited Disease*, 7th edn, McGraw-Hill, New York.

Part Two

Renal Investigations in Clinical Practice

Diagnosis of acute renal failure

Linda De Luca

Introduction

Acute renal failure (ARF) can be defined as a rapid deterioration, over hours or days, in baseline renal function resulting in retention of nitrogenous waste and presenting clinically as an elevation of serum urea and serum creatinine (Brenner and Lazarus, 1988). Overall mortality in the setting of ARF ranges from 15–60% and is related to the severity of renal failure and to its etiology (Hou *et al.*, 1983). It is therefore critical to make a rapid diagnosis so that therapy aimed at reversible causes may be initiated promptly. It remains clinically useful to divide the differential diagnosis of ARF into the three conventional categories of prerenal uremia, intrinsic renal disease including acute tubular necrosis (ATN), and postrenal uremia (Table 9.1).

It is notable that almost 90% of cases of community-acquired ARF have a reversible cause either prerenal or postrenal (Kaufman et al., 1991; Feest, Round and Hamad, 1993). Common causes of prerenal uremia in this setting are vomiting, diarrhea, diuretics, glycosuria, congestive heart failure, gastrointestinal bleeding and sepsis. The most common causes of intrinsic renal disease (11% of community-acquired ARF) are drug-induced (e.g angiotensin-converting enzyme (ACE) inhibitors), glomerulonephritis secondary to an infectious etiology (e.g. endocarditis) or vascular disease (e.g. atheroembolic). Mortality is high in this group at 55% compared with 7% in prerenal uremia and 42% in postrenal uremia.

In a hospital setting, almost 80% of patients with ARF have either prerenal ischemia or established ATN secondary to decreased renal perfusion (hypovolemia, congestive heart failure, sepsis, postoperative ischemia), or nephrotoxic insult (contrast media, aminoglycosides, ACE inhibitors). Mortality in this group of patients can be as high as 64% (Werb and Linton, 1979; Hou *et al.*, 1983).

An understanding of the most common causes of ARF in both the community and hospital environments, and of the potential impact of prevention and early intervention is important in our approach to the

Prerenal

Decreased effective circulatory volume
- Fluid loss: renal, gastrointestinal, dermal (e.g. burns)
- Redistribution or third space loss: sepsis, hypoalbuminemia (nephrotic), liver failure, pancreatitis, trauma, gastrointestinal obstruction
- Decreased cardiac output: myocardial ischemia, heart failure, pulmonary embolism

Vascular
- Renal artery stenosis
- Thrombosis
- Atheroemboli
- Vasculitis
- Altered autoregulation, e.g. prostaglandin inhibitors, ACE inhibitors

Intrinsic renal

Glomerular disease
- IgA nephropathy
- associated with low serum complement levels: lupus nephritis, postinfectious (e.g. endocarditis), cryoglobulinemia – mixed essential or associated with hepatitis B or C
- Normal serum complement: Goodpasture's disease, hemolytic uremic syndrome, Wegener's granulomatosis, microscopic polyarteritis, idiopathic necrotizing glomerular nephritis, Churg–Strauss syndrome

Interstitial nephritis
- Drugs (see Table 9.4)
- Infiltrative, e.g. lymphoma
- Granulomatous, e.g. sarcoidosis, tuberculosis
- Infectious, e.g. pyelonephritis or systemic infection (fungal, bacterial, parasitic)

Tubular injury
- Ischemic (prolonged prerenal)
- Toxic: drugs (e.g. aminoglycosides), contrast media, metals, poisons (e.g. ethylene glycol), pigment (e.g. myoglobin)
- Metabolic: hypercalcemia, light-chain nephropathy
- Crystal: uric acid (tumor lysis), oxalate crystals, acyclovir, suphadiazine

Vascular
- Atheroemboli
- Cortical necrosis
- Renal vein thrombosis

Postrenal

Intrinsic
- Urethral stricture
- Prostatic hypertrophy or cancer
- Bladder tumors
- Calculi
- Papillary necrosis

Extrinsic
- Retroperitoneal fibrosis
- Malignancy

Table 9.1
Causes of acute renal failure

patient with ARF. However, in addition, making a diagnosis of ARF invariably requires careful attention to history, physical examination, evaluation of urinary sediment and urinary indices, judicious use of other laboratory tests, use of radiological procedures and, in some cases, use of renal biopsy when diagnosis remains elusive or confirmation of clinical suspicion is required prior to therapeutic intervention.

Clinical presentation

HISTORY AND PHYSICAL EXAMINATION

Establishing the presence of ARF involves documentation of a recent fall in glomerular filtration rate (GFR). In a patient presenting for the first time without a record of previous serum creatinine concentrations, chronic as opposed to acute renal failure may be suggested by a long-standing history of hypertension, diabetes, pyelonephritis, and symptoms of nocturia, hematuria, proteinuria and uremia (e.g. pruritis, peripheral neuropathy). However, even in the setting of chronic renal failure, potentially reversible causes of an acute fall in GFR need to be considered.

Diagnosis in a patient with ARF must begin with a thorough history followed by physical examination looking for features suggestive of either prerenal uremia, intrinsic renal disease or postrenal uremia (Brady, Brenner and Lieberthal, 1996).

Prerenal uremia

Prerenal uremia is suggested by a history of decreased oral intake, thirst, dry mucous membranes, rapid weight loss, vomiting, diarrhea, hematemesis, melena, fever, extensive skin burns, use of diuretics or glycosuria. All of these lead to an **actual** decrease in intravascular volume as a cause of decreased renal perfusion. A decrease in, **effective** circulating volume is suggested by a history of cardiac disease with symptoms of congestive heart failure; hypoalbuminemia with ascites and peripheral edema secondary to cirrhosis of the liver or nephrotic syndrome; intra-abdominal disease such as pancreatitis or intestinal obstruction with possible third space fluid losses; sepsis or shock with peripheral vasodilatation. A history of recent trauma or arterial catheterization, especially if in the presence of atheromatous vascular disease, raises the possibility of embolic (e.g. cholesterol) or thrombotic disease of the renal vasculature (Black, 1987). Renal artery stenosis, especially if bilateral or if unilateral in a solitary kidney, may predispose to ARF secondary to thrombotic occlusion or prerenal insults. In the presence of a decrease in effective circulating volume or renal artery stenosis, renal autoregulatory mechanisms are active to maintain both renal blood flow and GFR (Figure 9.1). In this setting, use of prostaglandin inhibitors (e.g. non-steroidal anti-inflammatory drugs) or ACE inhibitors (Hricik *et al.*, 1983) will interfere with autoregulatory mechanisms, allowing a drop in renal blood flow and GFR, and contributing to prerenal uremia or leading to ischemic ATN. Recent use of antihypertensive medication resulting in a significant drop in blood pressure may also decrease renal blood flow, leading to renal ischemia.

Physical examination looking for evidence of a prerenal insult involves careful assessment for signs of volume depletion or of a decreased effective circulatory volume secondary to third space loss, sepsis, heart failure or liver disease. In some cases, it may be necessary to measure central venous pressures or pulmonary artery pressures directly for a more accurate assessment and to guide fluid resuscitation. Presence of abdominal or

Fig. 9.1

Compensatory mechanisms in the maintenance of renal blood flow (RBF) and glomerular filtration rate (GFR). (a) Normal effective circulating volume: normal RBF and GFR. (b) Decreased effective circulating volume or renal artery stenosis: prostaglandins dilate the afferent arteriole and angiotensin II constricts the efferent arteriole resulting in a slight decrease in RBF, an increase in intraglomerular pressure (P*glom*), and a maintained or slightly decreased GFR. (c) Same clinical setting as in (b): non-steroidal anti-inflammatory drugs (NSAIDs) and ACE inhibitors block the compensatory mechanisms resulting in a more pronounced drop in renal blood flow, decreased P*glom* and a significant fall in GFR.

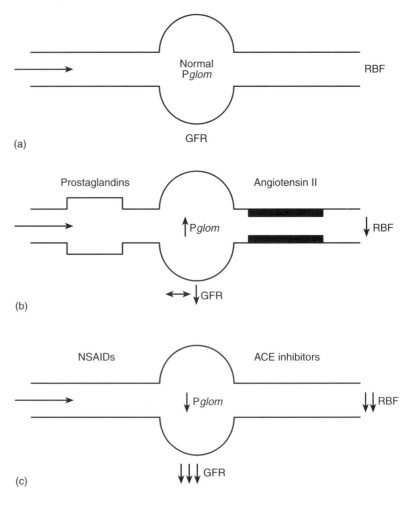

femoral bruits, as well as evidence of peripheral vascular disease, may raise suspicion of renal vascular disease such as renal artery stenosis, atheroembolism or thrombosis.

Intrinsic renal disease

History taking pertinent to a diagnosis of **intrinsic** renal disease focuses on identifying ingestion of a drug(s) that is possibly responsible either for toxic renal tubular damage or interstitial nephritis, and on identifying symptoms that are suggestive of multisystem disease, which may involve the renal glomerulus or renal vasculature.

Intravenous drug use or a recent history of invasive procedures (e.g. dental or urologic) if associated with fever and chills is highly suggestive of postinfectious glomerulonephritis. Recent use of drugs such as antibiotics and non-steroidal anti-inflammatory agents, for example, may lead to allergic interstial nephritis (Table 9.2) (Cooper and Bennett, 1987; Cameron, 1988; Neilson, 1989). Aminoglycosides, chemotherapeutic agents, contrast media or ethylene glycol, for example, are among the agents that can cause ARF by direct tubular toxicity or crystal-induced renal tubular damage. A history of a prolonged or severe prerenal insult suggests the possibility of established ischemic ATN. This is particularly true if renal failure persists after volume repletion and normalization of effective circulatory volume. Symptoms such as a low grade fever, migratory polyarthritis, weight loss, abdominal pain, shortness of breath, pleuritic chest pain, epistaxis, hearing loss or hemoptysis are highly suggestive of the presence of a multisystem disease such as a vasculitis (e.g. polyarteritis nodosa, Wegener's granulomatosis or hemolytic uremic syndrome) or other immune-mediated diseases such as systemic lupus erythematosus or cryoglobulinemia (mixed essential or associated with hepatitis C viremia). A history of long-standing microscopic hematuria or intermittent gross hematuria may suggest the presence of IgA nephropathy, which is sometimes associated with a rapidly progressive decline in renal function.

Physical examination involves searching for manifestations of multisystem disease. Uveitis or iritis may be associated with vasculitis, and scleral icterus with liver disease. Sinusitis and nasal septum deformities may suggest Wegener's granulomatosis. On examination of the skin, a butterfly facial rash may suggest systemic lupus erythematosus; purpuric lesions, a vasculitis; a maculopapular rash, an allergic drug reaction; and needle marks, intravenous drug use possibly resulting in postinfectious glomerulonephritis or hepatitis C-associated cryoglobulinemia (D'Amico and Fornasieri, 1995). Respiratory and cardiovascular findings of pulmonary hemorrhage or edema, pleural or pericardial friction rubs, and murmurs may suggest multisystem disease; however, these may also be due to retention of nitrogenous waste and volume overload, which are often present in renal

Table 9.2
Drug-induced acute renal failure*

Type	Causes
Ischemic acute tubular necrosis	Prostaglandin inhibitors
	Angiotensin-converting enzyme inhibitors
	Cyclosporin A; FK 506
Toxic (direct, tubular) acute tubular necrosis	Aminoglycosides; foscarnet
	Amphotericin B
	Radiocontrast media
	Heavy metals, e.g. cisplatin, lead, lithium
	Solvents, e.g. ethylene glycol, toluene
	Insecticides; herbicides (e.g. paraquat)
	Amphetamines; heroin
Interstitial nephritis	Penicillins; cephalosporins
	Sulfonamides; rifampicin
	Allopurinol
	Diuretics: thiazides, frusemide
	Non-steroidal anti-inflammatories
	Cimetidine
	Diphenylhydantoin (phenytoin)
Intratubular obstruction secondary to crystal formation	Acyclovir
	Sulfadiazine
	Methotrexate
Intratubular obstruction due to retroperitoneal fibrosis	Methysergide

*Source: Cooper and Bennett, 1987; Cameron, 1988; Neilson, 1989.

failure. The clinical manifestations of severe peripheral edema and hypertension seen in nephrotic syndrome should lead to a suspicion of ischemic ATN or renal vein thrombosis as possible causes of rapid deterioration in renal function.

Postrenal failure
Postrenal failure is suggested by a history of:

- renal calculi
- prostatic hypertrophy or cancer
- urethral strictures

- bladder, pelvic or abdominal malignacy.

Previous abdominal or pelvic radiation therapy can be a cause of retro-peritoneal fibrosis with bilateral ureteric obstruction. Diabetes, analgesic nephropathy and sickle cell disease are associated with papillary necrosis. Symptoms associated with obstruction may include gross hematuria, frequency, dysuria, weak urinary stream, and abdominal or flank pain.

Clinical examination involves a search for the presence of a palpably enlarged prostate gland, bladder distension, pelvic or abdominal masses and adenopathy. Urinary bladder catheterization is an important diagnostic maneuver if bladder outlet obstruction is suspected.

Evaluation of urinary indices and urinary sediment

Urinary indices (Table 9.3) provide us with laboratory data that are useful, although not definitive, in differentiating between prerenal disease and established ATN or other intrinsic renal disease. Our use of these data is based on the knowledge that in the absence of established renal disease, the renal tubules maintain their ability to conserve sodium and water in the presence of a decreased effective circulating volume (Rose, 1994). Hypovolemia is a potent stimulus for the release of the antidiuretic hormone (ADH) (via volume-sensitive receptors in the left atrium and carotid sinuses). ADH acts via the cortical collecting ducts to increase water reabsorption. This results in an increase in urine osmolality to 1.5 times (or greater) that of serum (Miller *et al.*, 1978; Rose, 1987). A urine osmolality above 500 mosmol/kg is highly suggestive of prerenal disease with maintenance of renal tubular function. In contrast, a urine osmolality of less than 350 mosmol/kg suggests the loss of concentrating ability seen in ATN. There can be considerable overlap, however, with values of less than 500 mosmol/kg seen in prerenal disease.

	Prerenal state	**Established ATN**
Urine osmolality	> 500 mosmol/kg	< 350 mosmol/kg
Urine Na concentration	< 20 meq/l	> 40 meq/l
FENa	< 1%	> 2%

ATN, acute tubular necrosis; FENa, fractional excretion of Na.

Table 9.3
Urinary indices in acute renal failure

A decrease in effective circulating volume also results in avid sodium (Na) reabsorption in the proximal tubule and, under the influence of aldosterone, distally. Therefore, in prerenal disease, the urine Na concentration is usually low at less than 20 meq/l. Because of loss of tubular function, ATN is usually associated with a urine Na greater than 40 meq/l (Miller *et al.*, 1978). There can, however, be considerable overlap due to variability in water reabsorption. A patient who is volume depleted, for example, will be avidly reasorbing water in addition to Na, resulting in a higher and misleading urine Na concentration. It is for this reason that the fractional excretion of Na (FENa) may provide a more useful tool for differentiating between prerenal states and established ATN (Miller *et al.*, 1978; Steiner, 1984). The FENa attempts to correct for differences in water reabsorption. It is calculated as follows:

$$\text{FENa} = \frac{\text{urine Na} \times \text{plasma creatinine}}{\text{plasma Na} \times \text{urine creatinine}} \times 100$$

The FENa is usually less than 1% in prerenal disease and greater than 2% in ATN.

It should be remembered that prerenal disease may coexist with chronic intrinsic renal disease. In this setting, all of the above urinary indices may not accurately reflect the prerenal state due to the presence of chronic tubular dysfunction.

Urinalysis (Table 9.4) provides valuable diagnostic information (see also Chapter 3). In prerenal diseases it is mostly normal. There may be a few

Table 9.4
Urinary sediment in renal disease

Urinary sediment	Renal disease
Red blood cell casts	Glomerulonephritis, proliferative Vasculitis, small vessel Rarely ATN Rarely interstitial nephritis
White blood cell casts	Interstitial nephritis Pyelonephritis
Granular, pigmented casts 'muddy brown'	Acute tubular necrosis

Crystals:
  uric acid
  calcium oxalate
	Tumor lysis syndrome
	Ethylene glycol ingestion

Bland sediment	Prerenal uremia Postrenal uremia

hyaline casts, one or two white or red cells but no significant hematuria, no significant proteinuria and no cellular casts. Postrenal failure is also usually associated with a bland urinary sediment unless a tumor or calculus is a source of hematuria. In ATN, urine is usually positive for blood with small amounts of protein, and the sediment contains epithelial cells, epithelial cell casts and pigmented (muddy brown) granular casts (Plate 26). Absence of these findings, however, does not necessarily exclude the presence of ATN. Significant proteinuria (more than 1–2 g/l), hematuria, fragmented red blood cells, and red cell casts are highly suggestive of glomerular disease, either primary or secondary to infection or vasculitis (Plate 27). White blood cell casts are seen in interstitial nephritis, either infectious or allergic (Plate 28). The presence of urinary eosinophils, detected by either Wright's or Hansel's stain of the urine, may be indicative of allergic interstitial nephritis (Nolan, Anger and Kelleher, 1986; Sutton, 1986; Ruffing *et al.*, 1994). Since these stains may not always be very sensitive, absence of eosinophils by no means excludes this diagnosis. In addition, eosinophils have also been seen infrequently in vasculitis, prostatitis and renal ather-oemboli. The presence of urinary eosinophils is therefore compatible with interstitial nephritis, but it is not specific and a diagnosis must be made considering the clinical picture as a whole.

The presence of crystals in the urine may also be useful. Uric acid crystals may be seen in acute renal failure secondary to tumor lysis syndrome, and calcium oxalate crystals may be seen in renal failure secondary to ethylene glycol poisoning (Plate 29).

Two things must be remembered in relation to routine dipstick testing of urine. Firstly, a positive reading for blood may not differentiate between hemoglobin or myoglobin, and in the absence of red blood cells on microscopy, the possibility of rhabdomyolysis with myoglobinuria or of hemoglobinuria should be considered. Secondly, the routine dipstick is able to detect negatively charged albumin but not positively charged para-proteins such as myeloma proteins or light-chains. Multiple myeloma and light-chain deposition disease are frequently associated with glomerular lesions leading to albuminuria, accounting for the positive reading on a dipstick. If either of these diseases is a possibility based on clinical presentation, then a urine immunoelectrophoresis is required (p. 37).

Other laboratory investigations

Serial measurements of serum urea and creatinine are indicative of the rate of deterioration in renal function, are important in patient care and may help to differentiate between prerenal disease and established ATN based on, for example, the response to volume repletion or correction of other prerenal insults. Measuring serum electrolytes is also important for patient management and may provide clues to diagnosis. An extremely high serum potassium, especially if not in keeping with the severity of the renal dysfunction, may suggest tissue injury and rhabdomyolysis. An elevated serum creatine phosphokinase and myoglobinuria are confirmatory. The presence of an elevated anion gap (Table 9.5) should lead to a search for possible toxic ingestion. Ethylene glycol, for example, is metabolized to oxalic acid, which increases the anion gap. Ethylene glycol also adds to the serum osmolality causing a gap between the measured and calculated osmolality (Table 9.5). Serum ethylene glycol levels can be measured and oxalate crystals may be found in the urine (Plate 29).

A full blood count measurement may be helpful. The presence of anemia may suggest chronic renal failure or acute renal failure secondary to vasculitis or blood loss. The presence of thrombocytopenia along with a peripheral smear showing fragmented red cells is suggestive of a thrombotic microangiopathy, such as hemolytic uremic syndrome, or sepsis, such as bacterial endocarditis. The presence of eosinophilia may suggest an allergic reaction causing interstitial nephritis, although its absence does not exclude it.

An elevated antistreptolysin-O titer or positive blood cultures raise the suspicion of postinfectious glomerulonephritis. In this case, complement

Table 9.5

Use of the anion and osmolar gaps in diagnosis of acute renal failure

Anion gap acidosis	**Osmolar gap**
Definition	**Definition**
H ion accumulates with anion other than Cl causing a decrease in HCO_3 without an increase in Cl, thereby increasing the anion gap	Measured plasma osmolality minus calculated osmolality is increased (should be zero)
Causes	**Causes**
Ketoacidosis	Ethanol
Lactic acidosis	Ethylene glycol
Poisons: methanol, ethylene glycol, salicylates, paraldehyde	Methanol
	Mannitol
Renal insufficiency	**Calculation**
Calculation	P Osm − C Osm = 0 calculated
Na − [HCO_3 + Cl] usually equals 9–13 meq/l	osmolality = (2 × plasma Na) + glucose + urea (mmol/l)

levels (C_3) may be decreased (p. 48). Complement levels may also be decreased in systemic lupus erythematosus or cryoglobulinemia (p. 50). The cryoglobulinemia may be either essential or secondary to hepatitis B or C positivity (p. 47). A serum protein electrophoresis with immunofixation or quantitative measurement of immunoglobulins is important to rule out the presence of light-chains or myeloma proteins (p. 59). An elevated IgA level may suggest IgA nephropathy.

Over the past few years, our ability to detect the presence of anti-neutrophil cytoplasmic antibodies (ANCA) (p. 55) has been extremely helpful in facilitating the diagnosis of small vessel vasculitides such as Wegener's granulomatosis and microscopic polyarteritis, which lead to a rapidly progressive necrotizing glomerulonephritis (Hagen *et al.*, 1993; Kallenberg *et al.*, 1994; Falk and Jennette, 1997). Cytoplasmic ANCA (c-ANCA) is an autoantibody usually directed against neutrophil proteinase 3. Most p-ANCA (perinuclear ANCA) are directed against myeloperoxidase. Combining indirect immunofluorescence to determine the pattern of staining (c-ANCA or p-ANCA) with ELISAs specific for the major auto-antigens (PR-3 and MPO, respectively) is of great value in the diagnosis of small vessel vasculitis. This is discussed more fully in Chapter 4.

Radiographic studies

The main reasons for using radiological procedures in the diagnosis of acute renal failure are to assist in the differentiation of acute from chronic renal failure and to rule out the presence of obstruction. Renal ultrasonography is perhaps the most useful investigation to help provide answers to both those questions (Kaye and Pollak, 1982; Jeffrey and Federle, 1983; Denton, Cochlin and Evans, 1984). Small kidney size is highly suggestive of chronic renal failure. It is important to remember, however, that even in this setting acute renal failure may be superimposed on existing chronic disease. Chronic renal failure secondary to diabetes or amyloid may be associated with normal sized or even large kidneys on ultrasound examination. Ultrasonography is highly effective at diagnosing hydronephrosis, with a sensitivity greater than 98%. It must be remembered that attributing the presence of acute renal failure to obstruction should involve demonstration of bilateral hydronephrosis or hydronephrosis of one kidney in the presence of a contralateral small, and therefore presumably end-stage, kidney. Ultrasonography may also identify the presence of renal calculi or papillary necrosis, ureteral dilatation and a full and distended urinary bladder. If the reason for or site of obstruction is not clear, then cystoscopy and retrograde pyelography or antegrade pyelography via a nephrostomy tube may be required.

A unilaterally enlarged kidney in the presence of nephrotic syndrome may lead to suspicion of renal vein thrombosis, which would require duplex sonography or, ideally, as the gold standard, venography for confirmation (p. 64).

Duplex ultrasonography may also be useful in the diagnosis of renal artery stenosis as a potential cause of rapid and progressive deterioration in renal function (Textor and Canzanello, 1996). Arteriography may be needed, however, to confirm a diagnosis of renal artery occlusion secondary to emboli or thrombosis, particularly if the occlusion is believed to be recent (one to three hours), in which case thrombolytic therapy and heparinization may prevent renal infarction. A nuclear medicine renal scan can demonstrate absence of renal blood flow, segmental areas of infarction or maintenance of renal blood flow with delayed function consistent with ATN. Digital subtraction angiography, magnetic resonance angiography and angiography using carbon dioxide are newer, potentially less nephrotoxic, imaging techniques undergoing evaluation (p. 66).

Renal biopsy

A diagnosis of the etiology of ARF can usually be made on the basis of clinical and laboratory evaluations, and renal biopsy may not be required. There are, however, several instances where a biopsy is necessary (see also Chapter 7). In cases where an initial diagnosis of ATN or suspected interstitial nephritis was made, or where offending agents have been discontinued and prerenal factors corrected and yet renal failure persists longer than expected, a renal biopsy may become necessary to confirm a diagnosis, establish correct therapeutic options and predict the potential for recovery (Richards *et al.*, 1994). A renal biopsy is also indicated in the presence of suspected glomerular disease without an obvious cause such as endocarditis. The biopsy may reveal the presence of glomerulonephritis with immune complex deposition, as seen in systemic lupus erythematosus, or few immune deposits and a necrotizing glomerulonephritis, as seen in the small vessel vasculitides such as Wegener's granulomatosis or microscopic polyarteritis. The biopsy in these cases will both confirm the need for therapy with immunosuppressive agents and, in some cases, help to predict the outcome based on the extent of established sclerosis and obsolete glomeruli. A patient with a suspected vasculitis, in whom infection has been ruled out and who is too ill for renal biopsy, should be treated on the basis of history, and clinical and laboratory findings since morbidity and mortality without treatment may be high.

Conclusion

The morbidity and mortality associated with ARF is high. The etiology of the renal failure in the majority of patients, both from the community and in hospital, will be prerenal or postrenal, and it is therefore crucial to establish a diagnosis and implement therapy aimed at correcting prerenal factors and relieving the obstruction. Other patients will present with intrinsic renal disease due to established ATN from prolonged prerenal failure or other toxic insults, interstitial disease related to a drug or toxin, or glomerular disease, either primary or associated with a systemic illness. It is important to establish a diagnosis rapidly in these cases too, so that offending agents may be discontinued and appropriate supportive and therapeutic maneuvers initiated. Making such a diagnosis requires careful history-taking and physical examination looking for evidence of prerenal or toxic insults, and the possibility of obstruction or multisystem disease. Urinalysis and urinary indices will help to differentiate between prerenal disease, established ATN or glomerular disease. Other laboratory investigations will help in diagnosis, and renal ultrasound will allow estimation of renal size and serve to rule out obstruction. Therapeutic trials such as fluid challenge, improvement in cardiac output, removal of offending agents and bladder catheterization should be initiated. A renal biopsy may be necessary to establish the diagnosis if no cause is apparent or if renal function does not recover as predicted.

Acknowledgment

I would like to record my sincere thanks to Frances Andrus, medical laboratory technologist in the Division of Nephrology, Department of Medicine at the London Health Sciences Center, Victoria Campus, London, Ontario, Canada, for the pictures of urinary sediment.

References

Black, R.M. (1987) Vascular diseases of the kidney, in *Pathophysiology of Renal Disease*, 2nd edn (ed. B.D. Rose), McGraw-Hill, New York, pp. 353–60.

Brady, H.R., Brenner, B.M. and Lieberthal, W. (1996) Acute Renal Failure, in *The Kidney*, 5th edn (eds B.M. Brenner and F.C. Rector, Jr), W.B. Saunders, Philadelphia, p. 1222.

Brenner, B.M. and Lazarus, J.M. (eds) (1988) *Acute Renal Failure*, 2nd edn, Churchill Livingstone, New York.

Cameron, S. (1988) Allergic interstitial nephritis: clinical features and pathogenesis. *Q. J. Med.*, **66**(250), 97–115.

Cooper, K. and Bennett, W.M. (1987) Nephrotoxicity of common drugs used in clinical practice. *Arch. Intern. Med.*, **147**, 1213–18.

D'Amico, G. and Fornasieri, A. (1995) Cryoglobulinemic glomerulonephritis: a membranoproliferative glomerulonephritis induced by hepatitis C virus. *Am. J. Kid. Dis.*, **25**(3), 361–9.

Denton, T., Cochlin, D.L. and Evans, C. (1984) The value of ultrasound in previously undiagnosed renal failure. *Br. J. Radiol.*, **57**, 673–5.

Falk, R.J. and Jennette, J.C. (1997) ANCA small-vessel vasculitis. *J. Am. Soc. Nephrol.*, **8**(2), 314–22.

Feest, T.G., Round, A. and Hamad, S. (1993) Incidence of severe acute renal failure in adults: results of a community based study. *Br. Med. J.*, **306**, 481–3.

Hagen, E.C., Ballieux, B.E., van Es, L.A. *et al.* (1993) Antineutrophil cytoplasmic antibodies: a review of the antigens involved, the assays, and the clinical and possible pathogenetic consequences. *Blood*, **81**, 1996.

Hou, S.H., Bushinsky, D.A., Wish, J.B. *et al.* (1983) Hospital-acquired renal insufficiency: a prospective study. *Am. J. Med.*, **74**, 243–8.

Hricik, D.E., Browning, P.J., Kapelman, R. *et al.* (1983) Captopril-induced functional renal insufficiency in patients with bilateral renal-artery stenosis or renal-artery stenosis in a solitary kidney. *N. Engl. J. Med.*, **308**, 373.

Jeffrey, R.B. and Federle, M.P. (1983) CT and ultrasonography of acute renal abnormalities. *Radiol. Clin. North Am.*, **21**, 515–25.

Kallenberg, C.G.M., Brouwer, E., Weening, J.J. and Cohen Tervaert, J.W. (1994) Antineutrophil cytoplasmic antibodies: current diagnostic and pathophysiological potential. *Kid. Int.*, **46**, 1–15.

Kaufman, J., Dhakal, M., Patel, B. and Hamburger, R. (1991) Community-acquired acute renal failure. *Am. J. Kid. Dis.*, **17**, 191–8.

Kaye, A.D. and Pollak, H.M. (1982) Diagnostic imaging approach to the patient with obstructive uropathy. *Semin. Nephrol.*, **2**, 55–73.

Miller, T.R., Anderson, R.J., Linas, S.L. *et al.* (1978) Urinary diagnostic indices in acute renal failure: a prospective study. *Ann. Intern. Med.*, **89**, 47–50.

Neilson, E.G. (1989) Pathogenesis and therapy of interstitial nephritis. *Kid. Int.*, **35**, 1257.

Nolan, C.R. III, Anger, M.S. and Kelleher, S.P. (1986) Eosinophiluria – a new method of detection and definition of the clinical spectrum. *N. Engl. J. Med.*, **315**, 1516.

Richards, N.T., Darby, S., Howie, A.J. *et al.* (1994) Knowledge of histology alters patient management in over 40% of cases. *Nephrol. Dial. Trans.*, **9**, 1255–9.

Rose, B.D. (1987) *Pathophysiology of Renal Disease*, McGraw-Hill, New York, pp. 16–17.

Rose, B.D. (1994) *Clinical Physiology of Acid–base and Electrolyte Disorders*, 4th edn, McGraw-Hill, New York.

Ruffing, K.A., Hoppes, P., Blend, D. *et al.* (1994) Eosinophils in urine revisited. *Clin. Nephrol.*, **41**(3), 163–6.

Steiner, R.W. (1984) Interpreting the fractional excretion of sodium. *Am. J. Med.*, 77, 699.

Sutton, J.M. (1986) Urinary eosinophils. *Arch. Intern. Med.*, **146**, 2243.

Textor, S.C. and Canzanello, V.J. (1996) Radiographic evaluation of the renal vasculature. *Curr. Opin. Nephrol. Hypertens.*, **51**, 541–51.

Werb, R. and Linton, A.L. (1979) Aetiology, diagnosis, treatment and prognosis of acute renal failure in an intensive care unit. *Resuscitation*, 7, 95–100.

Further reading

Finn, W.F. (1990) Diagnosis and management of acute tubular necrosis. *Med. Clin. North Am.*, 74(4), 873–91.

Jennette, C.J. and Falk, R.J. (1990) Diagnosis and management of glomerulonephritis and vasculitis presenting as acute renal failure. *Med. Clin. North Am.*, 74(4), 893–908.

Mason, P.D. and Pusey, C.D. (1994) Glomerulonephritis: diagnosis and treatment. *Br. Med. J.*, **309**, 1557–63.

Thadhari, R. *et al.* (1996) Acute renal failure. *N. Engl. J. Med.*, **334**(22), 1448–60.

Chronic renal failure

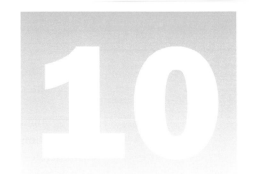

Patricia Campbell and Allan Murray

Patients with chronic renal failure are subject to complications as a result of the extrarenal manifestations of the underlying disease, the effects of treatment, and the secondary effects of renal failure on other organs. This chapter will review the laboratory investigations available to define the etiology and manage the complications of renal failure in clinical practice.

Diagnosis of the etiology of chronic renal insufficiency

When evidence of renal insufficiency is detected, usually by assay of the serum creatinine, an assessment should be made to determine if an acute or reversible cause of renal dysfunction is present (Chapter 9). The presence of a normochromic normocytic anemia, renal osteodystrophy, or small kidneys on renal ultrasound suggests renal disease is well established.

It is nevertheless important to establish a diagnosis of the cause of chronic renal failure. Over the past decade, clinical trials have identified promising therapeutic strategies for delaying the progression of chronic renal dysfunction, and in some cases for specifically treating the underlying disease. The general approach we take in our clinical practice to the diagnosis and management of patients presenting with typical renal syndromes is reviewed below.

THE ROLE OF URINALYSIS

In many cases the diagnostic decision tree used to evaluate a patient with evidence of chronic renal dysfunction starts with evaluation of the urinalysis and the amount of proteinuria found in a 24-hour urine collection. In general, the clinical syndromes may be divided into:

- little microhematuria (< 5 red cells/high power field) or proteinuria (< 150 mg/day)
- moderate to nephrotic range proteinuria (proteinuria > 3.5 g/d), with little microhematuria
- proteinuria and microhematuria.

The finding of an elevated serum creatinine and few red blood cells or little protein on the urinalysis suggests that the site of renal injury lies outside the glomerulus and does not involve an inflammatory process affecting the tubulointerstitial compartment of the kidney. Common non-inflammatory tubulointerstitial diseases include autosomal dominant and autosomal recessive forms of polycystic kidney disease, and medullary cystic disease. In this setting, imaging studies of the kidneys should be obtained to look for evidence of these diagnoses, and to exclude urinary tract obstruction. Injury to the glomerular capillary bed without rupture of the capillary basement membrane, as occurs in thrombotic microangiopathy, may present in this fashion. Consideration must also be given to diseases in which the principal target of renal injury is the extraglomerular vasculature. Such processes may be related to disorders of the large vessels, e.g. renal vascular disease complicated by ischemic nephropathy, disease of smaller arterioles due to atheroembolic events or hypertension, or of the peritubular capillaries such as sickle cell disease. These disorders are often characterized by secondary changes in the glomeruli with the appearance of focal glomerulosclerosis.

In contrast, a different set of diseases is suggested by the finding of proteinuria in the absence of microhematuria. The kidneys normally allow between 500 mg and 1 g of protein, of which one-third is albumin, to pass through the glomerular membrane per day. About 90% of this is reabsorbed by the tubular epithelial cells, which in turn excrete small amounts of Tamm–Horsfall and other proteins into the urine. In the normal state, 150–200 mg of protein is found in a 24-hour urine collection. Pathological proteinuria may result from a large filtered load of normal protein caused by glomerular disease, incomplete reabsorption of normally filtered protein caused by tubular epithelial cell injury, or increased excretion of abnormal protein. Urine protein electropheresis may be used to describe the sieving characteristics of the glomerulus based on the molecular weight and the relative amount of negatively charged protein present in the urine. In adults, this is rarely useful in clinical practice since, among the glomerular diseases, only minimal change nephropathy shows selective proteinuria. However, it is important to ensure that the urine protein is studied to exclude immunoglobulin light-chains found in multiple myeloma.

The quantity of proteinuria will often determine the degree to which the patient is evaluated. In most cases, proteinuria of > 2 g/d reflects significant glomerular injury and increases the risk of progressive renal failure. An estimate of the degree of proteinuria may be obtained from a spot urine sample by comparing the protein to creatinine ratio. The histological correlates of this clinical presentation range from relatively benign diseases such as minimal change disease, to membranous glomerulonephropathy, and focal and segmental glomerulosclerosis. Each of these pathological entities can be primary ill-understood renal disorders, or secondary to multisystem diseases including underlying malignancies or immunological disorders. The World Health Organization (WHO) class V variant of lupus nephropathy, for example, has the appearance of membranous injury on renal biopsy.

Diabetes mellitus, the most common cause of end-stage renal disease requiring dialysis in most industrialized countries, may also present in this fashion during the overt nephropathy phase of renal injury. In most cases a history of diabetes for 15 years, coupled with evidence of damage to the retinal microvessels is sufficient evidence of diabetic nephropathy to preclude further testing. In the older population, multiple myeloma may also present with renal amyloidosis, occasionally even in the absence of convincing monoclonal immunoglobulin peaks on serum electrophoresis.

In the third class of findings, the urinalysis shows the combination of microhematuria and proteinuria. Glomerular hematuria is suggested by the presence of a large fraction of dysmorphic red blood cells when examined under phase contrast microscopy, and a wide variation in the size of erythrocytes found in the urine. However, care must be taken to exclude extrarenal sources of bleeding. Extrarenal bleeding may be generated by nephrolithiasis, inflammation of the collecting system, or epithelial neoplasia. On rare occasions, coagulation defects may present with microhematuria.

If the proteinuria is heavy (> 2 g/d) or red blood cell casts are seen on urinalysis, a glomerular cause is strongly implicated. Since the identification of even one red blood cell cast signifies glomerular injury, it is important for the nephrologist to examine the urine carefully (Chapter 3). The histological correlates of glomerular microhematuria include forms of proliferative glomerulonephritis such as mesangial proliferative or membranoproliferative glomerulonephritis. In many cases it may be difficult to establish the tempo of the observed renal dysfunction for lack of previous documentation of renal function tests. Suspicion of acute glomerulonephritis should initiate a series of laboratory tests to identify the cause. The serological tests are described in Chapter 4. In most cases, renal biopsy is performed to establish a diagnosis (Chapter 7).

Table 10.1

Uses of renal biopsy in evaluating patients with chronic renal failure

- Guide management decisions
- Focus further investigations
- Provide prognostic information
- Material for clinical investigation

THE ROLE OF RENAL BIOPSY

A renal biopsy is the definitive test to establish the nature of glomerular injury. However, renal biopsy is usually uninformative when used to investigate chronic renal dysfunction due to extraglomerular diseases of the kidney, or when renal dysfunction is far advanced. Renal biopsy of native and transplant kidneys may be performed safely and, in selected cases, real-time ultrasound guidance has been used to perform percutaneous biopsy of single native kidneys with success.

In the setting of chronic renal dysfunction renal histology may determine the treatment strategy (Table 10.1). For example, the management options for membranous nephropathy include conservative measures or more aggressive therapy with cyclosporin or a combination of alkylating agents and corticosteroids. In addition, the biopsy may be used to suggest a range of underlying diseases that have been associated with given renal disorders. For example, membranous nephropathy may occur as an isolated entity, be related to an underlying malignancy, or as a manifestation of systemic lupus erythematosus (SLE). Immunofluorescence examination in the latter case usually reveals a characteristic 'full house' pattern of immunoglobulin and complement component deposits and distinguishes this secondary cause of membranous glomerular nephropathies (MGN) from other etiologies. Histological features of the biopsy material may thus focus subsequent management of the patient towards investigation and treatment of the underlying disease.

The renal biopsy may also provide prognostic information on the outcome of renal disease. Such information might have implications for any life decisions the patient may take, or might affect the patient's treatment by insurance companies. Moreover, histological confirmation of the diagnosis may assist the physician counseling a patient who is considering renal transplantation. Several disorders are known to recur in the kidney allograft and to have an effect on graft survival.

THE USE OF RENAL IMAGING TECHNIQUES

Renal ultrasound is the primary imaging technique used to evaluate patients with suspected chronic renal failure. Diseases characterized by abnormalities in renal structure, such as polycystic kidney disease (PKD), are easily diagnosed using this technique. Family members of an affected PKD patient may also be screened for the characteristic cysts, even at very early stages of the disease.

In other conditions, renal ultrasound provides information about the size of each kidney. A measurement of less than 9 cm on the long axis of the kidney suggests chronic renal scarring. Diffuse thinning of the renal cortex or increased cortical echogenicity are less specific indicators of chronic renal disease. Focal scarring is suggestive of segmental arterial occlusion or reflux nephropathy.

Marked differences in the size of the kidneys suggest an underlying structural abnormality, such as renal artery stenosis. Doppler examination of the renal arteries, nuclear imaging techniques, renal angiography, magnetic resonance angiography (MRA) or spiral computed tomography may all be used to evaluate native renal arteries.

Ultrasound examination is also a sensitive technique for detecting urinary tract obstruction, which is a common cause of renal dysfunction in the elderly male, typically due to bladder outlet obstruction by an enlarged prostate. The findings may include either mild or pronounced pelvicalyceal dilation, hydroureter, and an increased volume of urine in the bladder after micturition. The cause of ureteric obstruction may not be seen on ultrasound if retroperitoneal structures are inadequately visualized. In this situation, antegrade or retrograde pyelography, usually performed in conjunction with stent placement, localize the site of the obstructing lesion. Computed tomography (CT) or magnetic resonance imaging (MRI) provide better detail of the retroperitoneal tissue.

Conventional or high dose intravenous pyelography (IVP) has been largely displaced by ultrasonography in the investigation of chronic renal failure. IVP provides better resolution of medullary and calyceal structures than ultrasonography, but is less sensitive than CT or MRI techniques for identifying abnormalities in these regions. IVP is more sensitive than ultrasonography to detect medullary cystic disease or a cause of renal failure associated with papillary necrosis as the disorder underlying the renal dysfunction. The technique remains useful in the evaluation of nephrolithiasis that may accompany some causes of renal disease. Care must be taken, however, to ensure that the patient is well hydrated prior to the administration of contrast material so as to reduce the risk of acute renal failure.

Nuclear renal scans using either ^{99m}Tc DTPA (diethylenetriamine pentaacetic acid) or ^{99m}Tc MAG 3 (mercapto-acetyltriglycine) have a limited place in the evaluation of the cause of chronic renal dysfunction. A nuclear renogram may provide confirmatory evidence of urinary tract obstruction when the sonographic findings are equivocal. Parenchymal retention of the radionuclide following a challenge with frusemide in the setting of mild pelvicalyceal dilation on ultrasound is suggestive of an obstructed collecting system and warrants further investigation. Nuclear renal scans are more sensitive than ultrasound in the detection of focal regions of scarring caused by ureteric reflux, and hence may be used to diagnose reflux nephropathy. Finally, renal blood flow scans may be used to study lesions of the main renal arteries. However, as renal function deteriorates, the sensitivity of the captopril challenge test decreases, and most cases are best evaluated by direct angiography if renal artery stenosis is suspected. In some cases, segmental radiopenic areas on SPECT (single photon emission computed tomography) scanning may identify vascular occlusion of branches of the renal arteries.

ESTIMATING THE SEVERITY OF RENAL DYSFUNCTION

The glomerular filtration rate (GFR) is widely used as an index for the severity of renal disease. However, interpretation of several clinically available surrogate measurements of the GFR is fraught with pitfalls. Even the most sensitive measures of GFR may underestimate the degree of renal dysfunction since, for a time, GFR is maintained by increasing the glomerular capillary hydrostatic pressure (Pgc) and the filtration coefficient (K_f) of undamaged nephrons even as other nephrons are destroyed. This section will discuss the relative merits of the clinically available methods of determining GFR, and the utility of these measurements in the management of patients with chronic renal failure (Table 10.2).

The GFR cannot be directly measured in humans. In the laboratory setting, renal clearance of inulin, a marker that is both completely filtered by the glomerulus and unmodified by either additional tubular secretion or reabsorption accurately mirrors GFR. Alternative methods to assess GFR clinically have been developed, the most accurate of which use radioisotopes ^{99m}Tc DTPA or ^{51}Cr EDTA (ethylenediamine tetra-acetic acid) as renal filtration markers.

Table 10.2

Uses of accurate measurements of the glomerular filtration rate in patients with chronic renal failure

- Assessment of the effect of clinical interventions
- Accuracy of drug dosing
- Prediction of the time to dialysis
- Assessment of residual renal function in patients supported by peritoneal dialysis

For most clinical applications, estimates of GFR are based on the serum creatinine or the endogenous creatinine clearance. However, unlike inulin or radioisotopic techniques, creatinine is not a perfect filtration marker.

Creatine, the precursor of creatinine, is generated in the liver and exported to other tissues, principally the skeletal muscle, where it is actively taken up into myocytes. Creatine undergoes non-enzymatic dehydration to form creatinine, which is released to the extracellular compartment. Creatine and creatinine from ingested meats are also absorbed and may increase serum creatinine concentrations. Although creatinine is freely filtered by the glomerulus, both active tubular secretion and passive tubular reabsorption are thought to occur. In addition, creatinine has been shown to be excreted by the gut in the setting of advanced renal dysfunction.

Derivation of the GFR from the serum creatinine concentration or even from the creatinine clearance rests on several assumptions. First, that the serum creatinine concentration is in a steady state. Second, that the total pool of creatinine reflected by the muscle mass is normal or at least constant between determinations. Third, that the conversion of creatine into creatinine occurs at a constant rate. Fourth, that systematic errors in the renal and extrarenal excretion of creatinine are constant across a broad range of GFR.

Simple formulas have been derived to calculate the GFR based on the serum creatinine concentration. For example, the Cockroft–Gault (Cockcroft and Gault, 1976) equation is widely used:

$$\text{GFR (ml/min)} = \frac{[(140 - \text{age}) \times \text{ideal body weight (kg)}]}{[0.8 \times \text{serum creatinine (\mu mol/l)}]}$$

Nevertheless the complex metabolism of creatinine may lead to pitfalls in interpretation of the GFR based on serum creatinine concentrations. If the range of serum creatinine concentration is established from determinations in a normal population, variations in the size of the creatine pool or in the rate of creatinine synthesis in a given patient under study may lead to under- or overestimates of GFR. Moreover, changes in these parameters over time may lead to misinterpretation of trends in the GFR. Similarly, estimates of the rate of loss of renal function determined by plotting reciprocal serum creatinine versus time must be interpreted with caution. The chemical assay used to determine the creatinine concentration in body fluids may introduce additional error, particularly if the older chromogen-based assay methods are used.

Calculation of the creatinine clearance based on accurately timed 24-hour urine collection improves the accuracy of the GFR estimate. Creatinine clearance is calculated as follows:

$$\text{GFR (ml/min)} =$$

$$\left(\frac{\text{urine creatinine (μmol)} \times \text{urine volume per minute (ml/min)}}{\text{serum creatinine (μmol/l)}} \right) \times 1000$$

An assessment of the accuracy of the timed urine collection may be made since daily creatinine production is about 175–250 μmol/kg/d ideal body weight for males and 135–175 μmol/kg/d ideal body weight for females. As the GFR declines, the fraction of total creatinine excretion accounted for by tubular secretion rather than glomerular filtration increases. In this setting, creatinine clearance measurements may overestimate true GFR by as much as twice (Table 10.3).

Cimetidine has been used to improve the accuracy of GFR estimates in patients with moderately advanced renal dysfunction. Cimetidine inhibits the secretion of creatinine by the proximal tubule, presumably by out-competing creatinine for binding to an exchange protein. After loading a patient with 800–1200 mg cimetidine and allowing time for drug equilibration, a three-hour timed urine collection allows the calculation of the creatinine clearance corrected for tubular creatinine secretion.

The limitations of endogenous creatinine-based techniques have been demonstrated in two clinical scenarios:

- chronic liver disease
- solid organ transplant recipients.

Glomerular filtration rate, defined by inulin clearance, has been found to vary widely despite normal serum creatinine values in patients with acute or chronic liver disease. The discrepancy between serum creatinine estimates of GFR and inulin clearances appears to be caused by impaired hepatic production of creatine. Significantly, even 24-hour urine collections for

Table 10.3
Effect of renal dysfunction on the relative fraction of tubular secretion to total excretion of creatinine*

GFR range (ml/min)	> 80	40–80	< 40
Patients (n)	42	50	81
GFR (mean ± SD) (ml/min)	113 ± 32	60 ± 7	22 ± 9
Ccr (mean ± SD) (ml/min)	134 ± 45	94 ± 23	42 ± 18
Ccr − GFR (ml/min)	21	34	20
Ccr/GFR (ml/min)	1.16	1.57	1.92

*Source: Shemesh et al., 1985.
GFR, glomerular filtration rate; Ccr, creatinine clearance.

creatinine clearance determinations may grossly overestimate GFR. These observations have implications for the correct dosing of drugs and in monitoring the effect of clinical interventions used to manage salt and water excess in these patients. Moreover, they suggest that the hepatorenal syndrome, frequently a cause of death in the setting of cirrhosis, may have an insidious onset that is difficult to recognize if the serum creatinine is the only test used to estimate GFR.

The serum creatinine also fails to reflect accurately changes in GFR of the renal allograft recipient over weeks or months. This is mainly due to a decrease in muscle mass and creatinine generation. Immunosuppressive regimes that include prolonged exposure to corticosteroids are likely responsible for muscle atrophy, but intercurrent illness due to opportunistic infection may play a role in some patients. Because the rate of creatinine generation tends to fall in parallel with the decrease in graft function, little change in the serum creatinine may be observed. The creatinine clearance, as in other settings with significant impairment of GFR, also overestimates graft function, and these observations should be considered when evaluating the effects of chronic rejection or cyclosporin toxicity in this population.

The timing of initiation of renal replacement therapy, either dialysis or transplantation, is usually based on an assessment of the GFR. Uremic symptoms tend to develop when the GFR falls below 10 ml/min, and this is generally considered to be the threshold for initiation of dialysis. Transplantation may be performed before dialysis is started in patients whose GFR is projected to fall to this level within six months. Nevertheless, in clinical practice the GFR is often very low before elective hemodialysis is initiated.

Assessment of the adequacy of dialysis

ASSESSMENT OF ADEQUACY IN HEMODIALYSIS

Adequate dialysis is defined as the amount of dialysis below which an increase in patient morbidity and mortality is seen. The criteria for defining adequate dialysis may be based solely on urea kinetic modeling (UKM), or it may include clinical parameters such as the response to erythropoietin, nutrition, and uremic symptoms. The uremic toxins that contribute to the increased morbidity of hemodialysis patients have not been identified, but the products of protein degradation are thought to play a role. Urea is easily measured and is thought to be a good substitute marker for the lower molecular weight uremic toxins. An increase in urea clearance is associated with an improvement in uremic symptoms, and blood urea levels correlate with dialysis outcome.

Urea kinetic modeling

UKM was developed to analyze the data from the National Co-operative Dialysis Study (NCDS) (Lowrie *et al.*, 1981). It attempts to describe the changes in urea concentration that occur during and between hemodialysis sessions. The mathematical model is then used to prescribe dialysis and to calculate the dose of dialysis delivered. UKM is limited by its design and assumptions. First, the variable volume single pool (VVSP) model reflects only small molecule transfer. Second, it assumes that the urea concentration in the blood is equal in all the various body compartments, that urea removal during dialysis is uniform, and that the interdialytic weight gains and urea generation are constant.

Pre- and postdialysis serum urea measurements are required for UKM. However, equilibrium of urea distribution between the extracellular and intracellular compartments after a hemodialysis session does not occur by the time the postdialysis blood sample is drawn. The postdialysis serum urea concentration is therefore lower than the urea concentration in total body water, and the amount of urea removed is overestimated by the mathematical model. This anomaly is most marked for high flux, high efficiency dialysis. In addition, inaccuracies in calculating the urea removal may occur if the postdialysis sample is taken while the blood pump is running. The blood should be drawn after dialysis is finished to avoid recirculation of dialyzed blood into the arterial side, which falsely lowers the postdialysis urea concentration.

Measurement of serum urea concentrations between dialysis sessions reflects urea generation (G). Single pool kinetics are appropriate here since urea accumulates slowly, thus allowing time for it to diffuse evenly across intra- and extracellular compartments.

Clinical situations where the transfer of urea is slow, such as in patients with poor skin perfusion or poor cardiac output, are not suited to single pool models. Two- and three-compartment models have been developed. However, the more complicated models require frequent blood sampling and sophisticated computer software to perform the analysis. Currently, it is impractical to use these models routinely, but centers that perform high efficiency dialysis should use a two-compartment model, since this more accurately predicts the changes in urea concentration during dialysis, in order to obtain a more accurate measure of urea removal.

The amount of dialysis delivered is reflected by the urea clearance during dialysis. This is calculated using the formula Kt/V which measures the intensity of dialysis (Kt) in relation to the patient's weight (V).

To write a dialysis prescription it is reasonable to target a Kt/V of 1.2 using the VVSP model.

t = time on dialysis in minutes
V = the volume of distribution of urea in ml, i.e. $0.6 \times$ body weight (in kg) $\times 1000$
K = clearance of the dialyzer and usually refers to the urea clearance

To select a dialyzer for Kt/V = 1.2, first calculate the required urea clearance, K:

$$K = \frac{1.2 \times V \ (\text{ml})}{t \ (\text{min})}$$

$$K = \frac{1.2 \times 0.6 \times \ \text{weight} \times 1000}{t \ (\text{min})}$$

For a given time of 240 minutes and a patient weighing 70 kg

$$K = \frac{1.2 \times 0.6 \times 70 \times 1000}{240}$$

$$= 210 \ \text{ml/min}$$

The clearance of the dialyzer depends on the surface area of the dialysis membrane and the blood flow through the dialyzer. The urea clearances specified by manufacturers are often generated using saline rather than blood and may overestimate urea clearance in the clinical setting. Calculations using a value of 80% of that stated by the manufacturer will generally correct for this. Alternatively, the dialyzer mass transfer coefficient (K_oA) can be calculated. Using the manufacturer's urea clearance at a given blood flow, the K_oA can be determined (Figure 10.1). The *in vivo* clearance is calculated by finding the urea clearance at the prescribed blood flow and the K_oA (Figure 10.2).

The initial dialysis prescription is used as a first approximation in the provision of adequate dialysis. The residual renal function is not usually included in the calculation of Kt/V since the renal function decreases after starting dialysis. The dose of dialysis actually delivered to the patient must be confirmed and reassessed periodically by UKM since the flow characteristics of the dialysis access or patient characteristics such as weight may change.

Numerous formulas for calculating the Kt/V have been developed, but these are often complicated and require the use of computers. Simpler formulas have been introduced that enable the physician to do a simple bedside calculation using the pre- and postdialysis urea concentration.

Fig. 10.1
To determine K_oA find the urea clearance on the x axis and then on the y axis find the K_oA at the chosen blood flow. This is based on the manufacturer's stated urea clearances using either water or saline solutions. The 200 ml/min blood flow should not be used at urea clearances > 170 ml/min (dotted line). (Source: Daugirdas and Depner, 1994.)

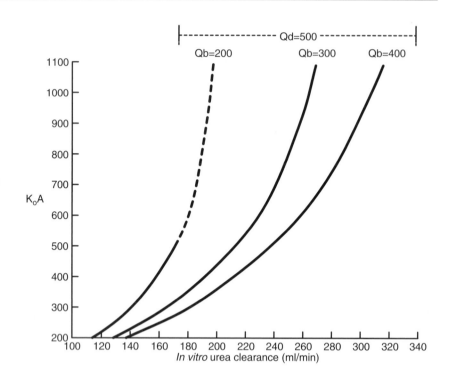

Fig. 10.2
Select the line corresponding to the K_oA value obtained in Figure 10.1. For a given blood flow rate listed on the x axis, the *in vivo* blood water urea clearance is found on the y axis. Corrections for blood water, blood pump calibration error and cardiopulmonary recirculation have been made. This gives approximately 20% reduction in the urea clearance when compared with the *in vitro* clearances. (Source: Daugirdas and Depner, 1994.)

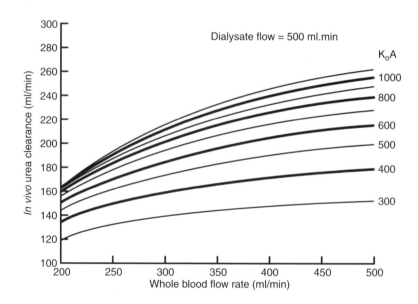

The urea reduction ratio (URR) or the percentage reduction in urea (PRU) is a simple calculation. It does not, however, take into account the values for urea clearance that are achieved with ultrafiltration and any residual renal function.

U_{post} = postdialysis urea concentration
U_{pre} = predialysis urea concentration

$$URR = \frac{U_{pre} - U_{post}}{U_{pre}}$$

$$PRU = 100 \times \left(1 - \frac{U_{post}}{U_{pre}} \right)$$

Figure 10.3 shows the relationship between the URR and Kt/V using the data from the NCDS.

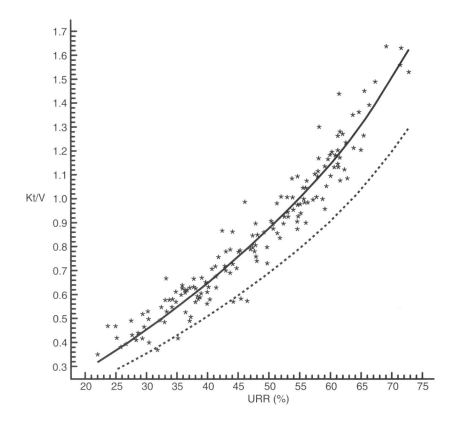

Fig. 10.3
Comparison of the NCDS data with the use of an equation to estimate the Kt/V from the URR. The solid line represents the line of best fit through the data from the NCDS; the dashed line represents the results of calculations using the equation Kt/V = $-\ln (1 - URR)/100$. (Source: Lowrie and Lew, 1991.)

Bedside calculations for Kt/V have been derived. If no ultrafiltration or urea generation occurs, then the concentration of urea (U) would fall during dialysis with a constant (K).

$$U_{post} = U_{pre} \, e^{(-Kt/V)}$$

and Kt/V can be calculated from the pre- and postdialysis urea:

$$\frac{Kt}{V} = \ln\left(\frac{U_{post}}{U_{pre}}\right)$$

$$= -\ln R$$

This formula does not, however, take into account the urea lost through ultrafiltration and the urea generated during dialysis. Garred, Canaud and McCready (1994) developed this formula to take these measures into account.

$$\frac{Kt}{V} = \frac{-\ln R + \dfrac{3\Delta BW}{BW}}{1 - 0.01786t}$$

t = duration of dialysis minutes; ΔBW is the weight loss due to ultrafiltration; BW is body weight;

$$R = \frac{U_{post}}{U_{pre}}$$

Daugirdas and Depner (1994) have a similar method:

$$Kt = -\ln\left(R - 0.008t - \frac{\Delta BW}{BW}\right)$$

Both of these formulas can be used to calculate the Kt/V at the bedside with a pocket calculator.

The gold standard for assessing urea clearance during dialysis measures the total amount of urea removed. This requires the collection of the total dialysate volume and the direct measurement of the dialysate urea concentration. This method is expensive and, because of the large volumes of dialysate, it is not practical for routine assessment of urea clearance. The recent introduction of a device to sample dialysate for urea determination at set intervals promises to be a more accurate method of measuring urea removal during dialysis than the conventional method.

Factors affecting the adequacy of hemodialysis

If the prescribed dose of dialysis is not delivered, several possible causes should be addressed before the dialysis prescription is changed. A review of the dialysis record from the day the blood samples were drawn will determine if the blood work represents a typical dialysis session. For example, specific questions would include the following.

- Did the patient dialyze for the full time prescribed?
- Were there any problems with the access, i.e. inability to increase pump speed, frequent blood pump alarms, or poor blood supply?
- Did the patient develop hypotension requiring a reduction in the ultrafiltration rate?

Dialyzer surface and volume affect the clearance. A reduction in the efficiency of the dialyzer may be seen if a high hematocrit causes clotting of the dialysis membrane, and hence a loss of surface area. This problem is seen commonly in patients treated with erythropoietin.

Another important variable for efficient urea removal is the blood flow through the dialyzer, hence good access performance is essential. Poor arterial supply or persistently elevated or increasing venous pressures may result in high blood recirculation and should be investigated further.

Recently it has been suggested that current recommendations for the dialysis prescription may still provide inadequate solute removal. A US collaborative study (Flanigan and Lim, 1996) compares the impact of long versus short dialysis sessions and high versus low flux dialysis modalities. The recommended dose of dialysis may change as a result of this study.

Recirculation

Dialysis access recirculation exists when dialyzed blood returns to the access by the venous limb then re-enters the arterial limb, returning to the dialyzer instead of the circulation. Dialysis access recirculation greater than 10% will impair urea clearance during a dialysis session. Several factors contribute to recirculation:

- venous stenosis or any outflow obstruction
- poor arterial supply
- high blood volume
- malposition of the needles
- increased length of dialysis lines.

To determine whether recirculation exists, arterial, venous and systemic blood samples are drawn. In the past the systemic sample was taken from a peripheral limb. However, this technique may not accurately reflect true blood recirculation in the dialysis access. Recently the concepts of cardio-pulmonary recirculation and venovenous dysequilibrium have been introduced to challenge the conventional method of assessing dialysis access clearance. To reduce the impact of these problems, a second sample is drawn instead from the afferent limb, when the risk of blood from the venous side contaminating the afferent sample is minimal. This can be done by either a low-flow or stop-flow technique. Access recirculation may also increase as dialysis progresses due to volume depletion and subsequent changes in cardiac output. Blood should be drawn soon after dialysis has begun for an accurate measurement of recirculation (Table 10.4).

Hemodialysis access recirculation can also be measured by an online monitor. This electronic device measures changes in conductivity. A bolus of hypertonic saline is injected into the venous limb altering the conductivity when compared with the arterial blood. In the presence of recirculation, part of the bolus will recirculate through the arterial line and can be detected by the change in conductivity at the arterial line sensor.

An angiogram of the access should be performed if significant dialysis access recirculation at the prescribed blood flow is found. Stenosis of the venous anastomosis may be corrected by angioplasty. Repeated problems such as clotting or poor supply are indications for surgical revision.

ASSESSMENT OF THE ADEQUACY OF PERITONEAL DIALYSIS

A peritoneal dialysis prescription of four 2 l exchanges per day is no longer standard for every patient. The dialysis prescription should be individualized to the patient and calculations of adequacy of dialysis should be performed.

Table 10.4

Technique for estimating hemodialysis access recirculation

- Perform the test after approximately 30 min of treatment and after reducing the ultrafiltration rate
- Draw dialyzer afferent and efferent samples
- Immediately reduce blood flow to 50 ml/min
- Draw systemic sample from arterial line after sufficient time has passed to clear 150% of the volume between the arterial needle and the sampling point, but no later than 30 s after the blood flow was reduced*

*At a blood flow of 50 ml/min, 12.5 ml will be cleared from the arterial line in 15 s.

Measurements of adequacy include the Kt/V or weekly creatinine clearances. Peritoneal dialysis is best suited to the patient with residual renal function, and renal urea clearance may contribute significantly to the total urea clearance.

The major difference between peritoneal dialysis and hemodialysis is that the former provides continuous and the latter intermittent solute clearance. In continuous ambulatory peritoneal dialysis (CAPD) the serum urea and creatinine concentrations are steady, whereas in hemodialysis there are high peaks before and troughs immediately after each dialysis session. If uremic toxicity is related to the high peak of urea, a lower Kt/V may be required for peritoneal dialysis to achieve the same outcome (Figure 10.4). Figure 10.4 shows the relationship between the amount of dialysis for CAPD and hemodialysis, and the onset of uremic symptoms.

Weekly clearances of larger molecules such as vitamin B_{12}, inulin, and β_2-microglobulin are greater for CAPD than for standard hemodialysis. Inadequacies of CAPD therefore relate to poor small molecule clearance. Creatinine was initially proposed as the solute marker for CAPD, and a clearance of 50 l/week for peritoneal dialysis was felt to be adequate. Others have used urea as the solute marker for adequacy. Gotch (1990) calculated the range of adequate dialysis for CAPD to be a Kt/V of 1.75–2.1 based on a daily nPCR (normalized catabolic rate, see p. 196) of 0.8–1.2 g/kg and a blood urea nitrogen (BUN) of 60–80 mg/dl (21–28.6 mmol/l). The authors of the recent CANUSA study (Churchill, Taylor and Keshaviah, 1995) have recommended a target creatinine clearance of 60–70 l/week, and a minimum Kt/V of 2.

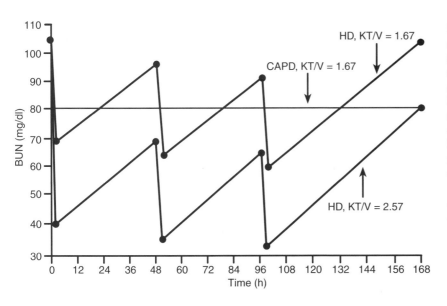

Fig. 10.4
A Kt/V of 1.67 in CAPD gives a maximum urea concentration of 80 mg/dl. Although a similar Kt/V in hemodialysis gives the same time-averaged concentration for urea, the high peaks > 80 mg/dl mean that adequate dialysis is not provided. A Kt/V of 2.57 is required to avoid a maximum urea of 80 mg/dl in hemodialysis.

To calculate the adequacy of peritoneal dialysis, dialysis and renal urea clearance are measured. Urine and dialysate are collected for 24 hours and urea concentrations are measured. A blood sample to determine serum urea concentration is also required during this period. From these data the Kt/V can be calculated.

In CAPD, V is assumed to be synonymous with total body water and is estimated from a suitable nomogram like the Watson nomogram or by using the formula $0.58 \times$ actual body weight (aBW) for men and $0.55 \times aBW$ for women.

Dialysis urea clearance, Kt, is calculated from the urea concentration in plasma (P) and a 24-hour collection of dialysate (D).

$$Kt = \frac{\text{volume dialysate} \times \text{dialysate urea}}{\text{Plasma urea}}$$

$$Kt/V \text{ (daily)} = \frac{(V \text{ dialysate} \times D/P)}{V \text{ body water}} \times 7 = \text{weekly } Kt/V$$

For example, consider a 66.5 kg patient on CAPD exchanging four times a day, V is the urea distribution space in the body or ideal body weight (IBW) $\times 0.58$.

$$
\begin{aligned}
\text{Drain volume} &= 10\,l \\
\text{Dialysate to plasma urea} \quad D/P &= 1 \\
Kt/V &= \frac{(10 \times 1)}{40} \\
&= 0.25 \text{ (daily) or } 0.25 \times 7 \text{ (weekly)} \\
&= 1.75 \text{ (weekly)}.
\end{aligned}
$$

The residual renal urea clearance is calculated from the 24-hour urine specimen. In this example, if the renal urea clearance is 1 ml/min or 14 l/week, then:

$$
\begin{aligned}
\text{total urea clearance} &= \text{dialysis} + \text{renal clearance} \\
&= 70 + 14 = 84 \text{ l/week} \\
Kt/V \text{ (weekly)} &= 84/40 = 2.1
\end{aligned}
$$

An alternative measure of the adequacy of peritoneal dialysis is the weekly creatinine clearance:

Weekly creatinine clearance
= daily clearance × 7
= daily drain volume (l) × D/P (creatinine) + urine creatinine clearance × 7 (normalized to $1.73m^2$ body surface area)

Estimates of the residual renal function may be more accurate if an average of the urea and creatinine clearances is used, since the creatinine clearance will overestimate the residual renal function. Others advocate direct measurements of GFR using exogenous filtration markers.

If dialysis is not adequate, a peritoneal equilibration test (PET) can be done to assess the peritoneal membrane characteristics and adjust the prescription (Table 10.5; Figure 10.5). The results are plotted into the graphs as shown in Figure 10.5. From these graphs the patient is classified according to the glucose transport characteristics of the peritoneal membrane. The patient with high transperitoneal glucose transport will tend to have poor ultrafiltration but adequate dialysis, whereas those in the low glucose transport group are at risk of underdialysis and may benefit from high dose peritoneal dialysis or a change to hemodialysis.

CLINICAL PARAMETERS FOR ASSESSING ADEQUACY

Neurological symptoms such as fatigue, agitation, cramps, insomnia and headache should alert the nephrologist to the possibility that the patient may not be receiving adequate dialysis. There may be associated electroencephalogram (EEG) or electromyogram (EMG) changes, but unfortunately these tests do not correlate well with either symptoms or biochemical parameters and contribute little to the assessment of adequacy.

- Drain the overnight bag
- Infuse 2 l of 2.5% solution over 10 min and have the patient move around every 500 ml to ensure mixing with residual dialysate remaining in the peritoneal cavity. Take a sample of dialysate (T = 0)
- Draw a blood sample and a dialysate sample for creatinine and glucose concentration at 2 h
- At 4 h drain the fluid. Weigh the bag to calculate the ultrafiltration volume. A sample of dialysate is taken for creatinine and glucose concentration

Table 10.5
Peritoneal equilibration test (PET)

Fig. 10.5

This figure summarizes the PET test. First collect sample of either peritoneal fluid (PET) or serum at the specified times. Use the results obtained to calculate the D/P ratios for creatinine and glucose at the time points. Plot the results on the graph (3). Use the table (4) to determine the patient's membrane transport characteristics. (Source: Twardowski, 1989; Keshaviah, 1993.)

Peritoneal equilibration test (PET)

1. Collect patient samples

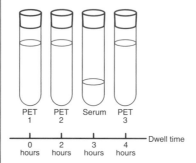

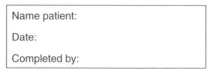

Name patient:

Date:

Completed by:

3. Plot to graph

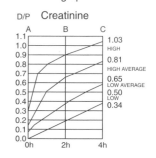

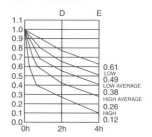

2. Calculations

a. Creatinine (D/P)

$$D/P = \frac{\text{dialysate concentration of corrected creatinine}}{\text{serum concentration of corrected creatinine}}$$

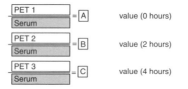

b. Glucose (D/DO)

$$D/PO = \frac{\text{dialysate concentration of glucose at 2/4 hours}}{\text{dialysate concentration of glucose at 0 hours}}$$

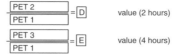

4. Diagnosis

Baseline PET prognostic value			
Solute transport	Predicted response to CAPD		Preferred dialysis
	UF	Dialysis	
High	Poor	Adequate	CCPD dry day CAPD dry night
High average	Poor–medium	Adequate	Standard CAPD or APD
Low average	Good	Adequate Inadequate	Standard CAPD High dose PD APD
Low	Very good	Inadequate	High dose PD Hemodialysis

Reference: Zbylut J.TWARDOWSKI. Clinical value of Standardized Equilibration Tests in CAPD Patients. *Current Concepts of CAPD Blood Purif.* 1989; 7:97–108.

Anorexia, nausea and vomiting are common gastrointestinal symptoms in the dialysis population. Endoscopy findings of gastritis and colitis may reflect underdialysis. Poor nutrition may also result from inadequate dialysis and this may be reflected in the monthly blood work as a low predialysis urea, hypoalbuminemia, and anemia that is refractory to erythropoietin. Inadequate dialysis leads to an increase in the morbidity and mortality of the dialysis population. The effects of inadequate dialysis may persist even after returning to improved dialysis.

Nutritional assessment of patients with chronic renal failure

Inadequate nutrition is a frequent problem in those with end-stage renal disease and has a strong association with patient morbidity and mortality. Poor nutritional status may reflect inadequate dialysis. Alternatively, patients may have co-morbid conditions that may adversely affect their nutrition despite good dialysis. Experimental evidence from rodent models of renal failure, and analysis of human patients with moderately advanced renal failure, indicate that protein metabolism is abnormal even when the GFR is > 25 ml/min. Systemic acidosis may account in part for some of the recognized abnormalities.

Various methods have been employed for assessing nutritional adequacy (Table 10.6). The dietary history and diaries are notoriously inaccurate, but they are relatively easy to do and provide an indication of the patient's intake. Anthropometric measurements are also easily applied and relatively inexpensive, but like the biochemical parameters are not sensitive enough to detect the early stages of malnutrition.

Efforts have been made to assess the nutritional status more comprehensively. The subjective global assessment grades nutritional status based on elements of the history and physical examination. A history of weight loss, poor dietary intake, gastrointestinal symptoms, and subjective energy level are assessed. The physical examination grades the loss of subcutaneous tissue or muscle mass, and extravascular fluid gain. A composite score is then generated. In general these clinical parameters are late manifestations of protein malnutrition. More sensitive methods include bioelectrical impedance and dual-energy X-ray absorptiometry.

The bioelectrical impedance assay (BIA) uses the principle of impedance to predict total body cell mass. Changes in impedance are seen with poor nutrition. Improved sensitivity may be achieved using multifrequency BIA techniques. Other techniques such as dual-energy X-ray absorptiometry have been used primarily in the research setting.

Table 10.6

Means of assessing the nutritional status of patients with chronic renal failure

Type of investigation	Testing for/method
● Dietary history	Interview, diary and three-day diet recall
● Anthropometric measurements	Mid-arm circumference, scapular skinfold thickness
● Subjective global assessment	
● Biochemical markers:	
long-term	Albumin, transferrin, creatinine
short-term	Prealbumin, urea, phosphorus, potassium
others	Ferritin, fibronectin, somatomedin and amino acids
● Bioelectrical impedance (BIA)	
● Percentage lean body mass	Creatine kinetics, BIA
● Dual-energy X-ray absorptiometry (DEXA)	
● Urea kinetic modeling	Protein catabolic rate (PCR) or the protein equivalent of nitrogen appearance (PNA)

ASSESSMENT OF NUTRITION IN PATIENTS WITH END-STAGE RENAL FAILURE

UKM indirectly measures daily protein consumption in the dialysis patient who is neither catabolic nor anabolic by calculation of the protein catabolic rate (PCR). The relationship between the Kt/V, the PCR, and the blood urea nitrogen is shown in Figure 10.6. Urea alone gives no indication about the patients well-being, whereas viewed together with Kt/V and the PCR, the patient's nutritional status and adequacy can be determined.

The PCR is derived from urea generation assuming 6.49 g protein is catabolized to produce 1 g of urea. The interdialytic generation of urea (G) can be calculated by measuring the postdialysis urea of one session and the predialysis urea of the next session. Not all protein is converted to urea; some is lost in feces and sloughed from the skin. This loss is estimated to be 0.17 g/kg/day.

$$PCR = 9.35 \frac{G}{BW} + 0.17 \quad \text{(Garred, Canaud and McCready, 1994)}.$$

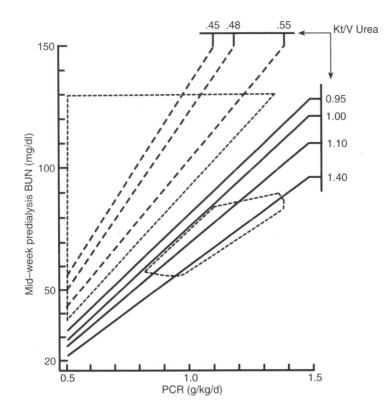

Fig. 10.6
PCR, mid-week dialysis BUN and Kt/V form a tight relationship. Values that fall within the dotted triangle are likely to represent patients who are inadequately dialyzed. Adequate dialysis is represented in the rhomboidal area. (Source: Lindsay and Spanner, 1989.)

A problem with the use of UKM to estimate the PCR is that inaccuracies in the calculation of Kt/V can overestimate G. To get around this, the normalized PCR (nPCR), i.e. the PCR normalized to urea body space (IBW × 0.58) rather than total weight, is used.

The term urea nitrogen appearance (UNA) has been suggested as a better term than urea generation as it reflects the net production or appearance of urea nitrogen in body fluids and all measurable outputs, e.g. urine, dialysate, fistula drainage.

$$UNA \ (g/d) = \text{urinary urea N} + \text{dialysate urea N} + \Delta \ \text{body urea N}$$
$$\Delta \text{Body urea N} = (U_{post} - U_{pre}) \times aBW_{pre} \times 0.58 + (aBW_{post} - aBW_{pre}) \times U_{post}.$$

If serum urea is expressed in mmol/l:

$$\Delta \text{Body urea N} = 0.028 \ [(U_{post} - U_{pre}) \times aBW \times 0.58 + (aBW_{post} - aBW_{pre}) \times U_{post}]$$

aBW is the actual body weight (kg).

0.58 is the fraction of body weight that is water.

In maintenance hemodialysis, UNA can be calculated using single pool kinetic models. Three blood samples are required: a pre- (U_1) and posturea (U_2), and a urea prior to the next dialysis session (U_3). The dialyzer clearance Kd is known. To calculate the V and UNA:

$$U_2 = U_1 \times e^{-(Kdtd/V)}$$

$$U_3 = U_2 + \frac{UNA \times t_{od}}{V}$$

td = time of dialysis

t_{od} = time between dialysis

Kd = dialyzer clearance either *in vivo* or calculated from K_oA; if unknown the equation can be solved for Kd/V or UNA/V.

These formulas are not suitable for patients with large volume changes during dialysis or residual renal function.

Estimation of protein intake from the UNA has been referred to as the PCR. This term is somewhat misleading, and protein equivalent of total nitrogen appearance (PNA) has been proposed as a term to replace PCR. PNA is calculated in the same way as the PCR.

$$PNA \ (g/d) = 6.49 \times UNA + 0.294V$$

The term 0.294V accounts for the average non-urea nitrogen losses. The regression equations relating UNA to PNA differ slightly between hemodialysis and peritoneal dialysis as described below.

Two point serum urea methods have also been developed to estimate PNA. These methods assume that the patient is in a steady state and calculate the average UNA over the duration of the weekly cycle that achieves the measured steady state predialysis and postdialysis urea (Kopple *et al.*, 1995). Garred, Canaud and McCready, 1994) developed the following formula to enable physicians to calculate the PNA using a pre- and posturea sample and the body weight:

$$PCR_n = \frac{0.018 \ (1 - 0.162R) \ (1 - R + \Delta BW/V)U_{pre}}{1 - 0.0003t}$$

t = treatment time

R = U_{post}/U_{pre}

V = Body weight × 0.58

In the chronic CAPD patient, the UNA can be calculated by:

$$UNA = (V_d \times DUN + V_u \ \Delta UUN)t + \Delta \ body \ urea \ N$$

V_d = dialysate volume
V_u = urine volume
DUN = dialysate urea nitrogen
UUN = urine urea nitrogen (g/l)
t = time of collection, usually 1 day.

Assuming the changes in body urea nitrogen are negligible, UNA can be estimated from:

UNA (g/d) = $(V_d \times DUN + V_u \times UUN)/t$
PNA (g/d) = $6.49 \times UNA + 0.294 \times V$ + peritoneal protein losses.

This formula has been simplified by Teehan, Schleifer and Brown (1994).

PNA (g/d) = 6.25 (UNA + 1.81) + 0.031 × aBW

1.81 g nitrogen/day = the average value from the literature for protein and amino acid nitrogen losses in CAPD patients.
0.031 g/kg/day = average value for non-urea losses.

A number of similar formulas exist. Generally the results are similar, but if the patient has severe protein loss from the peritoneum this may be underestimated in the latter formula.

Complications of renal disease

METABOLIC ACIDOSIS

Metabolic acidosis is a common complication of chronic renal disease. Daily hydrogen ion production is largely the result of the metabolism of protein. The underlying defect that accounts for the limited ability of the kidney to handle hydrogen ion production is thought to be related to a combination of both decreased excretion of ammonium ion in the urine and reduced ability to generate bicarbonate from organic anion metabolism.

Typically the degree of hypobicarbonatemia is mild to moderate (12–20 mmol/l) in the patient before dialysis is initiated. The serum anion gap, calculated as $((Na + K) - (Cl + HCO_3))$, is elevated > 16, and pH is maintained by hyperventilation in patients approaching end-stage renal disease. Nevertheless, acidosis in chronic renal failure has been implicated in the promotion of calcium loss from bone, worsening underlying renal osteodystrophy, and the development of a hypercatabolic state, exacerbating protein malnutrition. Correction of hypobicarbonatemia using $NaHCO_3$

has been advocated, although in the hemodialysis population no clear benefit of oral bicarbonate supplementation has been demonstrated.

Some causes of chronic renal dysfunction may be associated with disproportionately impaired acid excretion early in the disease process. These forms of metabolic acidosis, usually due to tubular injury, typically show hypobicarbonatemia and a normal serum anion gap. If the kidney responds appropriately to acidosis, the urine anion gap – a reflection of renal NH_4^+ production (calculated as urine $(Na + K) - Cl$) – should be more negative than -30, reflecting increased NH_4^+ excretion. In renal tubular acidosis type 1 and type 4 (pp. 16–18), the urine anion gap is neutral or even positive, reflecting inappropriately low NH_4^+ production. Note that as renal failure advances, total NH_4^+ production falls, but is thought to be maximal when considered at the single nephron level. In this case the lack of NH_4^+ production reflects an inadequate number of functioning nephrons.

HYPERKALEMIA

Hyperkalemia may develop in patients with chronic renal failure as the kidney function deteriorates, and reflects the inability of the kidneys to excrete the daily load of potassium. Hyperkalemia is exacerbated by a shift of potassium from the intracellular to the extracellular compartment as acidemia develops with decreasing GFR. In some cases, non-steroidal anti-inflammatory drugs or angiotensin-converting enzyme (ACE) inhibitors further impair the ability to promote potassium excretion in the urine by blocking the compensatory mechanisms recruited to handle potassium homeostasis as the GFR decreases.

ANEMIA

A normochromic normocytic anemia develops in most patients with chronic renal failure and is usually seen in proportion to the degree of decreased GFR. The anemia of renal failure is discussed in Chapter 5.

HYPERPHOSPHATEMIA, HYPERPARATHYROIDISM AND BONE DISEASE

Retention of phosphorus is an early feature of renal failure, and is thought to be a critical factor in the development of hyperparathyroidism as renal failure progresses. Hyperparathyroidism, in turn, accounts for significant morbidity through the development of osteitis fibrosa cystica, tendon rupture, and the deposition of hydroxyapatite in joints and blood vessels. Control of parathyroid hormone (PTH) secretion is complex; major

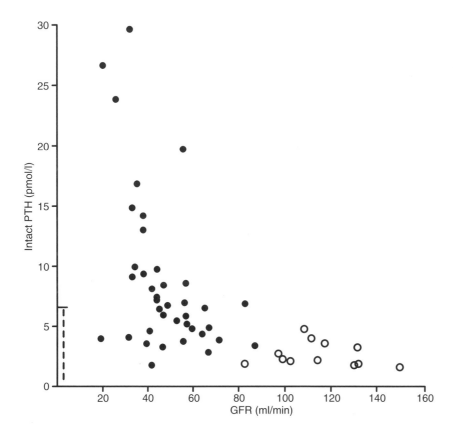

Fig. 10.7
Serum intact PTH levels are plotted against GFR. The open symbols represent values of normal individuals. The closed symbols are from patients with varying degrees of renal insufficiency. (Source: St John *et al.*, 1992.)

regulators of PTH synthesis have been identified as 1,25 hydroxy vitamin D_3 (1,25 $(OH)_2D_3$), serum ionized calcium, and phosphate concentrations acting either directly on the parathyroid glands or indirectly on 25 hydroxy vitamin D_3 hydroxylation. In early renal dysfunction levels of 1,25 $(OH)_2D_3$ have been found to be either normal or depressed by different groups. 1,25 $(OH)_2D_3$ plays an important role in the differentiation in the skeleton for osteoblasts and osteoclasts and it regulates the genes for osteocalcin and osteopontin. A decreased level of 1,25 $(OH)_2D_3$ reduces the absorption of calcium and phosphate from the gut.

Although PTH concentrations are found in the normal range in mild renal failure, investigators have found evidence for increased bone turnover, suggestive of relative hyperparathyroidism even at modest renal impairment. As shown in Figure 10.7, PTH has been found to be progressively elevated as the GFR decreases below normal.

While a consensus has developed that dietary phosphate should be restricted in early chronic renal failure, and that hyperphosphatemia requires treatment with phosphate binders, treatment with calcitriol in this

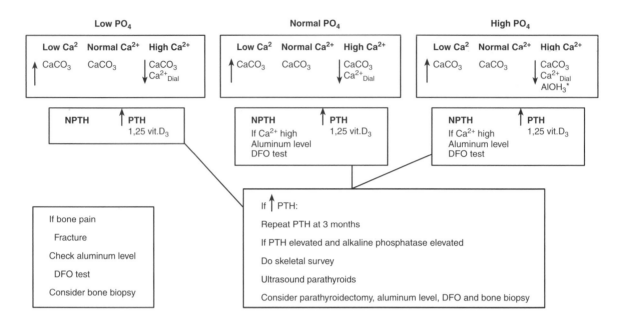

Fig. 10.8
A suggested algorithm for the management of renal osteodystrophy in the dialysis patient.
NPTH = < 4 times the upper limit of normal for the PTH; ↑ PTH = PTH level > 4 times upper limit of normal.
DFO = desferrioxamine.

setting may be the most effective measure to prevent the development of hyperparathyroid bone disease. Nevertheless, in uremic patients the effects of parathyroid hormone on bone turnover appear to be somewhat blunted. It has been suggested that the calcitriol dose should be titrated to maintain the PTH concentration at three to four times the normal range, since oversuppression of PTH may contribute to adynamic bone disease.

Several laboratory tests are available to assess the degree of hyperparathyroidism and high turnover bone disease. The initial assessment of metabolic bone disease involves measurement of the levels of:

- calcium
- phosphate
- alkaline phosphatase
- aluminum
- PTH
- $1,25 \ (OH)_2D_3$.

An algorithm for the evaluation of renal osteodystrophy is shown in Figure 10.8.

PTH

Previous methods of measuring PTH used antibodies directed against either the N- or C-terminal and did not distinguish between the inactive metabolites and the fully active hormone. As the metabolites accumulate in renal disease, this led to difficulty in interpreting results. Most centers now use an intact PTH (iPTH) assay such as the intact two-site immunometric assay (IRMA) or two-site immunochemiluminescence (ICMA). These methods are highly specific for iPTH and do not cross-react with C-terminal fragments; they therefore provide a more accurate reflection of bone turnover.

Alkaline phosphatase

Alkaline phosphatase is produced by the osteoblasts and thus the serum level has been used to reflect bone metabolism and to assess the extent of bony involvement. It is not specific and may be released from other sites such as the intestine or liver. Isoenzymes have been used to try to differentiate bone from liver alkaline phosphatase, but as the bone-specific alkaline phosphatase differs by post-translational modification that occurs in bone cells, the isoenzyme assays are unreliable and are therefore not routinely available.

Although the serum alkaline phosphatase correlates well with raised PTH levels and is indicative of high turnover disease, it is not specific. There is considerable overlap with other disease processes and it may not reflect the severity of disease as seen by X-ray or bone biopsy.

A number of other tests can be used to assess bone formation rates. These include measurement of the levels of osteocalcin, procollagen type, carboxy-terminal propeptide, somatomedin C, and tartrate-resistant acid phosphatase. These tests are not widely available and, although used by a few specialized centers, they are not generally used in the evaluation of metabolic bone disease.

Aluminum level

It is essential to measure the aluminum level in patients with end-stage renal function who have evidence of bone disease, since aluminum is a cause of low turnover osteodystrophy. In particular, if parathyroidectomy is planned to manage hyperparathyroidism, the aluminum load should be examined since aluminum osteodystrophy may be precipitated by the reduction in circulating PTH.

Skeletal fractures, especially of the rib, are common in patients with aluminum toxicity. Aluminum osteodystrophy may coexist with hyperparathyroidism and the X-rays may therefore be misleading. An aluminum level at the upper limit of normal ($> 60 \ \mu g/l$ or $188 \ nmol/l$) or a strong clinical suspicion of aluminum toxicity are indications for a desferrioxamine stimulation test (Table 10.7).

Patients should be closely monitored during administration of desferrioxamine as hypotension can develop. If hypotension does occur, stop or slow the infusion and resume it once the patient has stabilized again.

Hemodialysis	**Peritoneal dialysis**
• Draw baseline aluminum level	• Baseline aluminum level may be drawn at any time
• Give desferrioxamine at a dose of 5 mg/kg diluted in either normal saline or 5% dextrose over the last hour of dialysis	• The same dose of desferrioxamine is given either during the last hour of the dwell time or in the long day-time dwell for patients on a cycler
• Draw a second aluminum level at the start of the next dialysis session	• A second level is drawn 2 h after the infusion of desferrioxamine is completed

A rise in the serum aluminum concentration of > 50 μg/l or 1800 nmol/l following the desferrioxamine challenge suggests a heavy aluminum burden. Some centers use higher doses of desferrioxamine, and regimes of 15–40 mg/kg have been described. A bone biopsy should be done in situations where the results are equivocal.

In summary, blood tests are not sensitive or specific enough to determine the severity of metabolic bone disease, but do indicate which disease process is likely to be present. High phosphate, high alkaline phosphatase and elevated PTH levels are highly suggestive of secondary hyperparathyroidism, whereas a low normal PTH and low alkaline phosphatase would be more likely to indicate one of the low turnover states. Thus the blood tests are an important part of the evaluation of renal osteodystrophy and, together with further information obtained by radiography, can allow many diagnoses to be made and treatments initiated.

Radiographic investigations of renal osteodystrophy

A skeletal survey usually includes plain X-rays of the hands, chest (clavicles), the thoracic and lumbar spine and the skull. The classic findings in secondary hyperparathyroidism of bony erosions on the subperiosteal, intracortical or endosteal surfaces are usually not seen on X-ray until late in the proces. Plain X-rays are therefore not helpful in identifying patients with early hyperparathyroidism. Similarly, scintigraphy lacks both sensitivity and specificity and is not recommended in the investigation of renal osteodystrophy.

Subperiosteal resorption of the metaphysis of the radial side of the phalanx of the second or third digit are among the earliest findings. Tuft erosions of the distal phalanx are typical of uremic hyperparathyroidism and rare in primary hyperparathyroidism. Erosion is also seen at the medial ends of the clavicles and the lower end of the radius and ulna. Subchondral and periarticular erosions involving the hands, hips, patellofemoral joint or shoulder closely resemble changes seen in rheumatoid arthritis. Periosteal neostosis (new bone formation at the periosteal surface) is also seen in hyperparathyroidism. Osteosclerosis reflects the increase in the thickness and number of trabeculae in bone. The term 'rugger jersey spine' is used to describe the appearance of osteosclerosis in the vertebral bodies.

Brown tumors are more commonly seen in primary hyperparathyroidism and should not be confused with the cysts seen in dialysis-related amyloidosis. β_2-microglobulin cysts tend to be subchondral, and are also found in the phalanges, long bones, clavicles, and carpal and tarsal bones. They also tend to be larger, whereas brown tumors are smaller and are found in the skull or mandible.

Ultrasound examination of the parathyroid glands

Various methods of imaging the parathyroid glands have been used including ultrasonography, MRI, CT and Tl – Tc subtraction scintigraphy. Imaging may be helpful in assessing the number and size of the parathyroid glands in a patient who is being considered for surgery.

Bone density measurement

Examination of the bone density can be done by several methods such as photon absorptiometry and neutron activation. Photon absorptiometry, a non-invasive method for assessing bone mass, is a useful test to monitor the effect of therapy in patients with chronic renal failure. The measurements are usually made over the radius and ulna with a single beam, and the femur and vertebral bodies with a dual beam. These measurements provide information about the bone mass and risk of fracture, but do not identify the cause nor do the results correlate with the histological diagnosis. Bone loss in patients on chronic hemodialysis is largely related to the regions affected by renal osteodystrophy, and the bone density may be a useful tool for assessing these changes.

Bone biopsy

Bone biopsy is the gold standard in the diagnosis of metabolic bone disease. The indications for a bone biopsy are shown in Table 10.8. Bone samples are taken from the anterior iliac crest. Full histomorphometric and histodynamic studies with tetracycline labeling should always be done to ensure that as much information as possible can be obtained from the biopsy. Bone histomorphometry gives details about the percentage of bone that is calcified and uncalcified (the trabecular bone volume), the percentage of the trabeculae that are lined by osteoid, osteoblasts and osteoclasts.

Table 10.8

Indications for a bone biopsy in patients with chronic renal failure

- Severe bone disease
- Hypercalcemia with no obvious cause
- To assess aluminum content
- Prior to parathyroidectomy if there is a possibility of aluminum toxicity

Tetracycline localizes at the mineralization surface and its fluorescence can be detected by ultraviolet lights. Labeling with oral tetracycline at two time periods (double labeling) produces two separate stains on biopsy. From this the mineralization rate, bone formation rate, mineral apposition rate and the mineralization lag rate can be calculated. Suggested dosages are tetracycline 500 mg for two days, followed by an interval of 8–15 days. The second label is given for four days and a bone biopsy performed three to four days later. An alternative protocol starts with demeclocycline hydrochloride 150 mg twice a day for three days and then label 12 days later with tetracycline 250 mg twice a day for four days. The advantage of using two antibiotics is that each gives a different color on fluorescence and in patients with low bone formation rates the two stains can thus easily be distinguished.

Centers that routinely perform biopsies suggest that they should be performed more frequently as the various biochemical parameters do not distinguish well between the various types of renal osteodystrophy. Unfortunately, many centers do not have ready access to pathologists skilled in processing and interpreting the slides.

ASSESSMENT OF SEXUAL FUNCTION

Decreased libido, impotence and infertility are common problems among dialysis patients. Common causes of sexual dysfunction are shown in Table 10.9.

The initial assessment of a patient should include a review of the current medications. The sexual history prior to and after developing renal failure should be obtained. Men should be asked whether erection is achieved and maintained and whether they are able to ejaculate. Women should record a menstrual history.

Male impotence

In many patients, libido is unaffected but the ability to perform is compromised. Testosterone is mainly responsible for sexual desire rather than the ability to achieve and maintain an erection, which requires sympathetic and parasympathetic stimulation and involvement of the

Table 10.9
Some factors contributing to sexual dysfunction in patients with chronic renal failure and suggested methods of investigation

Factors	Action
Anemia	Measure the hemoglobin and hematocrit
Low estrogen or testosterone levels	Measure plasma estradiol or testosterone levels
High prolactin levels	Measure prolactin levels
Inadequacy of dialysis	Kt/V or URR
Medication	Review medication with patient
Vascular insufficiencies	Check peripheral pulses, listen for bruits
Co-morbid conditions, e.g. diabetes	Take a medical history
Neuropathies	Examine for evidence of neurological disease

Kt/V, intensity of dialysis/patient's weight; URR, urea reduction ratio.

peripheral nerves S2–4. A good arterial supply and an ability to restrict venous outflow are also essential.

Acute onset of impotence suggests either a recent change in medication or a psychological problem, especially if the patient describes normal morning erections. Organic impotence is usually gradual in onset. The patient may initially describe difficulty in maintaining erection and later an inability to achieve erection and a lack of nocturnal erections.

The examination is focused on the neurological system and the vasculature. The presence of femoral bruits or absent peripheral pulses indicates underlying vascular insufficiency. Peripheral neuropathy suggests neurological disease.

The nocturnal penile tumescence test (NPT) is often one of the first investigations of impotence. If this is normal, psychosocial factors should be considered.

Vascular disease is a major problem in the dialysis patient and this can contribute to impotence. The penile blood supply can be assessed by measuring the penile systolic pressure with a Doppler probe and comparing this with the brachial systolic pressure. This is known as the penile brachial index (PBI). Pharmacocavernosometry and pharmacocavernosography can determine the presence of vascular disease and whether angiography is indicated by measuring various parameters before and after intracavernous injections of papaverine and phentolamine. Arterial inflow and venous outflow restriction are probably adequate if rigid erection is achieved.

Assessment of neurological disease includes nerve conduction velocities along the pudendal nerve. These are impaired in patients with neuropathy, i.e. diabetics and others with peripheral neuropathies.

A low sperm count and motility is seen in semen analysis, and abnormal spermatogenesis occurs in patients with end-stage renal failure. Testosterone levels are often low, with high luteinizing hormone (LH) levels. Hyper-prolactinemia can be present in as many as 50% of males in chronic renal failure. Males with low levels of testosterone may benefit from taking testosterone replacement.

Ovarian dysfunction

Menstrual abnormalities are common in uremic women. Most patients are oligo- or amenorrheic. The precise cause is unknown, but is thought to be multifactorial. Hyperprolactinemia has been reported in up to 80% of women on dialysis, and this may be a factor in many cases, but some patients with amenorrhea have normal prolactin levels.

Postmenopausal women on dialysis have elevated LH and follicle-stimulating hormone (FSH) levels, indicating that the feedback loop between the ovaries and the hypothalamopituitary axis is intact. LH and FSH levels are often normal in the follicular phase but the mid-cycle surge in LH secretion is not seen. This may be partly due to the reduction in endogenous estrogen secretion, which fails to stimulate secretion of gonadotropin-releasing hormone (GNRH).

In summary, the LH, FSH, prolactin, estradiol and testosterone levels should be measured in patients who describe sexual dysfunction and/or menstrual abnormalities. Most of these hormonal changes will revert to normal after transplantation. An improvement in sexual function may occur after correction of anemia with erythropoietin therapy.

CARBOHYDRATE AND INSULIN METABOLISM

The kidney plays an important role in the regulation of insulin metabolism. Approximately a quarter of the insulin secreted by the pancreas is degraded by the kidney. A significant increase in the half-life of insulin is seen when the GFR is < 20 ml/min. The influence of renal failure on glucose metabolism is summarized in Table 10.10.

Chronic renal failure is associated with glucose intolerance secondary to insulin resistance and inappropriate release of insulin. A variety of toxins have been proposed as the mediators of impaired carbohydrate metabolism, but only a role for PTH is supported by experimental data. Secondary hyperparathyroidism decreases the secretion of insulin and thus contributes

- Mildly elevated fasting glucose
- Spontaneous hypoglycemia
- Fasting hyperinsulinemia
- Blunted response to intravenous insulin
- Reduced insulin requirements in diabetic patients
- Decreased peripheral sensitivity to insulin

Table 10.10
Abnormalities in glucose metabolism seen in patients with chronic renal failure

to impaired glucose tolerance. Insulin resistance is almost always present in uremic patients and appears to be at the level of skeletal muscle.

ABNORMALITIES IN THYROID FUNCTION

Abnormalities in thyroid function tests are common in patients with chronic renal disease. Low levels of T3 have been reported in 43% of euthyroid patients and may reflect decreased peripheral conversion of T4 to T3. Total and free T4 levels are reduced in 41% and 21%, respectively, of euthyroid patients with end-stage renal failure. Normal levels of free T4 are found in 88–97% of these patients if free T4 is measured by tracer equilibrium dialysis. Uremic patients rarely have elevated free T4 levels in the absence of hyperthyroidism.

The thyroid-stimulating hormone (TSH) level is the best means of differentiating between hypothyroidism and non-thyroid illness. A normal TSH level generally excludes hypothyroidism. Release of TSH from the pituitary is impaired in uremia, even in response to exogenous thyrotropin-releasing hormone (TRH), suggesting diminished responsiveness of the pituitary gland. Elevated TSH levels are found in 12% of euthyroid dialysis patients. Sick uremic patients with primary hypothyroidism have persistently elevated TSH, usually > 20 mU/l with reduced T4. TSH levels of 6.8–20 mU/l are more likely to be due to non-thyroid illness.

Primary hypothyroidism has been reported in up to 9.5% of patients with end-stage renal disease. An increased incidence of goiter has also been reported in patients with chronic renal failure. Excess exposure to iodine has been postulated as a contributing factor, but the evidence for this is controversial.

ADRENAL FUNCTION

Adrenal function can be assessed in the dialysis patient by the adrenocorticotropic hormone (ACTH) stimulation test. Although the baseline levels of cortisol in the uremic patient may vary, the adrenal glands' response to stimulation is not affected.

CARDIOVASCULAR COMPLICATIONS

Cardiovascular complications are a major cause of morbidity and mortality in patients with end-stage renal failure. Many patients have coexisting cardiovascular disease at the time of initiation dialysis. Left ventricular failure is the most common abnormality and may predispose to arrhythmias, diastolic dysfunction and congestive cardiac failure. Recent observations suggest that patients with chronic renal failure would benefit from more aggressive intervention in the predialysis period. Such measures include assessment of the conventional cardiac risk factors such as hypertension, smoking, hyperlipidemia and diabetes mellitus, and correction of anemia, although the effect of these interventions on cardiac disease in the renal population are largely unproved.

Hypertension has been identified as a major risk factor for progression of renal disease as well as the development of coronary artery disease. Control of hypertension is therefore a major goal of management in the predialysis period. Blood pressure measurements are performed routinely on dialysis, and continued control of hypertension is important in the prevention of long-term complications. New onset hypotension during the dialysis session may suggest underlying cardiac dysfunction. This warrants further investigation of ischemic heart disease and pericardial disease.

Investigation of the lipid profile of patients with chronic renal failure is also important since experimental evidence suggests that hyperlipidemia may have the effect of hastening the decline of renal function and the development of coronary artery disease and congestive cardiac failure.

The lipoprotein profile in patients with chronic renal failure resembles the type IV pattern, with elevated triglycerides contained in very low density lipoprotein (VLDL) particles and is found in an increasing fraction of patients as the GFR declines. Moreover, levels of apolipoprotein A, associated with high density lipoprotein (HDL) cholesterol, and apolipoprotein A/C-III ratios are also found to be depressed in end-stage renal disease patients, suggesting a defect in lipid catabolism. The elevated levels of Lp(a) found in patients with end-stage renal disease may represent an additional independent risk factor for the development of atherosclerotic complications.

Attention to a detailed evaluation of cardiovascular complications should be prompted by features of ischemic heart disease or left ventricular failure detected by the history and physical examination. However, limited routine laboratory investigations of the asymptomatic patient should be undertaken because of the high prevalence of heart disease in this population.

An electrocardiogram (ECG) should be carried out on every patient. Previous myocardial infarction, arrhythmias or left ventricular hypertrophy may be seen. A routine chest X-ray will give some indication if cardiomegaly and pulmonary edema exist. Consensus has not yet developed on the role of routine echocardiography in the assessment of patients with end-stage renal disease.

Symptomatic patients should be fully investigated. Echocardiography will determine valvular function, the ejection fraction, the presence of systolic or diastolic dysfunction and whether there is a dilated cardiomyopathy or concentric hypertrophy.

Symptoms of chest pain, or ischemic changes on the ECG are indications for further cardiac evaluation. Investigations may include exercise stress testing, stress [99m]technetium sestamibi (MIBI) or thallium scintiscans, and angiography. Conventional exercise testing is often difficult in renal patients who have limited exercise tolerance and bone pain, but persantin radionuclide imaging has reasonable sensitivity and specificity for the detection of coronary artery disease in the end-stage renal failure population.

ACQUIRED RENAL CYSTIC DISEASE (ACKD)

Over the years, chronic atrophic kidneys may develop cystic change. This acquired cystic kidney disease was initially thought to occur only in hemodialysis patients, but this has also been described in patients on peritoneal dialysis and predialysis. The incidence of renal cell carcinoma in ACKD has been reported to be between 5% and 25%.

Ultrasonographic screening is less sensitive than CT scanning, but also less expensive and should be the baseline investigation. It should detect ACKD and a large renal cell carcinoma, but may miss a small (< 1 cm) renal cell carcinoma. MRI scanning does not appear to be any better than CT scanning. Some investigators have recommended routine screening for acquired cysts and carcinoma by ultrasound or CT scanning. However, this is expensive and may not be cost-effective since many dialysis patients are likely to die of unrelated causes.

DIALYSIS-RELATED AMYLOIDOSIS

A major cause of musculoskeletal symptoms in the long-term dialysis population is related to deposition of β_2-microglobulin. In chronic renal failure, β_2-microglobulin is neither filtered nor catabolized. Levels therefore rise, and synthesis may also be increased by the use of incompatible membranes. Not all patients with elevated levels of β_2-microglobulin develop dialysis-related amyloidosis, indicating that other factors must be involved in the incorporatiion of β_2-microglobulin into amyloid fibrils. Collagen, P component and glycosaminoglycans have been identified as contributing factors.

Table 10.11

Radiographic and clinical features of dialysis-related amyloidosis

- Lesions with diameters >5 mm in wrists or >10 mm in shoulders and hips
- The joint space next to the lesion is normal
- Increase of defect diameter of >30% per year
- At least two joints affected

Any joint may be affected, but carpal tunnel syndrome is probably the most frequent manifestation. Shoulders, hips, knees and spine are also commonly involved. Tendon involvement is seen in trigger finger, tendon ruptures and flexor tendon fibrosis. Other organs such as the liver, gastrointestinal tract, heart, lung and endocrine glands may be affected.

Diagnosis usually depends upon history and X-ray findings (Table 10.11); biopsy and histological diagnosis is difficult and invasive. Nuclear medicine scans using ^{123}I-SAP have been used in a number of studies. However, this is a human protein and there are consequently some potential ethical issues associated with its use. [131]I β_2-microglobulin scans are more sensitive than radiological and clinical evaluation, and the recent substitution of ^{131}I with ^{111}In has decreased the exposure to radiation and improved optical resolution.

References

Churchill, D.N., Taylor, D.W. and Keshaviah, P.R. (1995) Adequacy of dialysis and nutrition in continuous peritoneal dialysis: association with clinical outcomes. *J. Am. Soc. Nephrol.*, 7(2), 198–207.

Cockcroft, D.W. and Gault, M.H. (1976) Prediction of creatinine clearance from serum creatinine. *Nephron*, **16**, 31–41.

Daugirdas, J.T. and Depner, T.A. (1994) A nomogram approach to hemodialysis urea modeling. *Am. J. Kid. Dis.*, **23**(1), 33–40.

Flanigan, M.J. and Lim, V.S. (1996) The NIH Hemo Study. *Semin. Dial.*, 9(1), 13–15.

Garred, L.J., Canaud, B.C. and McCready, W.G. (1994) Optimal hemodialysis. The role of quantification. *Semin. Dial.*, 7(4), 236–45.

Gotch, F.A. (1990) Application of urea kinetic modeling to adequacy of CAPD therapy. *Adv. Perit. Dial.*, **6**, 178–80.

Keshaviah, P. (1993) *Options in Renal Therapy: Assessing Dialysis Adequacy*, Baxter Healthcare Corporation, McGaw Park, Illinois.

Kopple, J.D., Jones, M.R., Keshaviah, P.R. *et al.* (1995) A proposed glossary for dialysis kinetics. *Am. J. Kid. Dis.*, **26**(6), 963–81.

Lindsay, R.M. and Spanner, E.A. (1989) A hypothesis: the protein catabolic rate is dependent upon the type and amount of treatment in dialyzed uremic patients. *Am. J. Kid. Dis.*, **13**, 382–9.

Lowrie, E.G. and Lew, N.L. (1991) The urea reduction ratio (URR). A simple method for evaluating hemodialysis treatment. *Contemp. Dial. Nephrol.*, 11–20.

Lowrie, E.G., Laird, N.M., Parker, T.F. and Sargent, J.A. (1981) Effect of the hemodialysis prescription on patient morbidity. *N. Engl. J. Med.*, **305**(20), 1176–81.

Shemesh, O., Golbetz, H., Kriss, J.P. and Myers, B.D. (1985) Limitations of creatinine as a filtration marker in glomerulopathic patients. *Kidney Int.*, **28**, 830–8.

St John, A., Thomas, M.B., Davies, C.P. *et al.* (1992) Determinants of intact parathyroid hormone and free 1,25-dihydroxy vitamin D levels in mild and moderate renal failure. *Nephron*, **61**, 422–7.

Teehan, B.P., Schleifer, C.R. and Brown, J. (1994) Adequacy of continuous ambulatory peritoneal dialysis: morbidity and mortality in chronic peritoneal disease. *Am. J. Kid. Dis.*, **24**(6), 990–1001.

Twardowski, Z.J. (1989) Clinical value of standardized equilibration tests in CAPD patients. *Curr. Con. CAPD Blood Purif.*, 7, 95–108.

Further reading

Ansari, A., Kaupke, C.J., Vaziri, N.D. *et al.* (1993) Cardiac pathology in patients with end-stage renal disease maintained on hemodialysis. *Int. J. Artif. Organs*, **16**(1), 31–6.

Caregaro, L., Menon, F., Angeli, P. *et al.* (1994) Limitations of serum creatinine level and creatinine clearance as filtration markers in cirrhosis. *Arch. Intern. Med.*, **154**, 201–5.

Depner, T.A. (1991) Urea modelling: the basics. *Semin. Dial.*, **4**(3), 179–84.

Gabay, C., Ruedin, P., Slosman, D. *et al.* (1993) Bone mineral density in patients with end-stage renal failure. *Am. J. Nephrol.*, **13**(2), 115–23.

Gotch, F.A. and Sargent, J.A. (1985) A mechanistic analysis of the National Cooperative Dialysis Study (NCDS). *Kid. Int.*, **28**, 526–34.

Halperin, M.L. and Jungas, R.L. (1983) The metabolic production and renal disposal of hydrogen ions: an examination of the biochemical processes. *Kid. Int.*, **24**, 709.

Hruska, K.A. and Teitelbaum, S.L. (1995) Renal osteodystrophy. *N. Engl. J. Med.*, **333**(3), 166–74.

Laidlaw, S.A., Berg, R.L., Kopple, J.D. *et al.* (1994) Patterns of fasting plasma amino acid levels in chronic renal insufficiency: results from the feasibility phase of the Modification of Diet in Renal Disease Study. *Am. J. Kid. Dis.*, **23**(4), 504–13.

Levey, A.S. (1990) Nephrology forum: measurement of renal function in chronic renal disease. *Kid. Int.*, **38**, 167–84.

Llach, F. (1995) Secondary hyperparathyroidism in renal failure: the trade-off hypothesis revisited. *Am. J. Kid. Dis*, **25**(5), 663–79.

Malluche, H.H. and Monier-Faugere, M.-C. (1994) The role of bone biopsy in the management of patients with renal osteodystrophy. *J. Am. Soc. Nephrol.*, **4**(9), 1631–42.

Milliner, D.S., Nebeker, H.G., Ott, S.M. *et al.* (1984) Use of desferoxamine infusion test in the diagnosis of aluminium-related osteodystrophy. *Ann. Intern. Med.*, **101**, 775–80.

Nankivell, B.J., Gruenewald, S.M., Allen, R.M. and Chapman, J.R. (1995) Predicting glomerular filtration rate after kidney transplantation. *Transplantation*, **59**, 1683–9.

Ritchie, W.W., Vick, C.W., Glocheski, S.K. and Cook, D.E. (1988) Evaluation of azotemic patients: diagnostic yield of initial US examination. *Radiology*, **167**(1), 245–7.

Rosenfield, A.T. and Siegel, N.J. (1981) Renal parenchymal disease: sonographic-histologic correlation. *Am. J. Roentgen.*, **137**, 793.

Sherman, R.A. (1993) The measurement of dialysis access recirculation. *Am. J. Kid. Dis.* **22**(4), 616–21.

Sobh, M., Moustafa, F. and Ghoniem, M. (1988) Value of renal biopsy in chronic renal failure. *Int. Urol. Nephrol.*, **20**(1), 77–83.

Wallia, R., Greenberg, A., Piraino, B. *et al.* (1986) Serum electrolyte patterns in end-stage renal disease. *Am. J. Kid. Dis.*, **8**(2), 98–104.

Working Group on Renovascular Hypertension (1987) Detection, evaluation, and treatment of renovascular hypertension. Final report. *Arch. Intern. Med.*, **147**(5), 820–9.

van Acker, B.A., Koomen, G.C., Koopman, M.G. *et al.* (1992) Creatinine clearance during cimetidine administration for measurement of glomerular filtration rate [see comments]. *Lancet*, **340**(8831), 1326–9.

Transplantation

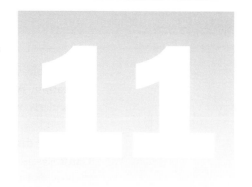

Siân Griffin and Ken Smith

Introduction

Renal transplantation is the treatment of choice for end-stage renal failure. Thirty years' experience has led to refinement of patient selection and assessment of donor–recipient compatibility, improvement in surgical techniques, and development of efficient immunosuppressive regimes. Consequently, both graft and patient survival have increased, with reduction in co-morbidity and improvement in quality of life. Diagnostic tests play an integral part of the pretransplant assessment of both recipient and donor. They play a vital role in the monitoring of graft function and immunosuppressive therapy, and in the diagnosis of problems occurring after transplantation.

Pretransplant assessment: recipient

NON-IMMUNOLOGICAL ASSESSMENT

All patients under consideration for renal transplantation require careful assessment, including history, examination and indicated investigations. Contraindications that preclude inclusion of a patient on a transplant waiting list should be detected early so as to avoid their coming to light only when the patient is called up as a potential recipient.

Age

Prior to the introduction of immunosuppressive regimes including cyclosporin A (CyA), transplantation in patients aged over 55 years was associated wth a significantly worse outcome than in younger patients. However, more recently the results in the two age groups have become comparable, and older patients are increasingly being considered for transplantation. A careful assessment of the presence of co-morbid conditions, particularly vascular disease, is essential.

Vascular disease

Cardiovascular disease remains the most common cause of death in both the dialysis and transplant patient populations, and may be indicated preoperatively by the presence of overt symptoms such as angina or intermittent claudication. All patients should be assessed by chest X-ray and electrocardiogram (ECG), with a subsequent stress test if there is any evidence of coronary artery disease. There should be a low threshold for referral for coronary angiography and appropriate surgical management prior to transplantation. The incidence of calcific aortic and mitral valve disease rises with both age and increasing duration of haemodialysis, and the severity of involvement should be accurately assessed by echocardiography. Left ventricular function may also be measured by echocardiography, as cardiac failure secondary to coronary artery disease, hypertension or chronic fluid overload is common in the dialysis population. End-stage diabetic nephropathy is the commonest diagnosis among British dialysis patients, and those in this group are at particularly increased risk for the development of vascular disease. Many units now have a policy of carrying out a stress test on all diabetics, and some will perform coronary angiography on all those over the age of 45–50 years, particularly if there is also a history of smoking. Patients with polycystic kidney disease are also at increased risk of severe atherosclerotic disease, partly because hypertension may predate the development of renal failure by many years.

Visualization of the peripheral vasculature by femoral angiography will allow transplantation on to the less diseased iliac artery, which is preferable in order to avoid the development of a steal syndrome and worsening symptoms of peripheral vascular disease postoperatively.

Measurement of serum cholesterol allows early detection of hypercholesterolaemia, which should be treated aggressively.

Malignancy

Common malignancies may be readily screened for at the time of pre-transplantation work-up. Breast and rectal examinations are performed as part of the general assessment. The presence of extensive skin damage due to sun exposure may be considered a relative contraindication to transplantation as the subsequent risk of malignancies is high. A cervical smear should be carried out in all women, and prostate-specific antigen measured in older men. All should have a chest X-ray. Early transplantation following treatment for malignancy is contraindicated due to the possible acceleration of recurrence; the procedure should be deferred for at least 12–24 months.

Infection

The prognosis of patients with the human immunodeficiency virus (HIV) receiving immunosuppression is poor and these patients should not be transplanted. Transplantation in any patient found to have a source of active sepsis must be deferred pending successful antimicrobial treatment.

Original renal disease

The underlying renal disease should be defined if possible. This will allow an estimate to be made of the risk of subsequent recurrence following transplantation (p. 232 and Table 11.2). The presence of diabetes lowers the threshold for investigation for coronary and peripheral vascular disease, as outlined above. Surgical factors are important for certain patients. The size of polycystic kidneys may necessitate nephrectomy to make room in the abdomen for transplantation. Patients with renal failure consequent on lower renal tract abnormalities, such as bladder dysfunction or outflow obstruction, will require a urological assessment and possible surgical correction prior to transplantation. The renal lesion in X-linked Alport's syndrome is due to the absence of the α5 chain of type IV collagen, and following transplantation there is the potential for these patients to develop antiglomerular basement disease with the autoantibody directed against the α5 chain. However, this is seen infrequently in clinical practice. For patients who have previously received a renal transplant, the cause of failure, whether technical or immunological, needs to be known. The risk of transplant rejection in subsequent grafts is higher in those with previous early acute rejection, and higher levels of anti-HLA antibodies will be present (see below).

IMMUNOLOGICAL

Human leucocyte antigens

The human leucocyte antigens (HLA) are a family of cell surface glycoproteins. They are encoded by the major histocompatibility complex (MHC), a cluster of genes on the short arm of chromosome 6, which are the most polymorphic group of proteins described in humans (Figure 11.1(a) and (b)). Class I molecules (HLA-A, B, C) consist of a single polypeptide chain in non-covalent association with β_2 microglobulin, whereas class II molecules (HLA-DR, DP, DQ) consist of an α and β chain (Figure 11.1(c). Both class I and II molecules bear a peptide binding groove into which peptides are placed by various specific transporter proteins in the endoplasmic reticulum, before transport of the MHC/peptide complex to the

Fig. 11.1(a)
Chromosomal organization of the human HLA genes. **(b)** Detailed chromosomal arrangement of HLA class II genes. (Figures 11.1(a) and 11.1(b) both redrawn from Taylor, C., The HLA System and its Nomenclature, in *Kidney Transplantation: Principles and Practice* (ed. P.J. Morris); published by W.B. Saunders, Philadelphia, 1994.) **(c)** Class I and Class II interaction with T-cell receptor CD8/CD4. (Redrawn from Terhorst, C. and Regueiro, J.R., T Cell Activation, in *Clinical Aspects of Immunology* (eds P. Lachman, D.K. Peters, F.S. Rosen and M.J. Walport); published by Blackwell Science, Cambridge, USA, 1993.)

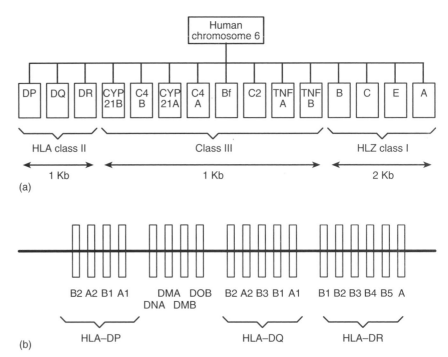

cell surface. T-lymphocyte activation is dependent on recognition by the T-cell receptor (TCR) of peptide in the context of self-MHC. The highly polymorphic nature of the HLA system enables an individual immune system to distinguish between self and non-self, and the interaction of T-cells with foreign antigenic peptides presented by self-MHC molecules enables the generation of an antigen-specific immune response.

Class I molecules are expressed on all somatic cells and present peptides derived from the degradation of endogenous proteins to CD8-positive T-cells. This MHC class has evolved to present 'endogenous antigens', predominantly those produced by intracellular organisms such as viruses and some bacteria. By virtue of their intracellular habitat, these would otherwise evade detection by the immune system. Presentation to CD8-positive T-cells allows a direct cytotoxic attack to be mounted on the infected cell.

Class II molecules are expressed on specialized antigen-presenting cells of the immune system, particularly dendritic cells, macrophages and B-cells. They present peptides derived from endocytosed exogenous antigens to CD4-positive T-cells. In addition to this constitutive expression, a number of other cell types such as endothelium can express MHC class II molecules when activated by cytokines such as gamma interferon (γIFN). Thus, local

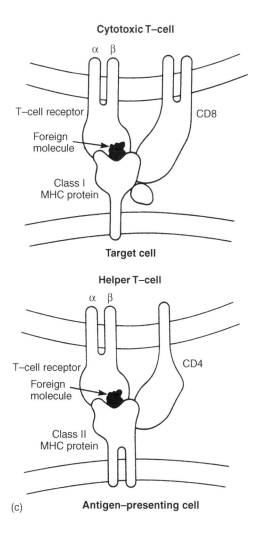

up-regulation of MHC class II molecules is a feature of many inflammatory reactions, serving to enhance presentation of exogenous antigen locally.

MHC polymorphism clearly did not evolve to allow transplant rejection! Rather, different polymorphisms allow binding of different antigenic peptides, and thus a large number of different MHC molecules allow a larger number of pathogens to be dealt with. The differences in the frequency of specific MHC polymorphisms seen between different human populations are thought to have evolved in response to the specific infective challenges that that population has faced.

An unfortunate 'side-effect' of MHC polymorphism is that the transplant recipient recognizes foreign MHC molecules as if they were self-MHC and peptide, that is as a 'pathogenic' challenge requiring disposal by an immune response. The TCR may interact with non-self MHC directly on foreign antigen presenting cells, and indirectly following their uptake, degradation and presentation by host antigen presenting cells. The indirect pathway of recognition additionally provides help for the production of alloreactive antibodies by B-lymphocytes. The direct interaction is thought to predominate during early transplant rejection against donor passenger antigen presenting cells, with the indirect interaction becoming more important later.

Graft rejection

Hyperacute Hyperacute rejection leading to immediate graft destruction results from preformed antibodies recognizing HLA class I determinants present on the vascular endothelium of the donor kidney, but will also be seen following blood group incompatible transplantation. Platelet activation leads to rapid graft thrombosis. Specific cross-matching between donor and recipient detects such antibodies and has dramatically reduced the incidence of hyperacute rejection. On the rare occasions when it now occurs it may usually be attributed to a technical or clerical error.

Acute Acute rejection episodes occur most frequently in the first three months after transplantation and are relatively uncommon after one year, when possible drug non-compliance should be considered as a cause. The renal interstitium is infiltrated with T-cells associated with monocytes and macrophages, often accompanied by tubular invasion and destruction. Vascular lesions of varying severity may also be present. The long-term prognosis is only affected in those whose response to rejection therapy is incomplete.

Chronic The gradual onset of 'chronic rejection' remains the most common cause of late graft failure regardless of the immunosuppressive regime. The process is influenced by both immunological and non-immunological factors, and an understanding of the mechanisms involved and identification of possible therapeutic targets is currently a major focus of transplantation research.

Events early on after transplantation undoubtedly influence long-term outcome, particularly HLA matching and episodes of acute rejection, although the prognosis is still good if the creatinine falls back to within the normal range after treatment. The creatinine level one month after transplantation gives a reliable indication of the expected lifetime of the graft, and despite the introduction of CyA this is little changed after the first year post-transplantation. The onset of chronic rejection may be identified clinically by the onset of a progressive, irreversible rise in creatinine, often associated with proteinuria. The histological appearances of arterial intimal fibrosis with T-cell infiltration, mesangial and glomerular expansion, tubular atrophy and interstitial fibrosis are characteristic. The relative contributions to this damage by persistent immunological challenge, associated inflammatory injury, ischaemic vascular damage and chronic CyA toxicity are not clear. Several experimental approaches have been taken to ameliorate the course of rejection and increase graft survival, such as reduction of cholesterol levels using HMG-CoA (β-hydroxy-β-methylglutaryl co-enzyme A) reductase inhibitors and prevention of microthrombotic events with salicylate and dipyridamole, but to date results have at best shown only modest effects.

HLA typing

Matching HLA type between donor and recipient helps the graft evade immune recognition and attack and thus improves graft survival (Figure 11.2). The initial calculations of survival improvement with HLA matching were carried out in patients receiving immunosuppression with azathioprine and prednisolone. The introduction of CyA has improved graft survival by 10–15% at one year and multicentre studies indicate that long-term survival is still enhanced by HLA matching. However, some single-centre studies have failed to demonstrate benefit in terms of graft outcome, although the clinical course in terms of rejection episodes may still be improved with matching.

Matching for HLA-DR has the greatest effect on graft survival, with HLA-B being the next most significant. HLA-A matching also has an

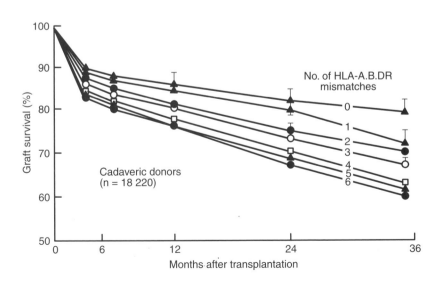

Fig. 11.2
Effect of HLA matching on survival: stepwise improvement with HLA matching. (Redrawn from Terasaki, P.I., Cecka, J.M., Lim, E. *et al.*, Overview, in *Clinical Transplants 1991* (ed. P.I. Terasaki); published by the UCLA Tissue Typing Laboratory, 1991.)

influence, but to a lesser extent than HLA-DR and HLA-B. Polymorphisms of HLA-C have been revealed recently, by sequencing rather than by serology, and presensitization has been associated with hyperacute rejection. HLA-DQ is in strong linkage disequilibrium with HLA-DR (the alleles are inherited together, homologous recombination between them being rare) and thus typing for it confers no advantage over typing for HLA-DR alone. HLA-DP is expressed at low levels (10% of HLA-DR) and has not been defined serologically. Polymorphisms in HLA-DP detected by sequencing have recently been shown to influence the outcome of second and subsequent grafts.

Methods of HLA typing

Serological   Differences between HLA antigens (polymorphisms) were first defined by the binding of antibodies in the sera of sensitized patients. That is, antisera were found that recognized HLA-A, for example, in some individuals but not others. The development of a large number of such antisera and their standardization at international meetings allowed definition of polymorphisms first in MHC class II and then in class I. Such standardized reagents are used to determine the HLA type of an individual by complement-dependent cytotoxicity assays on peripheral blood lymphocytes. The lymphocytes are labelled with a vital dye such as fluorescein diacetate or acridine orange, which is only taken up by viable cells and stains them green. They are then incubated with complement and a panel HLA-specific sera derived from patients following pregnancies. If an antibody binds to an HLA determinant on the lymphocyte cell surface, then the complement cascade is activated and the cell is lysed (p. 48). The dead cells are visualized by their loss of green staining and uptake of a red dye such as ethidium bromide. Serological studies have the advantage of being quick and relatively cheap to perform, but are less sensitive than the more recently developed sequence-based techniques.

Genetic analysis   Gene sequencing has revealed many MHC class I and II alleles that could not be distinguished by serological techniques. Direct DNA sequencing is too cumbersome to use routinely. Two polymerase chain reaction (PCR) techniques are currently in widest use. One involves amplification of, for example, all HLA-A genes using primers complementary to non-polymorphic regions. The PCR product is then blotted and probed with allele-specific oligonucleotides (PCR-SSO). The other technique uses primers designed to generate a PCR product only for a specific allele (PCR-SSP). The detection of these differences is of particular clinical relevance in bone marrow transplantation where graft versus host disease is a problem. Genetic analysis is now used routinely by 95% of UK laboratories for typing for HLA-DR.

Cross-matching

Once the HLA type of the potential donor and recipient have been identified, a cross-match is carried out to detect the presence of preformed antidonor HLA class I specific antibodies in the recipient serum. Sensitization to HLA antigens may develop following blood transfusion, pregnancy or previous transplantation. About 10% of patients awaiting a first transplant have preformed antibodies, compared with about 45% of patients awaiting regrafting. The presence of HLA specific antibodies may be detected by screening recipient serum against a panel of T-lymphocytes of known HLA type ('panel reactivity') to predict those to which a positive cross-match would occur. For patients on the transplant waiting list, repeat screening is carried out at a minimum of three-monthly intervals. Certain patients will be highly sensitized, with HLA class I antibody responses to a broad range of HLA specificities, reducing the chances of finding a suitable cross-match negative donor.

A B-cell cross-match to detect HLA class II specific-antibodies may also be performed as hyperacute rejection is possible in the presence of high titre HLA-DR specific antibodies.

Methods of cross-matching

Complement-mediated cytotoxicity assay   The complement-mediated cytotoxicity assay involves the incubation of the recipient serum with donor lymphocytes (usually derived from the lymph nodes or spleen) in the presence of rabbit complement. The cross-match is usually performed using both current and historical samples from the recipient. This reaction detects the presence of donor-specific anti-class I HLA antibodies, and if a current sample is positive for IgG this is an absolute contraindication to transplantation as almost all the grafts would undergo hyperacute rejection. A positive IgM cross-match is often due to non-HLA IgM, but if it is due to HLA antibodies it also precludes transplantation. The correlation between the cytotoxic cross-match and clinical outcome is excellent.

Flow cytometry   In sensitized patients and regrafts a more sensitive cross-match has proved beneficial, using the technique of flow cytometry (FC). FC will also detect antibodies that do not induce complement-mediated lysis, such as IgG4 and IgG2, which activate complement only weakly. The binding of antibodies in recipient serum to donor T-cells is detected by a secondary fluorescent-labelled antibody. FC analysis is carried out by passing a stream of cells through a laser. Those cells to which the dye has

Table 11.1

Investigations:
Pretransplant assessment

Type	Investigation
Haematology	Full blood count; clotting screen; ABO and Rh blood group typing
Biochemistry	Urea and electrolytes; liver function tests; calcium/phosphate
Immunology	HLA typing; screening for panel reactivity; donor lymphocyte cross-match
Virology	Hepatitis B and C; HIV; CMV IgG and IgM
Radiology	Chest X-ray; femoral angiography if at risk of PVD
ECG	Exercise ECG if past or current history of ischaemic heart disease or high risk coronary angiography if indicated (see text)
Echocardiogram	
Urological assessment if indicated	post-micturition bladder ultrasound; micturating cystogram; urodynamic studies

HLA, human leucocyte antigens; HIV, human immunodeficiency virus; CMV, cytomegalovirus; PVD, peripheral vascular disease.

bound will fluoresce, and a readout of cell number against fluorescence intensity is obtained. An FC cross-match is considered positive if there is an increase in lymphocyte fluorescence intensity greater than two standard deviations above that produced by a negative control.

A B-cell cross-match to detect the presence of antibodies to class II determinants may also be carried out, although the relevance of a positive cross-match in the context of renal transplantation remains to be established.

A summary of investigations indicated as part of the pretransplant assessment is given in Table 11.1.

Pretransplant assessment: donor

CADAVERIC

The majority of the transplants carried out in the UK are from cadaveric donors. These are usually obtained from patients with maintained cardiac output in whom the criteria for brain-stem death have been met, although organs are occasionally harvested from non-heart-beating donors. Once a potential donor has been identified and the relatives' consent obtained, the speed of arranging harvesting and transplantation becomes paramount in order to reduce the risk of complications in the donor and to minimize the warm and cold ischaemia times. The upper and lower age limits within which kidney donation is considered are flexible and are influenced by co-morbid conditions, particularly pre-existing hypertension in the more elderly donors. Transplantation of a very young and therefore small kidney is technically difficult and has an increased risk of vascular thrombosis. The presence of donor malignancy, unless it be a primary intracranial tumour, precludes transplantation due to the risk of dissemination in the immuno-suppressed recipient. Any sepsis and viral infection with hepatitis B,C or HIV must be excluded. The renal function should be normal or near normal, and consideration must be given to the drug treatment prior to harvesting, particularly the use of inotropes.

HLA typing and subsequent cross-matching once a suitable recipient is identified are carried out using lymphocytes derived from lymph node or spleen at the time of harvesting. A minority of units now carry out prospective donor typing before organ harvesting to minimize the cold ischaemia time. National organ sharing networks have enabled the rapid identification of the most suitable recipient.

LIVE

With the shortfall in available cadaveric kidneys, transplantation from living donors has been considered. Possible living donors may include blood group compatible family members and those with close emotional ties. The graft survival following transplantation from an HLA identical or haploidentical living donor is greater than following cadaveric transplantation, although the results following donation from an HLA mismatched donor have little advantage over a matched cadaveric transplant (Figure 11.3).

For patients with an unusual HLA type, a living donor may offer the best chance of successful transplantation. Living-related transplantation is, how-ever, discouraged for patients at high risk of recurrent disease. In addition to immunological assessment by HLA typing and cross-match with the potential recipient, donor glomerular filtration rate is measured and the contribution of each kidney to overall function estimated by DTPA (diethylenetriamine pentaacetic acid) scan. If split function is found to be slightly unequal then the kidney contributing least is transplanted, unless the split is marked, in which case further investigation of the underlying cause is indicated and immediate transplantation not possible. Renal anatomy may initially be visualized by ultrasound and the vasculature detailed by angiography. If possible, transplantation of a kidney with one

Fig. 11.3

Effect of haplotype matching in living-related donation. ((a) Redrawn from Cecka, J.M. and Terasaki, P.I., The UNOS Scientific Renal Transplant Registry – 1991, in *Clinical Transplants 1991* (ed. P.I. Terasaki); published by the UCLA Tissue Typing Laboratory, 1991. (b) Redrawn from Takemoto, S., Terasaki, P.I., Cecka, J.M. *et al.*, Survival of nationally shared, HLA-matched kidney transplants from cadaveric donors; published by the *New England Journal of Medicine*, 1992.)

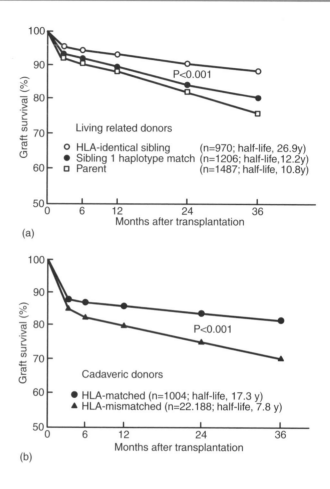

(a)

Living related donors
- ○ HLA-identical sibling (n=970; half-life, 26.9y)
- ● Sibling 1 haplotype match (n=1206; half-life,12.2y)
- □ Parent (n=1487; half-life, 10.8y)

P<0.001

(b)

Cadaveric donors
- ● HLA-matched (n=1004; half-life, 17.3 y)
- ▲ HLA-mismatched (n=22.188; half-life, 7.8 y)

P<0.001

renal artery is technically preferable to transplantation of a kidney with more than one.

Evaluation of transplant function

Close monitoring of the transplant recipient is essential in the immediate postoperative period. Hyperkalaemia is the most dangerous potential electrolyte abnormality and serum potassium should be measured on return to the ward from theatre and six to eight hours later. During the inpatient stay, most units will measure full blood count, urea and electrolytes daily, with predose CyA levels and liver function tests thrice-weekly. Following discharge, the frequency of monitoring is gradually reduced according to local policy. A baseline DTPA scan may be performed during the first week; it provides information on renal perfusion and may indicate the cause of dysfunction, as discussed below.

IMMEDIATE GRAFT DYSFUNCTION

Acute tubular necrosis

Acute tubular necrosis (ATN), with immediate anuria or following an initial polyuric phase, is the most common cause of immediate graft dysfunction after transplantation and is highly influenced by factors related to the donor. The mode of death is important, and ATN is more likely if the kidney was retrieved after cardiac arrest. The increased incidence of primary non-function associated with transplantation from non-heart-beating donors has led some centres to elect not to transplant kidneys from this source. Prior to death, inadequate fluid replacement, prolonged hypotension and inotrope dependency all increase the likelihood of subsequent ATN post-transplantation. Older kidneys are particularly susceptible to ATN. The method of harvesting is critical, with minimization of warm ischaemia essential, preferably with *in situ* perfusion of the kidneys. A good outcome following a cold ischaemia time of even up to 48 hours has enabled countrywide co-operation and sharing of donor organs to improve HLA matching, although prolonged cold ischaemia is also associated with a higher incidence of ATN. The diagnosis of ATN is often suspected from the history of the donor organ, particularly if the other kidney from the same donor has behaved similarly, and is strongly indicated if renal perfusion by isotope scanning is normal in the presence of immediate anuria (p. 92). If doubt remains, characteristic features are seen on renal biopsy.

Surgical complications

In adults, the donor kidney is transplanted extraperitoneally in the iliac fossa. The arterial supply is received by an end to end anastomosis between the donor renal artery and the recipient hypogastric artery, and venous drainage by anastomosis of the donor renal vein to the recipient iliac vein. In children, the kidney is transplanted retroperitoneally via a mid-line abdominal incision, and the renal vein anastomosed to the inferior vena cava. The donor ureter is implanted via a submucosal tunnel into the recipient bladder.

Arterial thrombosis is rare but may affect a branch artery, particularly if the procedure was technically difficult and involved the anastomosis of more than one renal artery. A major arterial thrombosis may present with a decline in renal function and hypertension, and although revascularization is theoretically possible if arterial occlusion is diagnosed rapidly (within one hour), graft nephrectomy is usually required. The diagnosis may be made by colour Doppler ultrasound or renal isotope scan. Gadolinium-enhanced nuclear magnetic resonance imaging (MRI) may be used to define segmental infarcts. The diagnosis of renal vein thrombosis, also rare, may similarly be made by ultrasound or isotope scanning.

A urinary leak due to failure of the ureteric anastomosis may occur occasionally, again following a technically difficult procedure. The resulting accumulation of fluid is most readily detected by ultrasound, as is upper tract dilatation consequent on ureteric obstruction due to clots.

Immunological factors

Hyperacute rejection causing immediate graft destruction may be recognized during surgery by the kidney becoming dusky and flaccid following reperfusion. If developing in the hours following surgery, the rejection results in vascular thrombosis, which may be demonstrated as above. If decreased renal blood flow is detected, renal angiography may demonstrate lack of perfusion throughout the kidney. Renal biopsy is characterized by a polymorphonuclear cell infiltrate, with vessel thrombosis and interstitial haemorrhage. There is no effective treatment, and graft nephrectomy is required.

EARLY GRAFT DYSFUNCTION

Mechanical

Arterial stenosis occurs more frequently in cadaveric donors than in living ones, and may be associated with a decline in renal function. On examination, a bruit may be heard over the transplanted kidney, and these patients frequently develop hypertension. Doppler ultrasound studies can be diagnostic in experienced hands, and subsequent angiography enables the localization of the stenosis and dilatation by angioplasty. As with native renal artery stenosis, a DTPA scan before and after a short acting angiotensin-converting enzyme (ACE) inhibitor such as captopril will also indicate the presence of a stenosis, but should be avoided if possible.

Ureteric stenoses are most commonly due to ischaemia and occur in the distal ureter as the distal blood supply is most vulnerable to disruption during harvesting. Ultrasound is the investigation of choice, with the opportunity of serial scans to demonstrate progressive upper tract dilatation. If a percutaneous nephrostomy is required, the level of stenosis may be determined by antegrade pyelography and ureteric stenting carried out. Surgical excision of the stenosed segment is often needed, with reimplantation of the remaining healthy ureter into the bladder. If the remaining ureter is too short, this may be anastomosed to the recipient ureter. Some groups insert ureteric stents, which are removed after a few weeks, to reduce the incidence of stenosis.

Ureteric ischaemia may also lead to necrosis and the formation of a urinary fistula. Prior to removal of the wound drain, the leaking urine will be collected and identified by the presence of high potassium and creatinine concentrations. Following drain removal, a urinoma may be identified by ultrasound, and the site of leakage by transcutaneous pyelography. If it is at the juncture with the bladder, surgical repair is required; if it is more proximal, non-operative intervention may be successful. The urine is drained via a percutaneous nephrostomy, and the wound is allowed to heal over a catheter inserted in the ureter at cystoscopy or percutaneously. A lymphocoele, resulting from recipient lymphatic leakage, may also cause a perinephric fluid collection and mimic a ureteric leak. These may be distinguished by their chemical composition: that of a lymphocoele is similar to plasma. Formal drainage is required if ureteric or venous function is compromised by obstruction, and reaccumulation may be treated surgically by intraperitoneal marsupialization.

Immunological

Accelerated rejection usually occurs within the first 10 days of transplantation and, as with hyperacute rejection, is thought to result from sensitization of the recipient to specific donor antigens. Decreased renal blood flow may be detected by Doppler ultrasound, and the presence of arteriolar thrombosis and patchy infarction can be demonstrated by angiography. Renal biopsy is characterized by severe necrotizing vascular lesions with a cellular infiltrate and areas of frank necrosis. No effective treatment is available, and graft nephrectomy is once again indicated.

The classic clinical presentation of acute rejection was with fever, hypertension and an enlarged tender graft. With modern immunosuppression this combination is now rarely seen, the usual first sign being a decline in renal function. Regular measurement of serum creatinine with prompt further investigation of any rise allows early treatment of the cause of graft dysfunction.

Renal biopsy is the gold standard method of diagnosing and determining the severity of rejection. Other non-invasive investigations, particularly ultrasound, will rapidly exclude most mechanical causes of a decline in function. A reduction in renal arterial blood flow in association with rejection may be detected by Doppler ultrasound or DTPA scan. Urine cytology and fine needle aspiration of the graft have been reported to be helpful by some groups and allow identification of the infiltrating cell population, but they are not in routine use.

The development of techniques for fine needle core biopsy has enabled safe and repeated sampling of the transplanted kidney with minimal risk of side-effects. Sufficient tissue is obtained for a detailed pathological review and readily allows rejection to be recognized and distinguished from the main differential diagnosis of CyA toxicity.

Drug-related

CyA The introduction of CyA has had a marked impact on short-term graft survival, although a disadvantage of its use has been attendant nephrotoxicity. This may manifest both early on after transplantation, and also later when chronic CyA toxicity may contribute to long-term graft dysfunction. CyA toxicity is the main differential diagnosis to rejection in most cases of early graft dysfunction when mechanical causes have been excluded. Toxicity is usually, but not invariably, associated with high trough levels between doses, but biopsy is frequently required to distinguish toxicity from rejection. Tacrolimus (FK506) has recently been approved for clinical use and is similarly associated with dose-dependent nephrotoxicity.

Trimethoprim The use of trimethoprim as a treatment for urinary tract infection or as prophylaxis against *Pneumocystis carinii* is occasionally associated with a transient rise in creatinine due to its decreased tubular secretion, which resolves following discontinuation of the drug.

Ganciclovir Ganciclovir, given as prophylaxis or treatment of cytomegalovirus (CMV) infection, may lead to a decline in renal function. Impaired function may also be associated with CMV infection itself, and the timing of the onset and recovery of function with respect to infection and the commencement of ganciclovir will often suggest the cause of rising creatinine. If it is the cause of impaired renal function, ganciclovir should be stopped unless it is required for severe CMV disease. Recovery of function occurs once the drug is stopped.

OKT3 OKT3 has occasionally been reported by some units to be the cause of an increase in serum creatinine. The cause for this is unclear and it has not been reported following the use of other monoclonal antibodies.

Others As with non-transplant recipients, renal function may decline consequent to treatment with non-steroidal anti-inflammatory drugs (NSAIDs), and a deterioration in function following the introduction of an ACE inhibitor is an indication to investigate for an underlying renal artery stenosis.

Infections

In the first month after transplantation, most infections (e.g. pneumonia, catheter- and wound-related sepsis, etc.) are similar to those occurring in a non-immunosuppressed surgical population. Their increased frequency in transplant recipients, however, emphasizes the need for technical care at the time of operation. Infections are occasionally transmitted with the graft and septic donors are therefore not used in order to reduce this risk.

Early urinary tract infections are frequently associated with the development of graft pyelonephritis and bacteraemia. Regular urine culture enables early diagnosis, not only of bacterial infection but also of that due to candida, before the onset of graft dysfunction.

As the cumulative dose of immunosuppression rises, so does the incidence of opportunistic infections. CMV infection is a principal cause of fever in the period of one to six months post-transplantation and may adversely effect graft function. Primary infection occurs when latently infected cells are passed from a seropositve donor to a seronegative recipient. Approximately 60% of such recipients will develop symptomatic CMV disease. Reactivation of disease in seropositive recipients occurs in approximately 20%, a figure strongly influenced by the type of immunosuppression received. The administration of antilymphocyte globulin (ALG) or OKT3 markedly increases the incidence of disease. Superinfection occurs in 20–40% when a seropositive recipient receives a seropositive graft, and the infection is due to CMV derived from the donor. Again, the incidence is influenced by the immunosuppressive regime, but whether this disease is more severe than that associated with endogenous reactivation is not known. In addition to causing symptomatic disease, the immunosuppressive effect of CMV itself further increases the host's susceptibility to opportunistic infections.

High dose oral acyclovir and hyperimmune CMV immunoglobulin have some success in preventing disease in high risk recipients, although their effect is reduced following treatment with ALG. Although an effective treatment for retinitis, ganciclovir is less useful for severe CMV-associated conditions such as pneumonitis. Prevention and early diagnosis of active CMV infection are therefore of prime importance following transplantation.

The diagnosis of acute disease in the early stages can be difficult as serological titres of anti-CMV IgM or IgG are not helpful. Viraemia is predictive of the development of CMV disease and usually precedes symptoms. The presence of CMV antigen in peripheral blood monocytes is rapidly detected by a binding assay of monoclonal anti-CMV matrix protein to fixed cells, although the assay may be negative if storage is prolonged. PCR detects CMV DNA and may be carried out using blood or tissue samples, providing the most sensitive means for detecting virus. The DEAFF (detection of early antigen fluorescent focus) test is a method of quick culture and can be carried out using urine, sputum or blood.

Fibroblast cells are incubated for 24–48 hours in the presence of the patient sample, and the expression of the CMV immediate early antigen is detected by a monoclonal antibody. Full culture of cells to the end point of a cytopathic effect takes 7–14 days. By performing these assays at weekly intervals in the early post-transplantation period, surveillance of patients at high risk of CMV disease is possible, allowing early and appropriate introduction of antiviral therapy.

Late graft dysfunction

Chronic rejection Both immunological and non-immunological mechanisms may contribute to chronic rejection and are discussed in greater detail above. The characteristic clinical presentation is with proteinuria and an inexorable decline in renal function; confirmatory renal biopsy is often not required.

Recurrent glomerulonephritis The original disease causing renal failure may recur in the graft following transplantation, although the course of recurrent disease is not invariably as severe as initial presentation. Caution should be exercised, particularly when considering live-related transplantation for a disease known to be at high frequency of recurrence. The development of haematuria, proteinuria or the nephrotic syndrome, or declining renal function will require renal biopsy to determine the cause. Table 11.2 indicates the frequency with which various glomerular diseases recur following transplantation.

Immunosuppression

Optimization of immunosuppressive regimes to balance the risk of rejection with that of toxicity continues to challenge physicians involved in the management of transplant recipients. The aim for each patient is to reduce the allograft rejection while preserving the ability to respond to pathogens. Regulation of T-lymphocyte activation and proliferation is central to the effects of the drugs used. There are several important drug interactions with both azathioprine and CyA that should be remembered when altering drug regimes. Therapeutic drug monitoring enables individual tailoring of dose to optimize survival while minimizing side-effects. The immunosuppressive drugs used have side-effects that are common to both as well as some that are specific to each drug. The recipient is rendered more susceptible to infections, both conventional and opportunistic, and to the development of malignancies, particularly skin cancers and those associated with a viral aetiology such as Kaposi's sarcoma, lymphoproliferative disease and carcinoma of the cervix. All patients should receive oral amphotericin lozenges as

Native disease	Recurrence (total)	Recurrence (graft lost)	Comments
Primary glomerular disease			
MCGN II	90%	10%	Clinical course of recurrence usually benign
FSGS	30%	15%	Recurs early; risk of recurrence in subsequent grafts 80%; caution if considering LRD
MCGN I	15%	5%	Present with recurrent nephrotic syndrome
IgAN/HSP	50%	Rare	Disease usually limited to mild proteinuria/haematuria
Anti-GBM	Rare	Rare	Provided transplanted in remission
Membranous	Variable		Recurs early with nephrotic syndrome; *de novo* disease may occur in graft (c. 2%)
Alport's syndrome	N/A		May develop anti-GBM antibodies directed against α5 chain type IV collagen (absent in X-linked Alport's)
Secondary glomerular disease			
Systemic vasculitis			
SLE	Rare	Rare	
Systemic sclerosis			
HUS	Variable		Recurrence unusual in sporadic HUS, variable in familial
Amyloid	20%	Unusual	
Diabetes	Inevitable	Unusual	Recurrent histological changes inevitable
Oxalosis			Early graft failure reduced by early transplantation and short period on dialysis; correction of enzyme defect by simultaneous liver transplant

MCGN, mesangiocapillary glomerulonephritis; FSGS, focal segmental glomerulosclerosis; IgAN, IgA nephropathy; HSP, Henoch–Schönlein purpura; GBM, glomerular basement membrane; SLE, systemic lupus erythematosus; HUS, haemolytic uraemic syndrome.

prophylaxis against fungal infections during their hospital stay, and co-trimoxazole for prophylaxis against *Pneumocystis carinii* for the first six months. Additionally, in patients with a history of tuberculosis, and in all those from the Indian subcontinent, treatment with isoniazid and pyridoxine should be considered while they are immunosuppressed.

Table 11.2
Renal diseases with significant risk of recurrence in transplant

CORTICOSTEROIDS

Relatively high-dose steroids are used around the time of transplantation, with the dose rapidly being tapered to a maintenance level of 5–10 mg/d, or even lower, with recent evidence suggesting that steroid withdrawal does not affect graft survival but does reduce the morbidity associated with prolonged treatment (especially in children). Corticosteroids have both a non-specific anti-inflammatory action, by reducing migration of immune effector cells, and a specific T-lymphocyte suppressive action by reducing the production of stimulatory cytokines. High-dose pulse intravenous corticosteroids are also used in the treatment of acute rejection. Regular monitoring of blood glucose is vital, particularly in the early post-transplantation period. Hyperglycaemia may initially require treatment with insulin, but usually resolves as the steroid dose is reduced. In the longer term, the incidence of osteoporosis is dose-related and is best avoided by early dose reduction, although bisphosphonates may also have a useful role in treatment. Bone densitometry will identify those patients at particularly high risk of osteoporosis, and some units will now perform this routinely to detect changes early and allow more aggressive treatment.

AZATHIOPRINE

Azathioprine is an antimetabolite and acts by inhibiting the synthesis of DNA and RNA. Actively dividing cells are those most susceptible to the effects of azathioprine, and lymphocytes are particularly sensitive when stimulated to replicate following antigenic challenge. Although useful for inhibiting primary immune responses, azathioprine has little effect in preventing acute rejection. The usual dose is 1.5–2 mg/kg, and its side-effects are predictable from its known effect on rapidly dividing cells. Nausea and dose-related myelotoxicity are the most common side-effects, and hepatotoxicity may also develop, progressing to chronic active hepatitis if azathioprine is continued. Frequent monitoring of the full blood count when the drug is first started and following an increase in dose enables early detection if leucopenia or thrombocytopenia develop. Once stable, three-monthly monitoring is sufficient. Macrocytosis may develop more insidiously. Derangement of liver function tests usually requires discontinuation of azathioprine.

CYCLOSPORIN A

The introduction of CyA to immunosuppressive regimes had a dramatic effect, improving the expected graft survival rate at one year by 15–20%. CyA is a cyclic peptide derived from a soil fungus. Following binding of the TCR to antigen, there is an increase in intracellular calcium, which is crucial for subsequent activation. CyA binds to a cytoplasmic receptor protein, cyclophilin, and the resulting complex binds to and inhibits calcineurin, a calcium- and calmodulin-sensitive phosphatase. Thus the phosphorylation of DNA-binding proteins is inhibited, including at least one that is responsible for binding the promoter sequence for interleukin-2 (IL-2), thus preventing completion of the activation cascade. Conversely, CyA enhances expression of transforming growth factor β (TGFβ), which may itself inhibit IL-2-stimulated T-lymphocyte proliferation. This enhancement of TGFβ production may mediate the renal fibrosis seen with CyA treatment.

The pharmacokinetics of CyA absorption and availability vary widely between individuals. There is a narrow therapeutic window for optimal immunosuppressive effect, and if levels rise above this then the risk of both acute and chronic nephrotoxicity increases sharply. The drug is usually given at 12-hourly intervals and plasma levels are monitored by measurement of trough levels in whole blood between doses. There is a linear relationship between the oral dose and the blood levels that enables predictable dose adjustment. Following a change in dose, a new steady state is reached in four half-lives, so there is no additional value in measuring levels more frequently than every 48 hours. An automated enzyme immunoassay technique has recently become available and is increasingly replacing previous methods for measuring CyA concentration, namely radioimmunoassay, high performance liquid chromatography and fluorescence polarization immunoassays. The oral preparation of CyA has recently been refined to achieve a more consistent concentration profile between peak and trough levels, and to deliver therapeutic trough levels earlier after initiation of therapy. The resulting more predictable immunosuppression has been associated with fewer acute rejection episodes during the first three months of treatment. The starting dose of CyA is usually 10–14 mg/kg/d, reducing, according to blood levels, to a maintenance dose of 3–6 mg/kg/d. In the early post-transplantation period, the aim is for a blood level of 150–300 ng/ml, which is later modified according to clinical indication.

Unfortunately, the major side-effect of CyA is nephrotoxicity. Acute reversible nephrotoxicity is associated with a reduction in intrarenal blood flow and increases the incidence of ATN. In patients with ATN, CyA is reduced and replaced with an increased dose of prednisolone, or occasionally with an anti-T-cell antibody preparation such as ALG or OKT3. A minority of units use anti-T-cell antibodies at induction and do not introduce CyA until later to reduce this risk of ATN. Chronic irreversible CyA toxicity is characterized by progressive renal dysfunction, with renal biopsy demonstrating tubular atrophy, interstitial fibrosis and glomerulosclerosis. Close monitoring of CyA levels enables minimization of the risk of toxicity developing, but it may occur despite levels within the therapeutic range. The minimal level to achieve optimal immunosuppression without nephrotoxicity remains undefined, although administration with other drugs has enabled the dose to be reduced.

Hypertension is the most common side-effect of CyA treatment. CyA may be associated with grand mal convulsions, particularly early on post-transplantation when doses are highest. The development of a burning pain in the hands and feet (acral dysaesthesiae), may necessitate a reduction in dose. Hypertrichosis may be particularly distressing for dark-haired women. Gingival hypertrophy is most pronounced in children and those with poor dentition. Optimum management and prevention require regular dental treatment.

MYCOPHENOLATE MOFETIL

Mycophenolate mofetil (MMF) was developed as an alternative agent to azathioprine. Most cell types have both *de novo* and salvage pathways for purine synthesis, although lymphocytes rely solely on *de novo* synthesis. The aim was to minimize side-effects by selectively inhibiting the final enzyme in the *de novo* pathway. Unlike the other immunosuppressants, both B- and T-cell responses are reduced. The side-effect profile is, in practice, similar to that of azathioprine. Gastrointestinal side-effects, which are responsive to either a reduction in dose or temporary cessation of treatment, are common. Three large co-operative studies (European mycophenolate mofetil study group, 1995; Sollinger, 1995; Tricontinental mycophenolate mofetil renal transplantation study group, 1996), two comparing additional MMF with prednisolone and CyA and one comparing triple therapy containing MMF with azathioprine, have shown a reduction in acute rejection rates during the first six months. The optimum dose is usually 2 g/day in divided doses. A higher dose produces no increased benefit in terms of fewer graft rejection episodes but is associated with a greater incidence of side-effects, which in practice occur at a similar rate to azathioprine. MMF may cause leucopenia, thrombocytopenia and macrocytosis, and measurement of the full blood count is recommended at least weekly initially and monthly for the first year of treatment. Blood glucose monitoring should be carried out to detect hyperglycaemia.

TACROLIMUS (FK506) AND RAPAMYCIN (SIROLIMUS)

In common with CyA, tacrolimus and rapamycin are derived from micro-organisms and exert their immunomodulatory effects by binding an intracellular receptor. They are both macrolide antibiotics, are structurally distinct from CyA, and bind to the tacrolimus (FK506)-binding protein (FKBP) family of immunophilins. As with CyA, the tacrolimus–

immunophilin complex then inhibits calcineurin, whereas the rapamycin–immunophilin complex inhibits signal pathways activated following binding of IL-2 to its cell surface receptor. As both drugs act through FKBP they are antagonists and there is no benefit in using both, although combination therapy with CyA and rapamycin may offer additional benefits compared with CyA alone. There is preliminary evidence that although similar one-year graft survival is achieved with treatment with either CyA or tacrolimus, tacrolimus is associated with fewer episodes of acute rejection and a longer predicted half-life of graft survival, without increases in attendant toxicity. Tacrolimus has also been used successfully as rescue therapy in patients with steroid- or antibody-resistant acute rejection. Treatment with tacrolimus is monitored by an enzyme immunoassay of trough levels in whole blood.

Although the incidences of hypertension and nephrotoxicity are similar to those with CyA, neurotoxicity is more common with tacrolimus, which does not produce gingival hyperplasia nor hirsutism. Impaired glucose tolerance and frank diabetes are more common than in patients receiving CyA. In the randomized tacrolimus trial in the USA (US multi-center FK506 kidney transplant group, 1996), the incidence of new-onset diabetes requiring insulin was 25% in the group receiving tacrolimus (40% in Blacks) compared with 5% of those receiving CyA. Children treated with tacrolimus are more susceptible to post-transplant lymphoproliferative disease and hypertrophic cardiomyopathy, which should be monitored with regular echocardiography. Experience with rapamycin is more limited, but nephrotoxicity is not a feature. Current trials of rapamycin are considering its use as an alternative agent to azathioprine.

ANTIBODIES

Both polyclonal and monoclonal anti-T-cell antibodies are available. They are used in the treatment of acute rejection refractory to steroids, when a response rate of up to 90% has been reported. As mentioned above their use at induction is favoured by some groups to delay the introduction of CyA. Their administration is commonly associated with flu-like side-effects, that are thought to be related to cytokine release. The subsequent risk of opportunistic infections and lymphoid malignancies is substantially increased.

ALG is produced by injecting animals such as horses or rabbits with human lymphoid cells and subsequently separating the immunoglobulin fraction for therapeutic use. Each polyclonal preparation contains a variable proportion of anti-T-lymphocyte antibodies, and prediction of a clinical response is therefore difficult. Side-effects are frequent and may consist of an anaphylactoid reaction by host antibodies to the foreign immunoglobulin, or result from contaminating antibodies with resulting thrombocytopenia, granulocytopenia or serum sickness. A host antibody response to ALG can render the treatment ineffective, and this can be monitored by sandwich ELISA (enzyme-linked immunosorbent assay).

OKT3 is a mouse monoclonal antibody directed against CD3, a constant component of the T-cell receptor responsible for transducing signals from the antigen-binding domain of the receptor to the cell interior. As a monoclonal preparation, standardization of dose is possible.

The total treatment period for acute rejection is 10–14 days, and monitoring of daily total, CD4- and CD8-positive T-cells by flow cytometry enables tailoring of the dose and avoidance of over-immunosuppression.

The use of monoclonal antibodies against other T-lymphocyte determinants remains experimental. Anti-CD4 antibodies can induce tolerance in rodents, although in larger animals, such as monkeys, tolerance is not achieved despite high doses. The prophylactic use of anti-CD4 in humans has had no influence on the number of rejection episodes or graft survival. Promising results have been achieved with the use of anti-CD11a in bone marrow transplantation in immunodeficient children, but it has not yet been used in immunocompetent adults. Early trials of an anti-IL-2 receptor antibody have shown a synergistic effect with CyA with reduction in the number of acute rejection events.

Surveillance for the long-term effects of immunosuppression

In addition to the increased susceptibility to infection and other side-effects of the drugs described above, the transplant recipient is in a high risk group for subsequent development of cardiovascular disease and malignancy due to a combination of metabolic and iatrogenic influences. By minimizing morbity due to these factors the life expectancy of the patient can be improved and hence the number of patients dying with a functioning graft can be reduced. Lifestyle recommendations form the starting point for optimization of patient and graft survival.

CARDIOVASCULAR DISEASE

A patient aged 35–44 years with end-stage renal failure has an increased relative risk of cardiovascular death of 70 compared with age- and sex-matched controls. This risk is further increased to 320 if the patient is also diabetic (source: European Dialysis and Transplantation Association; Raine, 1995). Smoking should be strongly discouraged and exercise recommended. Hypertension often predates transplantation and may worsen postoperatively due to CyA. The development of hyperlipidaemia is often multifactorial, and impairment of anti-oxidant mechanisms may result in increased atherogenicity by low-density lipoprotein (LDL). Lowering of serum cholesterol by HMG-CoA reductase inhibitors has also been suggested to influence the progression of chronic rejection, although there is an increased risk of myositis in patients also receiving CyA. There may be benefit in treating accumulated homocysteine with folic acid to reduce the associated vascular risk.

MALIGNANCY

Immunosuppression is associated with an increased risk of malignancy, particularly involving the skin. Sun exposure is a major risk factor for the development of all skin malignancies and patients are advised to avoid it. Basal cell carcinoma develops about three times more frequently than squamous, with melanoma the least common but associated with the worse prognosis. Although the majority of tumours develop on sun-exposed skin, regular total skin examination is vital to detect early operable tumours as the growth, particularly of squamous cell tumours, can be rapid and metastasis early. Kaposi's sarcoma may develop in an unusual visceral site, when discontinuation of immunosuppression may result in regression. In contrast to other skin tumours, the incidence of Kaposi's sarcoma appears to be higher in patients treated with CyA.

Lymphoproliferative malignancies are most common in patients treated with ALG, OKT3, or high dose CyA, and may develop in the first few months. Most of the lymphomas are of the non-Hodgkin's type and are associated with a high mortality. Epstein–Barr virus has been implicated in a minority of cases, when regression of lymphoproliferation may occur following withdrawal of CyA.

Carcinoma of the cervix is 14 times more common than in the general population, with a more rapid progression to invasive disease. Annual cervical smears are recommended for all female transplant recipients. Tumours of the gastrointestinal tract have been estimated to occur two to seven times more frequently, and those of the bronchus, breast and prostate at a similar rate to background.

Tumours have occasionally been inadvertently introduced with the transplanted kidney. Their course is aggressive, and if detected nephrectomy and cessation of immunosuppression are mandatory.

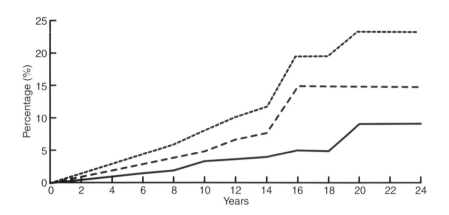

Fig. 11.4
Cumulative incidence of malignancy following transplantation, Manchester, UK. – – – Excluding skin; —— non-melanotic; . . . . all sites. (Redrawn from Johnson, R., Factors Affecting Graft Loss in *Transplantation '96: Maximising Patient Benefit in Transplantation* (ed. R.W.G. Johnson); published by the Royal Society of Medicine Press Ltd, 1996.)

The increased risk of malignancy is maintained after transplantation and long-term surveillance is mandatory (Figure 11.4). In high risk populations such as Caucasians living in Australia, the cumulative incidence of skin cancer is far higher than that shown in Figure 11.4.

BONE DISEASE

A normally functioning graft rapidly restores a normal calcium-phosphate balance in the recipient. Persisting hyperparathyroidism in a minority of patients requires subsequent parathyroidectomy. As detailed above, steroid-induced osteoporosis and avascular necrosis are best avoided by dose minimization.

HAEMATOLOGICAL COMPLICATIONS

The development of post-transplantation polycythaemia is best treated by regular venesection to maintain the haematocrit at less than 50%. ACE inhibitors may also usefully lower the haematocrit.

Conclusion

Renal transplantation has progressed in the past 30 years from being an experimental technique to an accepted and preferred mode of treatment. The drive to achieve graft tolerance with minimal disturbance to the overall host immunity has provided the impetus for a wide range of immunological research and subsequently increased understanding of immune mechanisms in a range of other settings. The use of diagnostic tests to monitor transplant recipients closely has contributed to this success, and their future role will be vital to achieve the aim of transplantation as an effective treatment for life.

References

Cecka, J.M. and Terasaki, P.I. (1991) The UNOS Scientific Renal Transplant Registry – 1991, in *Clinical Transplants 1991* (ed. P.I. Terasaki), UCLA Tissue Typing Laboratory, Los Angeles, pp. 1–11.

European mycophenolate mofetil study group (1995) Placebo-controlled study of mycophenolate mofetil combined with cyclosporin and corticosteroids for prevention of acute rejection. *Lancet*, 345, 1321–5.

Johnson, R. (1996) Factors Affecting Graft Loss, in *Transplantation '96: Maximising Patient Benefit in Transplantation* (ed. R.W.G. Johnson), International Congress and Symposium Series 217, Royal Society of Medicine Press, London, pp. 3–11.

Raine, A.E.G. (1995) Review article: Hypertension and ischaemic heart disease in rental transplant recipients. *Nephrol. Dial. Trans.* **10**(S1), 95–100.

Sollinger, I.I.W. for the US renal transplant mycophenolate mofetil study group (1995) Mycophenolate mofetil for the prevention of acute rejection in primary cadaveric renal allograft recipients. *Transplantation*, **60**, 225–32.

Takemoto, S., Terasaki, P.I., Cecka, J.M. *et al.* for the UNOS scientific renal transplant registry (1992) Survival of nationally shared, HLA-matched kidney transplants from cadaveric donors. *N. Engl. J. Med.*, **327**, 834–9.

Taylor, C.J. (1994) The Human Leukocyte Antigen (HLA) System and its Nomenclature, in *Kidney Transplantation: Principles and Practice*, 4th edn (ed. P.J. Morris), W.B. Saunders, Philadelphia, pp. 543–4.

Terasaki, P.I., Cecka, J.M., Lim, E. *et al.* (1991) Overview, in *Clinical Transplants 1991* (ed P. Terasaki), UCLA Tissue Typing Laboratory, Los Angeles, pp. 409–30.

Terhorst, C. and Regueiro, J.R. (1993) T Cell Activation, in *Clinical Aspects of Immunology*, 5th edn (eds P.J. Lachman, D.K. Peters, F.S. Rosen and M.J. Walport), Blackwell Science, Cambridge, USA, p. 450.

Tricontinental mycophenolate mofetil renal transplantation study group (1996) A blinded, randomized clinical trial of mycophenolate mofetil for the prevention of acute rejection in cadaveric renal transplantation. *Transplantation*, **61**, 1029–37.

US multi-center FK506 kidney transplant group (1996) One-year follow-up of an open label trial of FK506 for primary kidney transplantation. A report of the US multi-center FK506 kidney transplant group. *Transplantation*, 61, 1576–81.

Further reading

Abecassis, M.M., Koffron, A.J., Kaplan, B. *et al.* (1997) The role of PCR in the diagnosis and management of CMV in solid organ recipients. *Transplantation*, **63**(2), 275–9.

Austen, K.F., Burakoff, S.J., Rosen, F.S. and Strom, T.B. (eds) (1996) *Therapeutic Immunology*, Blackwell Science, Oxford.

Bennett, W.M., DeMattos, A., Meyer, M.M. *et al.* (1996) Chronic cyclosporine nephropathy: the Achilles' heel of immunosuppressive therapy. *Kid. Int.*, **50**, 1089–1100.

Colvin, R.B. (1996) The renal allograft biopsy. *Kid. Int.*, **50**, 1069–82.

Eriksson, B.-M., Zweygberg Wirgart, B., Claesson, K. *et al.* (1996) A prospective study of rapid methods of detecting cytomegalovirus in the blood of renal transplant recipients in relation to patient and graft survival. *Clin. Trans.*, **10**, 494–502.

Held, P.J., Kahan, B.D., Hunsicker, L.G. *et al.* (1994) The impact of HLA mismatches on the survival of first cadaveric kidney transplants. *N. Engl. J. Med.*, **331**, 765–70.

Olerup, O. and Zetterquist, H. (1992) HLA-DR typing by PCR amplification with sequence specific primers (PCR–SSP) in 2 hours: an alternative to serological DR typing in clinical practice including donor-recipient matching in cadaveric renal transplantation. *Tissue Antigens*, **39**, 225–35.

Opel, G. for the Collaborative Transplant Study (1988) The benefit of exchanging donor kidneys among transplant centers. *N. Engl. J. Med.*, **318**, 1289–92.

Peiris, J.S.M., Taylor, C.E., Main, J. *et al.* (1995) Diagnosis of cytomegalovirus disease in renal allograft recipients: the role of semiquantitive polymerase chain reaction. *Nephrol. Dial. Trans.*, **10**, 1198–1205.

Penn, I. (1993) The effect of immunosuppresion on pre-existing cancers. *Transplantation*, **55**, 742–7.

Soulillou, J.-P. (1994) Relevant targets for therapy with monoclonal antibodies in allograft transplantation. *Kid. Int.*, **46**, 540–53.

Starzl, T.E., Rosenthal, J.T., Hakala, T.R. *et al.* (1983) Steps in immunosuppression for renal transplantation. *Kid. Int.*, **23**(S1), 60–5.

Tait, B.D. (1993) Seeking the perfect match – HLA and transplantation. *Med. J. Aus.*, **159**, 696–700.

Taylor, C.J., Chapman, J.R., Ting, A. and Morris, P.J. (1989) Characterisation of lymphocytotoxic antibodies causing a positive cross match in renal transplantation. *Transplantation*, **48**, 953–8.

Hypertension

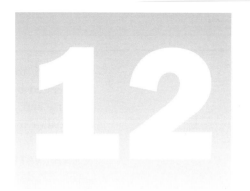

John Bradley

Investigations serve two main purposes in the hypertensive patient: to establish any treatable underlying cause for the hypertension; and to assess any organ damage that has already occurred as a consequence of the high blood pressure.

Most physicians perform the following investigations:

- urinalysis for blood and protein; if abnormal a mid-stream urine (MSU) test for cells, casts, proteinuria and evidence of infection, and a 24-hour urine collection to measure creatinine clearance and protein loss, should also be performed;
- blood urea, creatinine and electrolytes to assess renal function and look for the hypokalaemic alkalosis of Conn's or Cushing's syndromes (or diuretic therapy);
- 24-hour urine collection to measure vanillylmandelic acid (VMA) or 4-hydroxy-3-methoxymandelic acid (HMMA) output (to exclude phaeochromocytoma);
- electrocardiogram (ECG) to assess left ventricular size; if abnormal, a chest X-ray.

If the history or examination reveals evidence of cardiovascular or renal disease, or suggests an underlying cause, further investigations should be performed.

History and examination of hypertensive patients

SYMPTOMS

There are usually no symptoms of hypertension. It is important to establish whether patients have had blood pressure (BP) measurements taken in the past, and to ask about headaches or visual disturbance (in severe or accelerated hypertension), chest pain and intermittent claudication, family history, and any medication. Episodes of palpitations, headache, sweating and pallor may occur in phaeochromocytoma.

EXAMINATION

The blood pressure should be measured at rest. If it is high (systolic > 160 mmHg, diastolic > 90 mmHg), check it in both arms. Unless it is very severe, recheck on at least three separate occasions before considering treatment. A large cuff should be used in the 10% of the population whose arm circumference is over 33 cm. Phase 5 diastolic (disappearance) should be recorded together with the patient's posture and the arm used.

Mild or moderate hypertension usually gives no other abnormalities on examination. In long-standing or severe hypertension there may be evidence of left ventricular hypertrophy with an aortic ejection murmur and loud aortic second sound. The optic fundi may show evidence of retinopathy with arterial narrowing and arteriovenous narrowing (indicating atherosclerosis), haemorrhages and exudates. Papilloedema indicates the presence of malignant hypertension.

During the examination it is essential to think of less common causes:

- observe the face for evidence of Cushing's syndrome (usually due to steroid administration)
- examine for aortic coarctation: feel both radials and measure the blood pressure in both arms; look for radial–femoral delay, weak femoral pulses, and bruits of the coarctation and scapular anastomoses, which may produce visible pulsations.
- listen for an epigastric or para-umbilical bruit of renal artery stenosis
- feel for polycystic kidneys
- think of chronic renal disease, phaeochromocytoma (rare), and primary hyperaldosteronism (very rare).

Target organ damage

CARDIAC DISEASE

Left ventricular hypertrophy (LVH) may be present in even mild hypertension, and is associated with an increased risk of cardiac dysfunction, atherosclerosis, arrhythmias and sudden death. There is good evidence that treatment of hypertension results in regression of LVH. The diagnosis may be suspected from clinical examination and can be confirmed by ECG and echocardiography.

The characteristic finding on ECG is that the sum of the S wave in V_1 and R wave in V_5 or V_6 is greater than 35 mm. This may be associated with ST segment depression or T wave inversion ('strain pattern'). The chest X-ray may show cardiomegaly. Echocardiography is much more sensitive than the ECG. The left ventricular mass index (LVMI) is calculated from left ventricular (LV) wall thickness and LV internal diameters in systole and diastole. LVH is present if the LVMI is > 110 g/m^2 in women or > 131 g/m^2 in men.

RENAL DISEASE

The intricate relationship between blood pressure and the kidneys makes hypertension both an important cause and consequence of renal disease. Thus renal disease may develop as a result of hypertension, and hypertension is a common presenting problem in patients with renal disease.

Estimates of the prevalence of chronic renal failure due to essential hypertension vary widely from 0.002% to 20% of all cases of renal failure. These differences partly reflect the fact that the diagnosis of renal disease due to hypertension depends on the exclusion of other causes of renal failure. It is possible, therefore, that many cases of renal failure attributed to hypertension in fact have underlying renal disease. One consistent finding is that renal failure due to hypertension is much commoner in blacks than whites. Furthermore, within the black population there appears to be familial clustering of renal disease caused by hypertension, raising the possibility of a genetic susceptibility to hypertensive renal damage.

Renal failure is an invariable feature of accelerated hypertension in which acute severe hypertension is associated with gross intimal hyperplasia leading to occlusion of the lumen of the small arteries and arterioles within the kidney. Renal failure is a rapid consequence if the blood pressure is not controlled.

Identification of the underlying causes of hypertension

In over 90% of cases no specific cause is found, this hypertension is known as 'essential'. The aetiology in these cases is probably multifactorial. Predisposing factors include:

- increasing age
- obesity
- excessive alcohol intake.

Hypertension may be secondary to:

- renal disease
- endocrine disease: Cushing's syndrome; Conn's syndrome; phaeochromo-cytoma; acromegaly: hypertension is commoner in diabetics
- drugs: non-steroidal anti-inflammatory agents; contraceptive pill
- eclampsia
- coarctation of the aorta.

RENAL DISEASE AS A CAUSE OF HYPERTENSION

Although the prevalence of renal disease due to essential hypertension is unclear, high blood pressure is recognized to be a common complication of renal disease that may initially occur as a consequence of the disease and later become a reason for its progression. The mechanism by which hypertension is initiated and maintained in the presence of renal disease is complex. Activation of the renin–angiotensin–aldosterone system, retention of salt and water, abnormalities of the autonomic nervous system, reduced production of renal vasodepressor substances, and alterations in the structure and function of resistance vessels have all been implicated. Haemody-namically, the hypertension is maintained by an increased peripheral vascular resistance.

RENOVASCULAR HYPERTENSION

Ischaemia of the kidney due to renal artery disease is an important treatable cause of hypertension. Atherosclerotic renal artery disease accounts for approximately 70% of lesions, and occurs most commonly in elderly men. It is bilateral in 25% of cases, and usually results from a plaque in the first part of the renal artery. Fibrous renal artery disease occurs predominantly in young women, is frequently bilateral, and often involves the distal portion of the renal artery, giving rise to a beaded appearance in the artery. While both forms of renal artery stenosis are associated with hypertension, total occlusion of the renal artery and ischaemic atrophy of the affected kidney is commoner in atherosclerotic renal artery disease.

Angiotensin-converting enzyme (ACE) inhibitors provide an attractive means of reducing the blood pressure, but should be used with caution as renal perfusion in the presence of renal artery stenosis is dependent on angiotensin II. A decline in renal function following introduction of an

ACE inhibitor suggests a diagnosis of renovascular disease. Renal ischaemia should also be suspected in patients with refractory hypertension or unexplained renal impairment who have other evidence of atherosclerosis.

Renal arteriography remains the principal method of defining the anatomical lesion, although non-invasive techniques such as duplex ultrasonography (p. 66), magnetic resonance imaging (MRI) scanning (p. 66) and differential isotope renography before and after captopril administration (p. 93) may also provide useful information.

Considerable attention has been directed towards the management of patients with renal artery stenosis on the basis that correction of the arterial lesion, either by surgical revascularization or percutaneous transluminal renal angioplasty, may provide the potential to improve both blood pressure control and overall renal function.

PRIMARY ALDOSTERONISM (CONN'S SYNDROME)

Primary aldosteronism is thought to be present in 0.05–2% of hypertensive patients. It usually presents with moderate to severe hypertension, which may be resistant to treatment, and is characteristically accompanied by hypokalaemia, low plasma renin activity, and increased aldosterone excretion. If severe, the hypokalaemia may cause muscle pain and weakness, palpitations and polyuria. Metabolic alkalosis and relative hypernatraemia also occur.

The commonest causes are a unilateral aldosterone-producing adenoma or bilateral adrenal hyperplasia. Rarer causes are an aldosterone-producing adrenocortical carcinoma or gluocorticoid-suppressible hyperaldosteronism.

Screening for primary aldosteronism should be undertaken in patients with hypertension and spontaneous hypokalaemia, or severe hypokalaemia that is provoked by diuretics.

The diagnosis is confirmed by finding:

- hypokalaemia with an inappropriately raised 24-hour urinary potassium (greater than 30 mmol/24 h) in the presence of a low plasma potassium
- low plasma renin activity (upright plasma renin activity of less than 3.0 mg/ml/h)
- increased aldosterone levels in the presence of sodium loading: failure of urinary or plasma aldosterone levels to be suppressed after a high sodium diet for five days
- normal glucocorticoid levels.

Renin and aldosterone levels are affected by many antihypertensive drugs, particularly spironolactone and ACE inhibitors, and these should be stopped prior to measurement of these hormones.

If a diagnosis of hyperaldosteronism is confirmed, investigations should be performed to distinguish unilateral from bilateral adrenal disease. This is important to determine the appropriate therapy. Adrenal computed tomography (CT) scanning will localize 70–90% of adenomas. MRI may provide superior resolution for small adenomas (less than 1 cm diameter). If a unilateral lesion is found, surgical removal corrects hypokalaemia and often reduces blood pressure. In cases of bilateral adrenal hyperplasia, the hypokalaemia and hypertension usually respond to treatment with spironolactone or amiloride.

PHAEOCHROMOCYTOMA

Phaeochromocytomas, arising from chromaffin cells of the sympatho-adrenal system, account for fewer than 0.1% of cases of hypertension. However, diagnosis is important because the hypertension is potentially curable by resection of the tumour, and the prognosis without surgery is poor.

Phaeochromocytoma occurs equally in both sexes, and presents most commonly in middle age. About 10% are familial, of which 70% are bilateral. They may occur in the autosomal dominant multiple endocrine neoplasia syndromes MEN 2a (phaeochromocytoma, hyperparathyroidism and medullary carcinoma of the thyroid) and MEN 2b (in addition to features of 2a patients have a marfanoid appearance and intestinal ganglioneuromatosis). Phaeochromocytoma also occurs in neurofibromatosis and von Hippel–Lindau syndrome (p. 151). Most phaeochromocytomas secrete adrenaline and noradrenaline. Tumours arising in extra-adrenal tissue often secrete only noradrenaline because phenylethanolamine-*N*-methyl transferase, the enzyme that converts noradrenaline to adrenaline, is activated, primarily in the adrenal medulla and brain tissue.

Patients typically present with sustained or paroxysmal hypertension that is often resistant to treatment. Hypertension may be exacerbated by β-blockers, which allow unopposed α-adrenoreceptor stimulation. Severe headache, excessive sweating, anxiety, palpitations, tremor, heat intolerance, chest or abdominal pain, dizziness, seizures, nausea and bradycardia have all been described.

The diagnosis requires a high clinical suspicion followed by the demonstration of inappropriately high circulating urinary or plasma levels of catecholamines or their metabolites. Metabolites are usually measured as VMA (normal range up to 35 μmol/d) or metanephrines (normal range up to 5 μmol/d). Urinary catecholamines are now favoured in many centres as they are less prone to dietary interference. The level of urinary free noradrenaline is normally less than 290 nmol/d and adrenaline less than 90 nmol/d. Plasma catecholamine levels can be of value, particularly if measured while the patient is hypertensive, or during an episode when the patient is symptomatic.

Localization of the tumour is required prior to surgical resection; 90% of tumours are adrenal and can be identified by CT scanning (over 90% sensitivity) or MRI (almost 100% sensitivity). Extra-adrenal tumours are usually demonstrated by whole body MRI. In difficult cases ^{123}I-MIBG (meta-iodobenzylguanidine, a guanethidine analogue that localizes to chromaffin cells) can be used to visualize lesions. Venous sampling for catecholamine levels can also be used to confirm that a tumour is the source of catecholamine secretion.

PREGNANCY

Stroke volume and heart rate increase during pregnancy, leading to increased cardiac output. Blood pressure usually falls during early pregnancy as a result of reduced peripheral resistance, but rises towards non-pregnant values by term.

Pregnancy-induced hypertension has been defined as diastolic pressure of 110 mmHg or above, or two readings of 90 mmHg or above after 20 weeks in a previously normotensive woman (Davey and MacGillivray, 1988). Diastolic blood pressure above 90 mmHg before 20 weeks suggests chronic hypertension, which is confirmed if hypertension persists after delivery. Pre-eclampsia is defined as pregnancy-induced hypertension and proteinuria greater than 300 mg/24 h. It may lead, often rapidly, to the HELLP syndrome, characterized by:

- **h**aemolysis
- **el**evated liver function tests
- low **p**latelet count.

Pre-eclampsia affects about 5% of primiparae, but is less common in subsequent pregnancies.

DIABETES

Hypertension is commoner in diabetics than in non-diabetics. Possible reasons include:

- obesity

- increased sympathetic nervous stimulation and catecholamine production
- diabetic nephropathy
- insulin resistance and the associated hyperinsulinaemia.
  In patients with nephropathy, blood pressure control slows the decline in renal function. ACE inhibitors appear to have a specific renal protective effect that is independent of their antihypertensive action.

Implications for treatment of investigations

In patients with essential hypertension, antihypertensive therapy can achieve a significant reduction in stroke and coronary events, together with a reduction in both cardiovascular and overall mortality. The beneficial effect of antihypertensive therapy on renal function in acute severe (accelerated) hypertension is also well established. However, there is little evidence that treatment of mild and moderate hypertension prevents renal damage, although antihypertensive treatment does delay the development of renal insufficiency in diabetic patients.

The benefits of blood pressure control on renal function in patients with underlying renal disease are more clearly defined. Regardless of the cause of renal disease, once renal function is compromised a steady progressive fall in glomerular filtration rate is usually observed. The mechanisms underlying this progressive loss of renal function are unclear. Increased glomerular pressure (as a result of increased systemic blood pressure, or efferent arteriolar constriction as a consequence of increased angiotensin II levels), glomerular protein leakage, and lipid abnormalities have all been implicated. Whatever the mechanism, several studies (Brazy and Fitzwilliam, 1990) have shown that reduction of systemic blood pressure attenuates this progression. Furthermore, cardiovascular disease is the commonest cause of mortality in patients with chronic renal failure, and is likely to reflect an increased incidence of a number of factors including hypertension, lipid abnormalities, glucose intolerance and haemodynamic abnormalities (including left ventricular hypertrophy). Of these, hypertension is probably the most susceptible to treatment.

Thiazide diuretics, β-blockers, ACE inhibitors and calcium antagonists are all effective in reducing blood pressure in patients with early renal damage. The effects of these agents on lipid and glucose metabolism and both systemic and intraglomerular haemodynamic abnormalities should be taken into account when prescribing antihypertensive therapy for patients with renal disease. ACE inhibitors and calcium-channel blockers do not modify glucose or lipid metabolism, and have a favourable effect on LVA. These agents also have a potentially nephroprotective effect by reducing the increased renal vascular resistance that is typically associated with hypertension.

ACE inhibitors have the additional advantage of producing a fall in proteinuria in patients with both diabetic and non-diabetic renal disease. They should, however, be introduced with caution as they can reduce renal blood flow and precipitate acute renal failure, particularly in the presence of renal artery stenosis, by both reducing systemic blood pressure and interfering with intrarenal mechanisms for maintaining glomerular perfusion.

References

Brazy, P.C. and Fitzwilliam, J.F. (1990) Progressive renal disease: role of race and antihypertensive medications. *Kid. Int.*, **37**, 1113–19.

Davey, D.A. and MacGillivray, I. (1988) The classification and definition of the hypertensive disorders of pregnancy. *Am. J. Obstet. Gynecol.*, **158**, 892–8.

Further reading

Bouloux, P.-M. and Fakeeh, M. (1995) Investigation of phaeochromocytoma. *Clin. Endocrinol.*, **43**, 657–64.

Lewin, A., Blaufox, D., Castle, H. *et al.* (1985) Apparent prevalence of curable hypertension in the hypertension detection and follow up program. *Arch. Intern. Med.*, **145**, 424–7.

Whelton, P.K. and Klag, M.J. (1989) Hypertension as a risk factor for renal disease. *Hypertension*, **13**, 119–27.

Working group on renovascular hypertension (1987) Detection, evaluation, and treatment of renovascular hypertension. *Arch. Intern. Med.*, **147**, 820–9.

Young, W.F., Hogan, M.J., Klee, G.G. *et al.* (1990) Primary aldosteronism: diagnosis and treatment. *Mayo Clin. Proc.*, **65**, 96–110.

Pregnancy

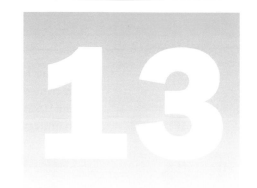

Lukas Foggensteiner

Renal disorders in pregnancy are relatively common and range from the benign, such as urinary tract infections, to rare events such as acute renal failure. Pre-eclampsia and eclampsia also have important renal manifestations. The investigation and management of renal problems in pregnancy follow the same general principles as in any other patient but there are certain physiological peculiarities of the pregnant woman that must be appreciated before many observations and test results can be meaningfully interpreted.

Normal renal and cardiovascular physiology of pregnancy

HAEMODYNAMIC CHANGES IN PREGNANCY

The profound haemodynamic changes seen in pregnancy are well described but their underlying causes remain obscure. Cardiac output is seen to rise very early and usually reaches a plateau at the end of the first trimester when it is raised by about 1.5 l/min. It then remains elevated for the duration of the pregnancy. This is associated with a rise in both resting pulse rate, of about 15 beats per minute, and left ventricular stroke volume. In the third trimester marked postural changes in cardiac output may be noted. In the supine position, compression of the inferior vena cava by the gravid uterus impedes venous return to the right heart causing a fall in cardiac output. Such postural phenomena confounded many early studies in the cardiovascular physiology of pregnancy before they were recognized and this must be borne in mind when reading some of the older literature.

The blood pressure in a normal pregnancy undergoes some well defined changes. Systolic blood pressure remains fairly constant throughout and should be the same at term as at baseline, usually less than 120 mmHg.

Diastolic blood pressure, on the other hand, falls progressively during the first trimester reaching a nadir at about 20 weeks. Typically the fall will be about 15 mmHg. A gradual rise towards baseline values is then seen in the remainder of the pregnancy.

GLOMERULOFILTRATION AND RENAL BLOOD FLOW

Significant changes in renal function are seen in the normal pregnancy. Studies of inulin clearance to measure the glomerular filtration rate (GFR) and paraaminohippuric acid clearance to measure effective renal plasma flow (ERPF) in pregnancy have shown marked increases in both of about 20–50% by the end of the first trimester. The fall in GFR and ERPF towards the end of pregnancy described in the past was due to measurements being taken in the supine position, where vascular compression reduces renal blood flow. The consequence of the raised GFR is a fall in serum creatinine to below prepregnancy levels. It is therefore important to realize that serum creatinine values in the normal range may represent pathological renal function. The creatinine should rarely rise above 80 µmol/l or the urea above 4.6 mmol/l.

Measurement of GFR can be performed in pregnancy by 24-hour urine collection for creatinine clearance estimation, although errors are particularly frequent in pregnancy when urinary frequency and nocturia can make accurate collection difficult. The alternative is to perform ^{51}Cr-labelled EDTA (ethylenediaminetetraacetic acid) clearance but the radiation exposure is rarely justified.

RENAL TRACTS IN PREGNANCY

Renal tract dilatation has long been recognized as a normal phenomenon in pregnancy. Dilatation of the renal calyces, pelves and ureters has been demonstrated to be present by ultrasound and intravenous pyelogram in about 90% of women in the third trimester. The ultrasound appearances are generally similar to those of ureteric obstruction but intravenous pyelograms reveal no evidence of delayed renal emptying. The cause of this phenomenon is almost certainly multifactorial, including hormonal effects on smooth muscle and direct compression of the ureters by the gravid uterus at the pelvic brim. In fact the ureteric dilatation stops abruptly just beyond this point. The right kidney and ureter are usually more dilated than the left, probably due to the slight dextrorotation of the normal uterus. Bladder capacity increases during pregnancy, but no significant post-micturition volume is seen. Ureteric reflux is only rarely demonstrable, although a diminution in the frequency of ureteric peristalsis is the norm. Most women will have some associated symptoms of frequency and nocturia during pregnancy. Although the changes in the renal tracts are of no consequence to the majority of women, it is possible that they account for the notable increase in cystitis and pyelonephritis seen.

Renal investigations in pregnancy

PROTEINURIA AND HAEMATURIA

Proteinuria in pregnancy is usually due to pre-eclampsia or eclampsia. Other renal causes, such as diabetic nephropathy, glomerulonephritides including minimal change nephropathy, renal amyloid and tropical diseases such as malaria or schistosomiasis, have all been described, however.

Screening for proteinuria is best done by means of a urine stick test. The test strips contain tetrabromophenol and a buffer to keep the pH of the strip around 3. Tetrabromophenol will change colour on exposure to proteins in an acid environment, and the colour change can then be read off the test strip. These tests are very sensitive to protein concentration as long as the urine is not very alkaline, and may detect as little as 150 mg/l of protein. Proteinuria on dipstick testing must always be followed up with a 24-hour urinary protein measurement. Protein excretion is usually below 200 mg/24 hours in fit gravidae, and rates above about 500 mg/24 hours are definitely abnormal. Excretion of more than 2 g/24 hours is almost always indicative of glomerular pathology, and rates in excess of 20 g/24 hours can occasionally occur. When evaluating proteinuria in pregnancy other features of pre-eclampsia should be sought. Haematuria must be looked for as it is not a feature of pre-eclampsia and generally indicates another pathology. Nephrotic syndrome in pregnancy can be treated conventionally with diuretics and intravenous albumin, although the latter is of unproven benefit.

Most urine stick tests include an assay for haematuria that is highly sensitive but may give false-positive results in the presence of free haemoglobin or myoglobin. If dipstick testing reveals haemoglobin, then urine microscopy must be performed. More than two red blood cells per high powered field is abnormal. In addition, microscopy allows the presence of red cell casts, indicating glomerular pathology, and white blood cells, indicating infection or other inflammatory processes to be seen. Possible causes include glomerulonephritides such as IgA nephropathy, systemic lupus erythematosus (SLE), renal calculi or, particularly in endemic areas, infections such as schistosomiasis.

RADIOLOGY IN PREGNANCY

Radiographic studies may be necessary in the pregnant patient with loin pain, haematuria, anuria or renal failure. The risk to the fetus of radiological procedures is generally lower than is popularly perceived, but must nevertheless always be balanced against the usefulness of the information obtained.

The risk of radiation exposure is very dependent on fetal maturity and can be divided into several phases. In the first two weeks after fertilization, the embryo is insensitive to teratogenic effects but sensitive to the lethal effects of radiation, which may lead to embryonic death and abortion. Diagnostic radiology should be avoided completely during this period. From 14 to 70 days' gestation, organogenesis takes place and the fetus is sensitive to the teratogenic effects of radiation. The degree of risk is proportional to the fetal dose received and is probably lower than one malformation per 2000 births for every cGy of radiation exposure. From 70 to 120 days' gestation, the teratogenic risks are much smaller and are mainly of central nervous system malformation. From 120 days' gestation to term the main concern is the unproven possibility of increased childhood malignancy. A plain abdominal radiograph results in a fetal radiation dose of about 0.05 cGy, an intravenous pyelogram about 0.3 cGy depending on the number of films taken, an abdominal and pelvic CT (computed tomography) about 2.2 cGy, but a renal CT only 0.025 cGy.

Renal ultrasound and magnetic resonance imaging (MRI) are thought to be completely safe. In general, radiation exposure in pregnancy should be kept to a minimum but may be justified in certain circumstances. The patient with loin pain and haematuria in whom one suspects renal calculi should initially have a renal ultrasound. A plain abdominal radiograph may be justified in the third trimester to demonstrate ureteric stones. If loin pain and renal impairment or anuria are present and renal tract obstruction is suspected, then an intravenous pyelogram will be necessary. Fluoroscopy will then be needed during the placement of ureteric or percutaneous stents.

Isotope studies such as ^{99m}Tc-DTPA (diethylenetriamine pentaacetic acid) scanning cause significantly less radiation exposure than an intravenous pyelogram and can give useful information about renal outflow obstruction, renal blood flow and tubular function. They may be justified in severe progressive renal impairment.

RENAL BIOPSY IN PREGNANCY

Renal biopsy is quite feasible in pregnancy but is rarely indicated because so few renal diseases have any specific treatments. In particular, biopsy has not proved useful in the diagnosis of pre-eclampsia and is not indicated in this context. In the case of nephrotic syndrome, minimal change nephropathy can be safely treated empirically with a course of steroids. Rare cases of rapidly progressive glomerulonephritis may require renal biopsy prior to immunosuppressive treatment. The outlook for the pregnancy in such cases is poor.

Renal conditions in pregnancy

HYPERTENSIVE DISORDERS

Given the importance of monitoring the blood pressure in pregnancy (and outside pregnancy for that matter), the practitioner should be aware of some of the practical problems that may be encountered. When measuring blood pressure with a mercury sphygmomanometer it is important to ensure that all observers use the same Korotkoff phase. In the UK, Korotkoff phase 5 (when the sounds disappear completely) is generally used and may be more reproducible than Korotkoff phase 4 (muffling of the sounds). In some young women, however, there is no Korotkoff phase 5 (sounds never disappear) and phase 4 must be used. The difference between the two phases may be up to 5 mmHg.

Another consideration is the use of appropriately sized cuffs. Blood pressure may be significantly overestimated in obese women if measured with a normal sized cuff. The woman's posture is also of consequence. In early pregnancy there is little difference in the values found for the systolic and diastolic pressure respectively, whether they are measured with the patient standing, sitting, supine or laterally recumbent. As the gravid uterus enlarges, however, it compresses the inferior vena cava and aorta at the pelvic brim when the patient is supine, causing a drop in venous return to the heart and a fall in systolic and diastolic blood pressure, usually by about 10%. Some may have falls in blood pressure of up to 30% with symptoms of hypotension. It is therefore important that the blood pressure is always measured in the same position, usually sitting or semirecumbent.

The definition of hypertension in pregnancy is, of necessity, arbitrary, and the blood pressure of any individual must be assessed in the context of prepregnancy levels if known. Usually, diastolic pressures above 75 mmHg in the second trimester, and above 85 mmHg in the third trimester, are considered suspicious. Equally important, though, is to recognize the significance of a rise in blood pressure. A diastolic pressure of 80 mmHg may be an indicator of pre-eclampsia in a woman with previous pressures of

Table 13.1

Hypertension in pregnancy

Class	Type of hypertension
I	Pre-eclampsia or eclampsia
II	Essential or chronic hypertension unrelated to pregnancy
III	Pre-eclampsia or eclampsia superimposed on chronic hypertension
IV	Transient or late hypertension of pregnancy with no other features of pre-eclampsia or eclampsia
V	Unclassified causes of hypertension

Source: American College of Obstetricians and Gynecologists.

50 mmHg. A diastolic incremental rise of 25 mmHg during pregnancy is considered abnormal.

Numerous classifications have been proposed for hypertension in pregnancy and the literature abounds with confusing and ill-defined terms. The classification produced by the American College of Obstetricians and Gynecologists (Working Group on High Blood Pressure in Pregnancy) is one of the most practical (Table 13.1).

Investigation usually involves hospital admission for careful and repeated measurement of blood pressure and to confirm hypertension. Continuous ambulatory blood pressure measurement has been advocated but often proves impractical. It is then important to distinguish pre-eclampsia from other causes of hypertension, as the management may be quite different. The time course of the hypertension is important to note. Elevated blood pressure in the first trimester usually reflects chronic hypertension and rarely pre-eclampsia.

PRE-ECLAMPSIA AND ECLAMPSIA

The syndrome of pre-eclampsia is by far the most common cause of hypertension and renal dysfunction in pregnancy. It is characterized clinically by the development of hypertension in the second half of pregnancy associated with oedema and proteinuria. Excessive weight gain is an early sign. Initially patients may be asymptomatic, but the condition may progress to multi-organ failure and fetoplacental damage. The development of neurological signs such as hyper-reflexia heralds the development of fitting and eclampsia.

The frequency of this condition in primigravidae lies between 0.7% and 3% depending on the diagnostic criteria used. Risk factors include first pregnancies, maternal history, multiple pregnancies, chronic hypertension and pre-existing renal dysfunction. Chronic hypertension imparts a three- to fivefold increase in the risk of pre-eclampsia, and the combination of renal impairment and hypertension doubles this.

The kidney is usually involved in pre-eclampsia, with proteinuria being a common feature. Increased renal sodium retention and nephrotic range proteinuria in addition to extrarenal endothelial cell damage lead to the oedema of the condition. A fall in the GFR is seen less frequently, but renal failure can develop. Renal biopsy is rarely indicated but when performed reveals a characteristic swelling of glomerular endothelial cells and the deposition of dense amorphous fibrin-derived material on the endothelial side of the basement membrane, which has been described as 'glomerular endotheliosis'.

Derangement of coagulation function is a major feature of the condition, and activation of intravascular coagulation may be seen. This is thought to be largely responsible for the end-organ damage seen in the lungs, liver, central nervous system (CNS) and kidney. Localized regions of cerebral anoxia due to small vessel thrombosis and small CNS haemorrhages are responsible for the fitting that defines the progression to 'full blown' eclampsia.

There is no specific test for pre-eclampsia and the condition remains a syndrome that is diagnosed if certain clinical or biochemical features are present. Specific diagnostic criteria have been proposed, and these are useful for epidemiological studies; but they are less useful for the practitioner concerned with the individual patient. The presence of two or more of the classically described clinical features of hypertension, oedema and protein-uria make the diagnosis likely, but these criteria alone have a low specificity. Certain biochemical and haematalogical investigations (Table 13.2) are often useful in strengthening the diagnosis, but none are specific in themselves.

Biochemical features	Haematological features
Hyperuricaemia	Deranged liver function tests
Thrombocytopenia	Raised plasma Von Willbrand factor
Proteinuria	Increased plasma fibronectin
Hypoalbuminaemia	Fall in plasma antithrombin III
Fall in glomerular filtration rate	Increased plasma fibrin degradation products
Proteinuria and hypocalciuria	Increased haematocrit

Table 13.2
Biochemical and haematological features of pre-eclampsia

Parameters of fetal health must also be taken into account as pre-eclampsia is a systemic condition that has a profound effect on the fetoplacental unit. When significant liver impairment is present, HELLP syndrome (haemolytic anaemia, elevated liver function tests and low platelets) may develop. HELLP syndrome is also caused by acute viral or drug-induced hepatitis, thrombotic thrombocytopenic purpura (TTP) or haemolytic uraemic syndrome (HUS), all of which can cause renal failure and form the main differential diagnoses in this context.

Of particular concern to the nephrologist are patients with pre-existing hypertension and/or renal disease, who are at high risk. Such patients should be carefully monitored with regular blood pressure measurement and urinalysis.

Treatment of pre-eclampsia is based on the fact that complete resolution of the condition usually occurs soon after delivery. The strategy is thus to maintain the pregnancy to such a time when delivery is deemed safe, usually around 34 weeks. The development of worsening coagulation defects, renal failure or neurological signs heralding eclampsia may force delivery to be induced early in the interests of the health of the mother. Hypertension is treated pharmacologically (see below).

CHRONIC HYPERTENSION

Pre-existing hypertension should ideally be treated before conception, but it is often only first detected when the blood pressure is measured in the first trimester. As mentioned above, it results in an increased risk of developing pre-eclampsia and patients should therefore be promptly treated and carefully monitored.

TRANSIENT HYPERTENSION OF PREGNANCY

This develops in the second half of pregnancy but has no other features of pre-eclampsia. Pre-eclampsia will develop in a proportion of patients, while in others the hypertension runs a benign course and resolves after delivery, although it is associated with essential hypertension in later life. Whether it represents an early form of pre-eclampsia is a matter of debate.

MISCELLANEOUS CAUSES OF HYPERTENSION IN PREGNANCY

Other causes of hypertension are rare but should be borne in mind. Phaeochromocytoma is known to occur in gravidae and has a very high fatality rate if unrecognized; it can be successfully treated pharmacologically.

Urinary vanillylmandelic acid (VMA) measurements should therefore always be made in severe hypertension. Electrolytes should be checked with the possibility of Conn's syndrome in mind, and renal artery stenosis or primary glomerulonephritis should not be forgotten as possibilities.

TREATMENT OF HYPERTENSION IN PREGNANCY

The practice of when and how to treat hypertension in pregnancy varies from place to place. Many begin treatment when diastolic pressure exceeds 90 mmHg, but most would agree that treatment is indicated when diastolic pressure exceeds 100 mmHg. The purpose of treatment in pre-eclampsia is to prevent the development of cerebral haemorrhage, which is a major cause of death in this condition. It should be noted that there is no evidence that treating hypertension alters the natural history of the other features of established pre-eclampsia, but the treatment of chronic or transient hypertension may retard the development of pre-eclampsia.

The repertoire of antihypertensive drugs with established safety profiles in pregnancy is relatively small but usually sufficient. In the UK, methyldopa is the drug of first choice, followed by β-blockers. Calcium antagonists, especially nifedepine, are also coming into more common use and appear safe and effective. Oral hydralazine is favoured in the USA and is safe. Angiotensin-converting enzyme (ACE) inhibitors are contraindicated as they are associated with intra-uterine death, oligohydramnios and fetal renal failure. For severe hypertension, intravenous treatment with hydralazine is safe and effective, as is labetolol, although there is less experience with the latter. Sodium nitroprusside has been used but can cause fetal cyanide poisoning. Intensive monitoring is necessary when any intravenous agents are used.

Aspirin, which inhibits thromboxane synthesis and thus reduces platelet aggregation, has been investigated as a potential agent for reducing the incidence of pre-eclampsia in high-risk populations. Despite early promising *in vitro* and *in vivo* results, recent large trials have shown no benefit (CLASP Collaborative Group, 1994).

URINARY TRACT INFECTIONS

Urinary tract infection (UTI) is one of the commonest medical problems that a pregnant woman may encounter, ranging from relatively benign cystitis to potentially life-threatening pyelonephritis. The majority of symptomatic infections occur in subjects with asymptomatic bacteriuria. The prevalence of asymptomatic bacteriuria in pregnancy is 4–7%, which is no different from that in non-pregnant sexually active women of similar age.

However the chances of this subgroup developing a symptomatic UTI during pregnancy are high, being of the order of 40%. The overall incidence of UTIs in pregnancy is therefore around 2%, although treating asymptomatic bacteriuria may reduce this. Diabetic women are particularly at risk.

The renal tract dilatation with reduced ureteric peristaltic activity and vesico-ureteric reflux that occur in pregnancy are probably largely responsible for the high rate of UTI, but other factors, such as the glycosuria and aminoaciduria, may be contributory. Screening for asymptomatic bacteriuria is usually performed in early pregnancy and treated if found. Such prophylactic treatment has been shown to reduce the risk of pyelonephritis in later pregnancy. The incidence of simple cystitis, however, is little altered.

Screening has been performed using leucocyte and bacteria nitrite urine stick tests, but these have a low sensitivity, particularly in pregnancy. Nitrate to nitrite conversion by bacteria requires urine to be in the bladder for about four hours, which may not occur with the urinary frequency seen in pregnancy. Furthermore, asymptomatic bacteria may be present without significant numbers of leucocytes in the urine. Contamination of the sticks with vaginal leucocytes may also result in false-positives. For these reasons, culture of a mid-stream urine specimen is preferred. This test is highly sensitive but not very specific owing to the frequent vulval contamination of the specimen. Careful collection is essential. If it is imperative to make a diagnosis, e.g. in a woman with an unexplained fever, and mid-stream urine culture is felt to be ambiguous, then suprapubic urine aspiration can be safely performed.

The treatment of UTIs in pregnancy differs from that of non-pregnant patients only in the choice of drugs, which must have an established safety record. Simple cystitis should be confirmed by culture (many pregnant women with dysuria and frequency will have sterile urine) and treated with oral antibiotics. Suspected pyelonephritis should be treated promptly with intravenous antibiotics before culture results are available. There is a high recurrence rate of pyelonephritis, and treatment courses of four to five weeks are recommended. The importance of treating asymptomatic bacteriuria and symptomatic UTIs is underlined by studies that have suggested that both are associated with fetal growth retardation and prematurity (Romero, Oyarzun, Mazor *et al.* 1989).

ACUTE RENAL FAILURE IN PREGNANCY

Renal impairment developing in pregnancy is unusual and renal failure requiring dialysis fortunately very rare. In the past, septic abortion and postpartum haemorrhage were the commonest causes. The frequency of these has fallen dramatically in developed countries; the incidence of acute renal failure requiring dialysis is less than one case per 10 000 births in the West. Pre-eclampsia and eclampsia now account for about half of cases. Antepartum or postpartum haemorrhage leading to shock and acute tubular necrosis or renal cortical necrosis account for about one-third of cases. Septicaemia, usually due to pyelonephritis, accounts for most of the rest. Other causes are very rare but several merit mention.

Rapidly progressive glomerulonephritis, lupus nephritis and various forms of systemic vasculitis have all been described as causing acute renal failure in pregnancy. Presentation may resemble that of pre-eclampsia, with proteinuria, hypertension and oedema. The presence of haematuria and red cell casts should be sought as this is highly suggestive of glomerulonephritis. Serological markers for SLE and vasculitis may prove very helpful in this context. Renal biopsy may be considered if renal failure is advancing rapidly.

Obstructive uropathy is well described in pregnancy and can progress to renal failure if untreated. It typically presents with loin pain and renal impairment, but not proteinuria. Bilateral ureteric obstruction due to renal papillary necrosis or renal calculi has been described, in which case haematuria may be present, but usually no such obstruction is seen and compression of the ureters between the uterus and pelvic brim is invoked. Diagnosis may be difficult due to the physiological dilatation of the renal tracts, which makes ultrasound of little use. An investigation such as an intravenous pyelogram or a DTPA scan is necessary to demonstrate functional ureteric obstruction. The diagnosis is important to make as the placement of percutaneous ureteric stents usually relieves the obstruction and reverses the renal failure.

Idiopathic postpartum renal failure occurs suddenly up to four weeks after an apparently normal and uncomplicated delivery. It has been called 'the postpartum haemolytic uraemic syndrome' as it shares many features with this and with thrombotic thrombocytopenic purpura. Maternal mortality is high and renal recovery rare.

Acute fatty liver of pregnancy is associated with renal failure in about 60% of cases but dialysis is required only rarely. This condition is primarily one of hepatic failure, but hepatorenal syndrome or acute renal failure due to hypovolaemia are frequent consequences.

The investigation and management of acute renal failure in pregnancy is much the same as in the non-pregnant (Chapter 9). Both haemodialysis and peritoneal dialysis have been successfully employed, but the former may be difficult in late pregnancy.

Fetal survival in the context of acute renal failure and dialysis in pregnancy is possible, but fetal mortality is substantial.

RENAL TUBULAR DYSFUNCTION

The rise in GFR results in a huge increase in work for the renal tubules, which have to reabsorb proportionally more solute. Certain substances exceed their renal tubular reabsorbtive threshold and appear in the urine, e.g. amino acids, nicotinic acid and folate. This is rarely of significance except perhaps in the very malnourished. The appearance of glucose in the urine in pregnancy can cause some diagnostic confusion. Two mechanisms account for the glycosuria, namely an unexplained reduced renal threshold for glucose and the increased filtered load. Glycosuria in pregnancy is almost the norm and therefore diabetics must not rely on urine tests, nor can urine dipsticks be reliably used as a screening measure. Capillary blood or plasma glucose levels should be employed instead.

PRE-EXISTING RENAL DISEASE AND PREGNANCY

Previous mention has been made of the increased risk of pre-eclampsia and eclampsia in gravidae with pre-existing renal disease. Such women run the additional risk of intrapartum worsening of renal function and increased incidence of fetal morbidity and mortality. In addition, fertility is related to the degree of renal impairment.

In general, the outcome of pregnancy in moderate to severe renal disease is relative to the degree of renal impairment rather than the precise renal diagnosis. As the degree of a woman's prepregnancy renal impairment increases, the rate of conception falls and the risk of hypertension and renal deterioration during pregnancy rises. Mild renal impairment with serum creatinine in the normal range has a good renal and obstetric prognosis. Up to 40% of women with moderate renal impairment and prepregnancy serum creatinine levels of 125–160 μmol/1 will suffer deterioration of renal function which is irreversible in about half. Prepregnancy serum creatinine levels of 160 μmol/1 or higher herald a worse prognosis, with over half the women suffering some irreversible impairment of renal function.

The main fetal complication in these groups is premature delivery, which is about six times the expected rate. With improving intensive care for newborns, however, the fetal survival is over 90%. Women with severe or dialysis-dependent renal failure have a low chance of conception and a high chance of early spontaneous abortion, with only 50% of fetuses surviving to term.

In general, if circumstances permit, women with moderate to severe renal impairment should be advised to await renal transplantation. Milder renal impairment poses more of a dilemma and an informed decision in the light of the patient's renal function, age, health and wishes should be sought. If pregnancy is desired, contraindicated drugs such as ACE inhibitors must be stopped and blood pressure brought under optimal control before conception. Haemoglobin levels and the calcium/phosphate balance should also be optimized. Once conception has occurred, careful follow-up by a renal physician and an obstetrician is mandatory.

PREGNANCY AND RENAL TRANSPLANTATION

Successful pregnancies after transplantation are now commonplace, and early concerns about immunosuppression therapy being a potential teratogenic risk have fortunately not been borne out. Outcome is related to prepregnancy renal function; when serum creatinine is < 180 μmol/l there is little risk of graft damage and fetal outcome is good, although hypertension is quite common. With worsening prepregnancy renal function, the risks of renal deterioration increase. The occasional patient will lose her renal graft and require dialysis during or soon after the pregnancy. Careful antenatal surveillance is therefore paramount, with frequent checks of renal function and strict control of blood pressure. Overall, the chance of a successful obstetric outcome is over 90%.

References

Clasp (Collaborative Low-dose Aspirin Study in Pregnancy) Collaborative Group (1994). A randomised trial of low-dose aspirin for the prevention and treatment of pre-eclampsia among 9364 pregnant women. *Lancet*, **343**, 619–29.

Romero, R., Oyarzun, E., Mazor, M. *et al.* (1989) Meta-analysis of the relationship between asymptomatic bacteriuria and pre-term delivery/low birth weight. *Gynecology*, **73**, 576–82.

Working Group on High Blood Pressure in Pregnancy (1990) National High Blood Pressure Education Program Working Group Report on High Blood Pressure in Pregnancy. *Am. J. Obstet. Gynecol.*, **163**, 1691.

Further reading

Broughton-Pipkin, F. (1995) The hypertensive disorders of pregnancy. *Br. Med. J.* **311**, 609–13.

Gallery, E.D. (1995) Hypertension in pregnancy. Practical management recommendations. *Drugs*, **49**(4), 555–62.

Jones, D.C. and Hayslett, J.P. (1996) Outcome of pregnancy in women with moderate or severe renal failure. *N. Engl. J. Med.*, **335**(4), 226–32.

Lindheimer, M.D. and Davidson, J.M. (eds), (1994) Renal disease in pregnancy. *Baillière's Clin. Obstet. Gynaecol*, **8**(2).

Robertson, E.D. (ed.). (1985) Renal disease in pregnancy. *Clin. Obstet. Gynecol*, **28**(2); 247–351.

Swanson, S.K., Hailman, R.L. and Eversman, W.G. (1995) Urinary tract stones in pregnancy. *Surg. Clin. North Am.*, **75**(1), 123–42.

Tan, J.S. and File, T.M. (1992) Treatment of bacteriuria in pregnancy. *Drugs*, **44**(6), 972–80.

Pediatric renal disease

14

Vikas Dharnidharka, Matthew Hand, Stephen Alexander and David Briscoe

Introduction

Renal disease is usually suspected in an infant or child when blood or protein is found on a routine urinalysis, or if decreased renal function is shown by routine blood chemistries. Any of these findings alarms the patient, the parents and the physician in charge of the patient, and often results in the performance of a large number of laboratory tests. While many of these tests will turn out to be normal, they do at least rule out serious conditions that might otherwise be overlooked. In this chapter we provide a systematic approach to the investigation of the more common renal diseases in children.

History and physical examination

A good history will guide the physician towards the correct diagnosis and will ultimately result in far fewer tests. Knowledge of a preceding or recurrent acute or chronic illness, weight gain and/or edema, changes in urine color and volume, aches and pains, skin rashes or joint pains will help in the provisional diagnosis of systemic disease resulting in acute nephritis or nephrosis. It is important to note any history of medication ingestion or recreational drug abuse, which is associated with acute or chronic interstitial nephritis. In addition, human immunodeficiency virus (HIV) nephropathy must be considered in the intravenous drug addict. In newborns, thorough knowledge of the pregnancy, prenatal ultrasound evaluation, birth history and invasive procedures (such as umbilical artery catheterization) will help in the diagnosis. Overall, a good history will help detect major or treatable problems while limiting the anxiety, energy and cost of a large number of unnecessary tests.

Physical examination should take into consideration height and weight percentiles and weight gain or loss. Significant chronic renal disease is usually associated with failure to thrive and developmental delay, whereas acute renal failure or acute nephrosis is usually associated with weight gain. Blood pressure should be assessed carefully on at least two separate occasions during the initial evaluation. Occasionally, physical examination will reveal evidence of a systemic disease, or may direct attention to the diagnosis. It is also necessary to consider dehydration as a factor in the disease process. Dehydration can be a cause of renal failure as well as a factor in the exacerbation of chronic renal failure.

Two important investigations that screen for patients who need more extensive investigation are:

- urinalysis
- serum urea and creatinine.

THE ABNORMAL URINALYSIS

A careful urinalysis is the most important tool in the evaluation of renal disease. Urine dipsticks are commonly used to screen the urine for evidence of leukocyturia, hematuria or proteinuria. Microscopic urinalysis will establish the characteristics of any cellular elements in the urine and may give hints about the nature of the underlying disease. In many of the glomerulonephritides, hematuria is accompanied by proteinuria and an abnormal urine sediment, with evidence of red blood cell casts and deformed red cells (classically spiculated) in the urine. In other renal diseases, hyaline, waxy or granular casts may be seen, or there may be evidence of crystalluria.

Hematuria is common and may originate from glomerular or nonglomerular sites, from the renal tubules, interstitium or lower tract (collecting systems, papilla, ureter and bladder). Hematuria may be the only finding in a patient with a urinary tract infection (UTI), or may be a subtle finding with a renal tumor or vascular lesion.

Proteinuria is more usually associated with diseases of glomerular origin and is considered a hallmark of many pediatric renal diseases. The child may be asymptomatic, or the proteinuria may be transient, such as in orthostatic proteinuria or in proteinuria associated with exercise or fever. On the other hand, even small amounts of proteinuria may be associated with significant underlying pathology.

SERUM UREA AND CREATININE

Renal function can be reliably assessed by evaluation of the serum urea and creatinine. Serum urea fluctuates such that it may increase dramatically in dehydrated states, in excessive nitrogen intake and in catabolic states. In contrast, the serum creatinine does not fluctuate as much and is a good indicator of renal function. A simple screen measurement of the serum creatinine is therefore a good reflection of the glomerular filtration rate. For instance, in our laboratory, a normally hydrated three-year-old should have a serum creatinine of less than 0.6 mg/dl (52 μmol/l). Thus, as a screen, if the serum creatinine is 1.2 mg/dl (105 μmol/l), we can predict that this represents a decrease in glomerular filtration rate of approximately 50%.

Urinary tract infections

UTIs are common in children, affecting at least 5% of girls and 2.5% of boys during childhood. While few children with recurrent UTIs progress to renal scarring, chronic pyelonephritis is still a major cause of end-stage renal disease and accounts for 15–20% of end-stage renal disease in adults. It is now established that high risk groups for progression to serious renal disease are:

- young children aged under five years with recurrent UTIs secondary to reflux nephropathy
- children with an underlying anatomical abnormality as a cause of reflux nephropathy (such as neuropathic/functional bladder disorders).

The presenting symptoms of UTIs are summarized in Table 14.1. In younger children, the symptoms of a UTI may be subtle. A high index of suspicion is necessary when evaluating a febrile neonate or infant. In general, a UTI should be considered in any child under five years of age with a fever. Indeed, UTIs may account for as much as 7.5% of all causes

Table 14.1
Presenting symptoms of UTIs

Infants	Older children	
	Cystitis	Pyelonephritis
Fever	Dysuria	High grade fever
Irritability	Low grade fever	Flank or loin pain
Poor feeding	Frequency, urgency	
Vomiting, diarrhea	Enuresis	

Table 14.2

Common causal organisms for UTIs in children

Gram-negative rods	Gram-positive cocci
Escherichia coli	Enterococcus
Klebsiella pneumoniae	Staphylococcus aureus
Proteus mirabilis	

of isolated fever in infants. Irritability, vomiting, diarrhea, poor feeding and a change in urinary pattern may all be symptoms of a UTI. Typically, patients are febrile, but they may also be asymptomatic.

In contrast, it is important to differentiate between cystitis and pyelonephritis in older children. High fever (> 38.5°C) and costovertebral angle tenderness suggest pyelonephritis. Suprapubic tenderness and mild symptoms of malaise favor a diagnosis of cystitis. Rarely, a child presents in hypertensive crisis with acute pyelonephritis.

The etiology of UTIs is summarized in Table 14.2. *E. coli* is the most common organism at all ages, *Enterococcus* is more usual in children under two years of age, and *Proteus mirabilis* infection is more common in boys under five years old.

INVESTIGATIONS

Urine culture remains the gold standard for diagnosis. In children, the method of collection is most important. Bag specimens have a high rate of contamination and are rarely useful unless culture negative. Older children may be able to provide a mid-stream sample after appropriate cleaning. In younger children, the preferred methods of collection include urethral catheterization or suprapubic aspiration. Rapid transport and plating are essential to avoid false-positive growth. Growth of $> 10^5$ colonies/ml of a single organism from a clean catch specimen or of $> 10^3$/ml from a catheter is strongly suggestive of a UTI. Any growth from a suprapubic specimen is considered positive.

Urinalysis alone is frequently helpful but not conclusive for the diagnosis of UTI, and microscopic analysis of the sediment may show the presence of white cells or bacteria. No one finding is highly sensitive or specific and any of these findings may be seen in other disorders. However, the combination of more than 10 white blood cells (WBC)/ml, bacteria by Gram stain, and a nitrite-positive urine has been found to yield positive and negative predictive values of > 88% and > 99%, respectively.

Overall, vesico-ureteral reflux (VUR) will be present in 30–40% of children with a documented UTI. VUR has been classified according to

Grade	Description of reflux
1	Reflux into ureter only
2	Ureter and collecting system involved; no dilatation
3	Mild calyceal blunting
4	More than 50% of calyces blunted; ureter tortuous
5	All calyes blunted; papillary insertions lost; ureter tortuous

*Modified from International Reflux Committee, Medical versus surgical treatment of primary vesicoureteral reflux; published by *Pediatrics*, 1981.

Table 14.3
International classification for grade of vesico-ureteral reflux (VUR)*

increasing order of severity into grades 1 through 5 (Table 14.3). VUR is partly genetically determined. It is present in 66% of offspring and 33% of siblings of patients with documented reflux.

Once a UTI has been documented, further investigations and treatment strategies depend on at least three factors:

- the age of the child
- a family history of UTIs or reflux nephropathy
- evaluation at time of presentation.

Age is an extremely important consideration. Renal parenchymal scarring due to reflux nephropathy occurs predominantly in the first five years of life. Thus, baseline investigations for young children should include one or more of the following:

- a renal ultrasound examination
- a voiding cystourethrogram
- a radionucleotide dimercaptosuccinic acid (DMSA) scan (or equivalent).

Since scarring may also occur even without reflux, some nephrologists obtain a renal scan in all young patients with a proven UTI. If performed at the time of active infection, renal ultrasound may reveal hydronephrosis, hydroureter or evidence of previous renal scarring.

After appropriate treatment has been completed, a follow-up urine culture should be confirmed to be negative. Current evidence suggests that adequate treatment of VUR includes frequent urine cultures while taking continuous low dose prophylactic antimicrobial therapy (usually grades 1 and 2), or surgical repair of the reflux (usually grades 4 and 5). Newer surgical techniques (such as the 'STING' procedure) have been developed and are effective at treating VUR. Future therapies include the development of vaccines to common organisms such as *E. coli*.

Hematuria and proteinuria

HEMATURIA

Hematuria is defined as more than five red blood cells per high power microscopic field on at least two of three consecutive urine specimens. The urine dipstick, which is the most common method used in diagnosis in most clinics, is too sensitive and can only be used as a screen. Upon referral, it is imperative first to perform microscopy to confirm diagnosis. Hemoglobinuria resulting from hemolytic anemias or myoglobinuria resulting from rhabdomyolysis may present as a positive dipstick for hematuria

The prevalence of hematuria in childhood is estimated at 0.4% of children aged between six and 12 years. A summary of the common etiologies of childhood hematuria is found in Table 14.4. It is clinically useful to distinguish between gross, painful hematuria (commonly due to urological causes), and painless hematuria, (suggestive of glomerular disease or a coagulation defect).

PROTEINURIA

In children, protein excretion varies with age and body surface area. There are three ways to document proteinuria:

- dipstick method
- random urine protein/creatinine ratio method
- specific quantitation.

Dipstick testing is accurate in a urine sample that is not too dilute. In general, if the specific gravity is > 1.015, a dipstick reading of $\geq$ 1+ is significant. Assessment of protein/creatinine ratios has been shown to be simple and accurate, avoids the problems of 24-hour urine collection, and correlates with more sensitive quantitative methods. In general, a protein/creatinine ratio of < 0.2 (mg/mg) is normal in children older than two years of age. A ratio of more than 3.0 (mg/mg) correlates with nephrotic range proteinuria. Nevertheless, the most sensitive way to quantify protein is by calculation of protein excretion in a timed 12 or 24-hour urine collection correlated to body surface area. For accuracy, the urine must be collected in the correct manner. Calculation of urine protein excretion is as follows:

- normal, ≤ 4 mg/m^2/h
- abnormal, > 4–40 mg/m^2/h
- nephrotic range proteinuria, > 40 mg/m^2/h.

A summary of common etiologies of proteinuria in childhood is given in Table 14.5.

INVESTIGATIONS OF HEMATURIA AND PROTEINURIA

Any preceding illness, such as an antecedent streptococcal infection or pharyngitis, recent gastrointestinal upset or diarrheal illness, or evidence of lower urinary tract symptoms, such as cystitis or renal colic, are likely to determine specific investigations in the initial evaluation. Attention should be given to recent rashes, arthralgias, arthritis, and fevers that occur in Henoch–Schönlein purpura or collagen vascular disease such as systemic lupus erythematosus (SLE). Obviously, it is important to note recent trauma, strenuous exercise or menstruation that may account for the hematuria. Pertinent history is critical in the screening for postinfectious glomerulonephritis or hemolytic uremic syndrome (HUS), as well as a simple UTI. A family member with hematuria, renal disease, renal calculi, polycystic kidney disease or collagen vascular disease renal failure will guide evaluation to that specific etiology. It is occasionally useful to assess urine specimens from parents and any other siblings, as this might help establish a diagnosis of benign familial hematuria (one needs to be cautious in this diagnosis). Upon physical examination, any mass detected requires radiological evaluation to determine whether it is a tumor, or a cystic or hydronephrotic kidney.

In order to plan appropriate investigations, it is important to be focused. Urinalysis and assessment of renal function is essential. A detailed urinalysis, enhanced by phase contrast, will help determine whether hematuria is of glomerular or non-glomerular origin. Some centers measure red cell size via automated counters. A urine culture is typically obtained at all initial visits. A renal ultrasound examination is a valuable investigation in the evaluation of non-glomerular hematuria to rule out structural abnormalities, renal calculi, renal vein thrombosis and tumors. In the event that all evaluations are normal, a work-up for hypercalciuria, and coagulopathies should be considered. A 24-hour calcium excretion or a spot urine calcium/creatinine ratio before and after modification of diet is fairly accurate (normal < 0.2 in mg/mg).

In the event that the child has hematuria associated with hypertension, edema and/or significant proteinuria, oliguria or decreased renal function,

Asymptomatic hematuria

1. Glomerulonephritis
   Evaluation should include antistreptolysin O (ASLO) titer, serum complement C_3 levels, IgA levels and erythrocyte sedimentation rate; differential diagnosis includes poststreptococcal glomerulonephritis and IgA nephropathy
2. Benign familial hematuria
   All family members should be screened for hematuria
3. Hypercalciuria
   Calcium/creatinine ratio (mg/mg) should be measured; if the ratio is greater than 0.3 on two consecutive occasions, reassess following test diets low and rich in calcium
4. Renal masses
   Renal ultrasound should be performed; differential diagnosis includes Wilms' tumor, cystic kidney disease and hydronephrosis
5. Sickle cell disease
   Persistent microscopic hematuria may be found; if symptomatic bleeding present consider diagnosis of acute papillary necrosis
6. Hereditary nephritis
   Usually associated with a family history of nephritis or deafness; audiogram should be performed to assess high tone deafness

Symptomatic hematuria

1. Urinary tract infection
   May need to rule out pyelonephritis or acute cystitis
2. Renal calculi
   Renal stones or nephrolithiasis is usually evident on renal ultrasound; when renal colic is present, intravenous pyelogram is the radiological examination of choice; CT scan may be indicated in complicated patients
3. Urethritis
   Gonococcal or non-gonococcal urethritis is suspected in high risk adolescents, or if any urethral discharge is noted on physical examination
4. Clot colic
   Renal colic may occur in the absence of renal calculi when clots of blood are passed down the genitourinary system; usual precipitating factors include trauma, but clot colic may occur spontaneously in cystic kidney diseases or may be associated with IgA nephropathy; investigations are the same as for urolithiasis.

Table 14.4 Differential diagnosis of hematuria

further laboratory evaluation is warranted at the initial encounter. This may include assessment of complete blood count, serum electrolytes, serum complement, streptozyme panel, IgA levels and throat culture. The results of these tests will help to rule out HUS and acute postinfectious glomerulonephritis. A follow-up evaluation of blood pressure, urine output and serum creatinine should be performed at frequent intervals. A renal ultrasound should be performed to rule out any anatomical abnormality.

Hematuria with hypertension, renal insufficiency and an active urinary sediment

1. Poststreptococcal glomerulonephritis

   Associated with a history of streptococcal infection, positive ASLO titer and/or streptozyme, low C_3 complement level; resolves with supportive care in almost all cases

2. IgA nephropathy

   Usually associated with a coincident upper respiratory tract infection and intermittent gross hematuria; investigations should include an IgA level, which is elevated in 50–60% cases; associated proteinuria and nephrotic syndrome are poor prognostic indicators

3. Focal and segmental glomerulosclerosis

   More commonly presents with associated proteinuria or nephrotic syndrome; serum complement levels are normal; poor prognosis if associated with renal insufficiency; represents a spectrum of clinical scenarios as a primary renal disease or as a secondary manifestation of a systemic disease

4. Rapidly progressive glomerulonephritis

   Requires immediate attention; investigations include early renal biopsy, serum antinuclear cytoplasmic antibodies (ANCA), antiglomerular basement membrane antibodies and serum complement levels; differential diagnosis includes ANCA-associated diseases (Chapters 4 and 7), systemic lupus erythematosus, Wegener's glomerulonephritis and poststreptococcal glomerulonephritis; treatment must be initiated early to avoid renal failure

5. Other nephritides

   Membranoproliferative and mesangial proliferative glomerulonephritis; diagnosis made following renal biopsy

6. Hemolytic uremic syndrome

   History of bloody diarrhea in most cases; diagnostic investigations include full blood count, blood smear, serum chemistries, serum lactate dehydrogenase or haptoglobin, and stool culture for *E coli* 0157

7. Renal vein thrombosis

   History of acute abdominal pain and hematuria, associated with neonatal umbilical catheters, inferior vena cava thrombosis in sick children and those with nephrotic syndrome, particularly membranous nephropathy; diagnosis by ultrasound and angiography; early intervention with thrombolytic agents within 24 hours may aid in resolution

Nephrotic syndrome

Nephrotic syndrome (NS) is defined as edema with massive proteinuria (greater than 40 mg/m^2/h), hypoalbuminemia and hyperlipidemia. In childhood, NS is usually idiopathic or congenital, although secondary NS due to infections (e.g. hepatitis, HIV, malaria and syphilis), malignancies (e.g. lymphoma) and drugs (e.g. penicillamine) is seen infrequently. Edema is the usual presenting symptom. This can be mild, usually localized to the

Table 14.5

Differential diagnosis of proteinuria

Isolated proteinuria
1. Orthostatic proteinuria
   Common in teenagers; assess proteinuria in morning and day-time urine
2. Persistent asymptomatic proteinuria
   Heterogeneous group of disorders; diagnosis made by exclusion; some progress to IgA nephropathy or focal and segmental glomerulosclerosis
3. Transient proteinuria
   Secondary to fever, exercise, cold, seizures; repeated sampling necessary to confirm transient nature of the proteinuria or temporal relationship to causative symptom

Nephrotic range proteinuria
1. Minimal change disease nephrotic syndrome
   Normal complement and renal function; responsive to steroid therapy
2. Focal segmental glomerulosclerosis
   Highly variable picture ranging from mild to severe proteinuria with active cellular sediment; usually progresses to end-stage renal disease
3. Membranoproliferative glomerulonephritis
   Variable picture; association with streptococcal infection or systemic diseases such as systemic lupus erythematosus; fluctuating complement levels common
4. Mesangioproliferative glomerulonephritis
   More benign course, similar to minimal change disease; usually responds to steroids
5. Membranous glomerulonephritis
   More common in adolescents secondary to viral hepatitis

Proteinuria with hematuria and active urinary sediment*
1. Postinfectious glomerulonephritis
2. IgA nephropathy
3. Systemic lupus erythematosus
4. Henoch–Schönlein nephritis
5. Hereditary nephritis
6. Interstitial nephritis

*See Table 14.4 and Chapter 3.

periorbital area or the feet. Hypertension and microscopic hematuria may be associated with NS. The incidence of NS has been estimated to be two to three new cases per 100 000 population per year, with a prevalence rate of 16/100 000/y. There is a slight male preponderance in early childhood.

Primary nephrotic syndrome has been classified into the following histological entities:

1. Minimal change disease (70–80% of cases)
2. Focal segmental glomerulosclerosis (5–10% of cases)
3. Membranoproliferative glomerulonephritis (5% of cases)
4. Mesangioproliferative glomerulonephritis (5% of cases)
5. Membranous glomerulonephropathy (2–3% of cases).

INVESTIGATIONS

A complete urinalysis is the best starting point. As described above, this yields important information not only on the degree of proteinuria, but also on the presence of associated hematuria or cellular casts. The urinary protein to creatinine ratio (in mg/mg as described above) or 24-hour urine protein excretion should be assessed for more definitive quantification. The selective protein index is the ratio of urinary IgG to urinary transferrin. An index of less than 0.1 is consistent with a diagnosis of minimal change disease. A less selective index suggests other causes. The blood tests used to assess the severity of nephrotic syndrome include: serum albumin; creatinine; cholesterol; and complement levels. Serum antinuclear antibodies (ANA), IgA, antistreptolysin O (ASLO), streptozyme, hepatitis serologies and HIV tests are necessary to confirm suspicions of underlying diseases such as SLE (ANA level) or poststreptococcal glomerulonephritis (ASLO). A renal ultrasound is usually not helpful.

NS is a relapsing disorder with a good overall prognosis. The majority of patients with minimal change disease can expect at least one relapse and the disease usually remits by adolescence. The incidence of minimal change disease in children is so high that, unless there are features to suggest otherwise, routine renal biopsy is not indicated. Most children are given a trial of steroid therapy. Other therapies used include cyclophosphamide, chlorambucil and cyclosporin.

Supportive treatment involves fluid and salt restriction during periods of edema. Fluids should be restricted to insensible losses plus urine output. This maintains euvolemia and minimizes interstitial fluid gain. Salt restriction is sometimes prescribed as aggressively as possible but a 'no added salt diet' is usually sufficient.

Failure to respond to steroid therapy after the first eight weeks is an indication for renal biopsy. Other indications for renal biopsy are active urinary sediment, renal insufficiency and/or hypertension, which are unusual in minimal change disease.

Hemolytic uremic syndrome

HUS comprises a triad of:

- microangiopathic non-immune hemolytic anemia
- thrombocytopenia
- uremia.

HUS is defined clinically by the presence, or absence or a prodrome of diarrhea (D+HUS or D–HUS, respectively). D+HUS typically occurs in epidemics and accounts for 90% of all cases. Causative organisms produce a *Shigella*-like toxin (SLT), also called a verotoxin (VLT). *E.coli* 0157:H7 has been found to be the most common organism in the USA associated with epidemic D+HUS. Other serotypes of *E. coli* and *Shigella dysenteriae* type 1 have also been associated with D+HUS mostly in countries outside the USA.

D–HUS may occur postpartum, post-bone marrow transplantation and in association with drugs, including cyclosporin and oral contraceptives. Rarely, it is caused by a variety of infectious agents, including pneumococcus, and viruses such as varicella or Coxsackie, or it may be associated with vaccines. Recurrent and familial forms of HUS are well documented in the literature.

The pathogenesis of HUS has been best characterized in D+HUS. SLTs bind to vascular endothelial cells through specific receptors that are thought to be more numerous on renovascular endothelium. Thus, endothelial cell injury is a central event in HUS and leads to a cascade of events including prostacyclin loss, local platelet activation and aggregation, and a thrombotic microangiopathy.

Often, the first suspicion of HUS occurs when a child with ongoing or resolving diarrhea becomes pale or has a drop in urine output. D+HUS typically occurs in late summer and is accompanied by a history of ingestion of incompletely cooked hamburger or unpasteurized apple juice or milk. A peripheral blood smear reveals evidence of fragmented red cells, schistocytes and burr cells, and there is thrombocytopenia. Assessment of urine output will be an indicator of the severity of the disease and the prognosis. If the urine output is good, the rate of rise of urea and potassium will be low, volume concerns will be diminished and dialysis will be less likely. On the other hand, if anuria is present, dialysis is usually initiated early in the disease process.

INVESTIGATIONS

Urinalysis demonstrates a variable amount of hematuria and proteinuria. A full blood count, reticulocyte count, serum electrolytes, glucose, urea and creatinine should be monitored regularly. Hyperglycemia may be indicative of pancreatic involvement and should be confirmed by assessment of the serum amylase and lipase. Assessment of serial lactate dehydrogenase (LDH) levels will determine the degree of hemolysis. Stool cultures will occasionally reveal the offending organism. A renal ultrasound is useful in anuric patients to assess renal blood flow.

Central nervous system (CNS) involvement is usually manifested by seizures and is associated with cerebral bleeds and cerebral infarction, which can be documented by imaging with a computed tomography (CT) or magnetic resonance image (MRI) scan. The possibility of bowel necrosis or perforation should be assessed in severely ill patients with symptoms of toxic colitis. Acute pancreatitis as well as transient or permanent diabetes mellitus are among the complications seen. A renal biopsy is rarely performed in D+HUS, but may be necessary to confirm the diagnosis in D−HUS.

Treatment involves supportive care, dialysis and plasmapheresis. Maintenence of fluid and electrolyte balances and administration of red cell transfusions are essential therapy. Occasionally, platelet transfusions are administered. Dialysis is indicated early in anuric patients and in those with rapidly rising urea and creatinine levels. Plasmapheresis is indicated in children with CNS involvement, but is rarely used in the absence of extrarenal manifestations. Certain features have been associated with a poorer prognosis. These include an elevated WBC count, prolonged anuria and multiorgan system involvement. Overall, more than 80% of patients will make a complete recovery. About 5–8% will progress to end-stage renal disease and there is a 5–10% mortality.

Hypertension

As in adults, hypertension in children can be divided into essential hypertension and secondary hypertension. The 'rule of thumb' for hypertension in children is that the greater the blood pressure and the younger the child, the more likely it is that there is a secondary cause for the hypertension. In order to evaluate hypertension in children one must:

- confirm the diagnosis
- investigate secondary causes of hypertension.

In order to confirm the diagnosis, it is important to ensure that the appropriate cuff size is used. The cuff should cover at least two-thirds of the

Table 14.6

Mean blood pressures in children*

Age	Male		Female	
	Systolic (mmHg)	Diastolic (mmHg)	Systolic (mmHg)	Diastolic (mmHg)
Newborn	72.7 ± 9.6	51.1 ± 8.9	71.8 ± 9.3	50.5 ± 8.4
1 year	93.6 ± 12.2	53.0 ± 9.0	93.0 ± 12.8	52.4 ± 9.2
3 years	93.5 ± 12.7	54.3 ± 9.4	92.6 ± 12.7	55.1 ± 9.8
5 years	94.3 ± 10.9	57.4 ± 9.7	94.1 ± 10.6	57.3 ± 9.9
10 years	101.9 ± 10.5	63.6 ± 9.5	101.8 ± 10.9	63.1 ± 9.9
12 years	105.8 ± 10.8	65.6 ± 9.8	107.5 ± 11.5	67.1 ± 9.7

*Figures represent mean ± SD. Source: reproduced from the Task Force Report on Blood Pressure Control in Children; published by *Pediatrics*, 1997.

upper arm. While exact measurements are not critical, it is advisable to use a larger cuff since a smaller cuff size will falsely elevate the blood pressure reading. Normal values for both systolic and diastolic measurements have been determined and nomograms are available for reference. Table 14.6 lists the mean systolic and diastolic blood pressures at different ages in childhood. In infants, the Korotkoff phase 5 sound is not audible, and so the Korotkoff phase 4 sound is used to determine the diastolic blood pressure. Once phase 5 becomes audible in older children it should be used as in the adult population. Significantly elevated blood pressure (BP) readings (diastolic BP ≥ 110 mmHg) are unusual but require immediate attention. Blood pressures elevated above the 95th percentile for age on at least three separate occasions are suggestive of hypertension and require evaluation. Ambulatory measurements are useful to differentiate transient hypertension, which is of minimal concern, from sustained hypertension, which will require further investigation and treatment.

The use of medication may be associated with marked elevations in blood pressure. Simple over-the-counter decongestants containing phenylephrine, ephedrine or other sympathomimetics may cause hypertension in older children that may persist for a few days beyond the discontinuation of the drug. Volume overload is a common cause in neonates.

Secondary causes of hypertension include intrinsic renal disease and renal scarring as a result of pyelonephritis and renovascular disease. Various syndromes such as Williams' syndrome and genetic diseases such as neurofibromatosis or tuberous sclerosis are associated with hypertension. In infants, congenital cardiac anomalies such as coarctation may result in elevated blood pressure in the upper limbs. A history of central umbilical catheters, bronchopulmonary dysplasia or renal ischemia may be noted in newborns, all of which may account for the renal disease or acute tubular necrosis. A family history of hypertension may suggest essential hypertension or familial causes of hypertension.

INVESTIGATIONS

Evaluation of hypertension should include investigation of renal function and serum electrolytes. A renal ultrasound including Doppler flow studies is helpful to rule out vascular anomalies. If renovascular disease is suspected, a renal scan should be performed with the use of captopril (an angiotensin-converting enzyme (ACE) inhibitor) to help in the assessment of differential renal blood flow. A renal angiogram with selective renal vein renin levels is helpful in the diagnosis of unilateral kidney disease, which might result in hypertension. Children who have persistent hypertension without evidence of renal disease should be evaluated for endocrine causes, including pheochromocytoma, primary hyperaldosteronism, 11-hydroxalase deficiency, and 3-β-hydroxylase deficiency, or central nervous system causes, including raised intracranial pressure and dysautonomia.

The treatment of hypertension in children is similar to that described for adults (Chapter 12). Betablockers, ACE inhibitors and vasodilator medications are used most frequently.

Congenital renal diseases

Congenital abnormalities of the genitourinary tract are rare. Some congenital diseases are of little concern, whereas others are associated with a high morbidity and mortality. Congenital renal disease may occur as a primary developmental abnormality, such as renal dysplasia, or as a feature of an associated structural anatomical abnormality such as occurs in the 'prune belly syndrome'. In general, developmental renal lesions usually occur in association with other congenital malformations or syndromes. Thus, any child with congenital renal disease must undergo a thorough evaluation for any other associated congenital malformation of the genitourinary tract as well as other organs.

In the next section, we discuss some of the more common structural renal lesions that occur in the newborn child. Congenital lesions that result in primary functional abnormalities (such as diabetes insipidus or renal tubular acidosis) are not considered as they are covered elsewhere in this book. Sporadic lesions that are reported to be associated with syndromes or ingestion of drugs during pregnancy are also not discussed.

RENAL DYSPLASIA AND HYPOPLASIA

Developmental abnormalities of the kidney result in a variety of structural and architectural abnormalities including renal dysplasia, renal hypoplasia, and horseshoe or duplex kidney. Renal dysplasia is defined as the failure of differentiation of renal tubules and the persistence of fetal mesonephric structures. Dysplastic kidneys show an abnormal architecture with poorly formed tubules and glomeruli, and the presence of cysts and extrarenal tissues (such as cartilage) within the parenchyma of the kidney. There is a strong association between renal dysplasia and obstructive uropathy. Obstruction at any site in the urinary tree may lead to dysplasia. Obstruction that results in unilateral dysplasia does not usually progress to renal insufficiency. Bilateral disease suggests a structural lesion in the lower genitourinary tract, and in a boy it may be associated with the presence of urethral valves. In the 'prune belly syndrome', urethral obstruction leads to bladder distention and severe hydroureter. The abdominal musculature is poorly developed and an excess of abdominal skin is found. Obstructive uropathy that results in renal dysplasia may be associated with a poorly developed or dysfunctional bladder. Bladder function tests will assess bladder volume and hypertonicity. The bladder may be the primary abnormality in the development of obstructive uropathy and renal failure.

Other causes of renal dysplasia include the cystic dysplasias (see below) and oligomeganephronia, which is characterized by the presence of fewer and larger glomeruli. In contrast to renal dysplasia, hypoplastic kidneys are smaller in size than normal, though normal in shape and architecture. Histological findings on renal biopsy are essentially normal.

The incidence of unilateral renal agenesis ranges from 1 in 400 to 1 in 1600 births. Unilateral agenesis is not usually of clinical concern as the child will be asymptomatic and renal function will usually remain normal. Bilateral renal agenesis occurs in approximately 1 in 7000 births and is usually fatal. Potter's syndrome (renal agenesis, oligohydramnios, flattened facies and pulmonary hypoplasia) is a cluster of clinical features associated with reduced renal output. This syndrome may occur in any circumstance where there is decreased urine output *in utero*.

Antenatal diagnosis of renal dysplasia/hypoplasia may be made by intrauterine renal ultrasound. Oligohydramnios is frequently assessed to determine whether early delivery of the infant will be beneficial. There is no treatment available for the underlying condition. After birth, assessment of renal function is performed by serial creatinine estimations and radionucleotide scanning of the kidney. Therapy is therefore directed to preservation of residual renal function, and treatment of chronic renal failure. Most infants with renal compromise as a result of renal dysplasia/hypoplasia will eventually require dialysis and renal transplantation.

CYSTIC KIDNEY DISEASES

A variety of cystic kidney diseases can present in childhood as either inherited diseases or developmental abnormalities. The common inherited diseases are autosomal dominant polycystic kidney disease (ADPKD) and autosomal recessive polycystic kidney disease (ARPKD). Developmental cystic diseases also occur in multicystic dysplastic kidney disease (MCDK), medullary cystic disease, and in cystic diseases associated with the phakomatoses, primarily tuberous sclerosis.

Polycystic kidney disease

Polycystic kidney disease (PKD) is the commonest of the renal diseases characterized by cysts in the kidney. As illustrated in Table 14.7, PKD is subdivided into ARPKD (also known as 'infantile' polycystic kidney disease) and ADPKD (previously known as 'adult' PKD). ADPKD is the most common inherited human kidney disease.

ARPKD appears to have two different clinical patterns, the first presenting in the newborn period and the second presenting later in childhood. The estimated incidence of ARPKD is one to two per 10 000 population, with a female predominance. The severely affected newborn has marked hypertension and a large abdomen with palpable smooth kidneys; the characteristic Potter's facies may also be present. In many newborns, there is a variable degree of renal failure and pulmonary hypoplasia, which can be life-threatening. Evaluation of infants with suspected ARPKD includes a thorough family history, renal function tests, hepatic and renal ultrasounds

ARPKD*	ADPKD†
Large hyperechogenic kidneys, stable in size throughout life	Kidneys slightly enlarged, increasing in size with age
Variable sized cysts present early in life	Discrete cysts, increasing in size and number with age (> three needed for diagnosis)
Hepatic disease including dilated biliary ducts and progressive hepatic fibrosis	Liver cysts may be present; no evidence of hepatic fibrosis
Kidneys smooth on palpation	Kidneys bosselated
Hypertension prominent in newborn period	Hypertension later in life

*Autosomal recessive polycystic kidney disease.
†Autosomal dominant polycystic kidney disease.

Table 14.7
Differential diagnosis of polycystic kidney disease

and, for definitive diagnosis in most cases, renal and hepatic biopsies. An excretory urogram typically demonstrates poor renal function as collection of contrast in the collecting tubule reveals typical linear streaks in a 'spokewheel' pattern. If the diagnosis of ARPKD is made at an older age, the presentation may be with liver abnormalities predominating. Diagnosis is confirmed by biopsy and histology. Classic liver biopsy findings include biliary duct ectasia, duct dilation and fibrosis.

No specific treatment is available for PKD. Renal concentrating defects, hypertension and progressive renal and hepatic deterioration require symptomatic therapy. In ARPKD, the kidneys may become large enough to cause respiratory distress, necessitating their removal even though renal function is normal. Many children will benefit from kidney transplants. Patients with ARPKD may require combined liver and kidney transplantation.

Glomerulocystic disease

Glomerulocystic disease is polycystic kidney disease with prominent glomerular involvement. Interestingly, glomerulocystic disease has been found in patients with a family history of ADPKD. A linkage to chromosome 16 in infants with glomerulocystic disease born to mothers with ADPKD suggests the disease may be an infantile form of ADPKD. The clinical picture can be similar to that of other forms of polycystic kidney disease. Patients may be asymptomatic or have chronic renal failure. Large palpable kidneys and hypertension may be present. Glomerulocystic disease is associated with syndromes such as trisomy 13 (Patau's syndrome), Zellweger syndrome and tuberous sclerosis. Not uncommonly, a renal biopsy is required for diagnosis.

Multicystic dysplastic kidney disease

Typically, the etiology of the multicystic dysplastic kidney (MCDK) is related to obstruction at the ureteropelvic junction or to improper interaction between the metanephric blastema and the ureteric bud. MCDKD can be unilateral or bilateral. If both kidneys are affected, the infant may present at birth with oligohydramnios, amnion nodosum, pulmonary hypoplasia and Potter's facies. In many cases, the cysts are unilateral and the affected kidney has little or no function. The evaluation of children with MCDKD should include renal function testing, evaluation of the associated hypertension and renal ultrasound. In addition, a DMSA scan and a voiding cystourethrogram should be obtained in view of the high incidence of VUR in affected and unaffected contralateral kidneys. If there is evidence of obstructive uropathy, medical or surgical treatment should be initiated. Severe hypertension, recurrent infections and a poorly functioning kidney are indications for nephrectomy.

CONGENITAL NEPHROTIC SYNDROME

Congenital nephrotic syndrome (congenital NS) is defined as the onset of nephrotic syndrome within the first three months of life. It is an extremely rare disorder and is often fatal. It represents a heterogeneity of kidney diseases, either primary or secondary, which are classified solely on the basis of histology. The most frequent histological finding is infantile microcystic disease, characterized by cyst-like dilation of the proximal tubules. This disorder is more common in Finland or in children of Finnish ancestry, where the inheritance pattern is reported to be autosomal recessive with a gene frequency of 1.2 in 10 000 births. Congenital NS may also occur as a result of other diseases, including diffuse mesangial sclerosis, or as a secondary manifestation of congenital infections such as congenital syphilis, cytomegalovirus and toxoplasmosis. Congenital NS may also be associated with other congenital malformations in the Drash syndrome (pseudo-hermaphroditism, Wilms' tumor and congenital NS). Pertinent history includes the presence of a large placenta (up to one-third of body weight), low birth weight and an elevated maternal amniotic α-fetoprotein level. The infant usually presents with severe incapacitating NS and hypo-gammaglobulinemia.

In the postnatal period, there is early onset of edema with proteinuria developing into the nephrotic syndrome. In addition to massive proteinuria and hypoalbuminemia, congenital NS results in urinary losses of immunoglobulins leading to a high infant mortality from infection. The mortality can be as high as 80% by one year of life. As a result of the immense protein losses there is also loss of thyroid hormones, anticoagulants (such as antithrombin 3) and other low molecular weight proteins, all of which can lead to additional medical problems. Evaluation involves careful assessment of electrolytes, albumin, immunoglobulins and blood anticoagulant levels as well as renal function. Risk of infection is high and a thorough work-up for sepsis is necessary with any fever. A renal biopsy must be performed in order to define the histological lesion. In high-risk individuals, evaluation of pregnancies is possible with maternal serum and amniotic α-fetoprotein assays. An elevated level in the second trimester is a reflection of proteinuria *in utero*. This test is highly sensitive in high-risk families, so termination of the pregnancy may be offered where infants are shown to be affected.

The treatment of children with congenital nephrotic syndrome is very challenging and requires a multidisciplinary team approach in a specialized center familiar with the complications that are frequently encountered. Daily albumin infusions are often needed to maintain clinical stability. Since the risk of death from infection is high, management is very aggressive and includes frequent immunoglobulin infusions and may necessitate early nephrectomy to reduce protein and immunoglobulin losses, with dialysis and transplantation at an early age.

Renal failure in neonates

Renal failure is defined as the cessation of kidney function with or without changes in urine volume. Arbitrarily, oliguria is defined as a urine output of less than 1 ml/kg/h and anuria is defined as a urine output of less than 0.5 ml/kg/h. Acute renal failure is separated into three major categories: prerenal; renal (intrinsic); and postrenal. While the causes of each of these categories are discussed elsewhere (Chapter 9), several clinical situations that result in acute renal failure in the newborn child are considered below. Pertinent investigations are noted.

DELAYED MICTURITION

Most newborns urinate within 24 hours of birth. Failure to pass urine by 48 hours after birth is abnormal. Evaluation includes careful physical examination of external genitalia for congenital malformations, assessment of renal function and a renal ultrasound examination. Evaluation should include assessment of blood flow to the kidney by Doppler flow ultrasound, arteriogram if an umbilical arterial line is present, or radionucleotide scan.

HYPOTENSION/SHOCK

Newborns are susceptible to undergo severe ischemic insults associated with abruptio placentae, meconium aspiration and shock. Severe respiratory distress or sepsis may result in hypotension that requires fluid and inotropic resuscitation. These newborns are likely to develop renal failure and acute tubular necrosis. Evaluation involves careful assessment of fluid input and output, serum and urine electrolytes and renal function. Ultrasound assessment of renal blood flow is necessary in anuric infants. Dialysis may be necessary if the blood urea generation rate is high or if severe electrolyte abnormalities develop.

CONGENITAL MALFORMATIONS/POSTOPERATIVE

Infants born with severe cardiac disease generally develop an associated prerenal failure as a result of poor perfusion of the kidneys. Following cardiac surgery, these infants may develop acute tubular necrosis, requiring careful monitoring of fluids, electrolytes and renal function. Dialysis may be necessary. Infants born with intra-abdominal malformations such as gastro-schisis are also prone to develop renal failure. These infants develop prerenal uremia as a result of severe fluid losses, and compromised renal perfusion as a result of a tense abdomen.

INVESTIGATIONS

The diagnosis of acute renal failure in the newborn is based on differentiating prerenal, renal and postrenal disease by laboratory values. Prerenal uremia reflects the body's attempt to maintain intravascular volume and renal perfusion. The kidneys conserve free water and sodium. In contrast, in intrinsic renal disease, the tubules are unable to conserve sodium or free water.

Laboratory investigation of acute renal failure is discussed in Chapter 9 and includes assessment of blood electrolytes, blood urea, blood creatinine, blood calcium, blood phosphorus and blood osmolarity, and urine electrolytes, urine creatinine and urine osmolarity. A renal ultrasound, with Doppler flow study of the renal vessels, is critical in pediatric patients, particularly neonates. The renal ultrasound will evaluate anatomic, obstructive, and vascular causes of acute renal failure. Radionuclide renal scans and intravenous pyelograms are rarely necessary or helpful. The presence of serum free myoglobin and urinary myoglobin is an early indicator of renal failure in an asphyxiated baby. Use of the serum creatinine level is limited in newborns as the serum creatinine values in the first 24 hours of life reflect maternal renal function and so are similar to adult values. Over the subsequent two weeks the creatinine level falls to 0.3–0.4 mg/dl in normal babies. Serial creatinine measurements will thus provide an indication of the baby's intrinsic renal function. If the creatinine fails to fall or rises, this is suggestive of intrinsic renal dysfunction.

Specific aspects of treatment of acute renal failure were discussed in Chapter 9 and are similar in adults and children. In children, careful management of fluid and electrolytes is mandatory. Peritoneal dialysis is the preferred mode of dialysis in very small infants. The development of small bore catheters and dialysis machines capable of handling low blood flow rates and ultrafiltrates has made hemodialysis and continuous venovenous hemofiltration a feasible option for very small infants and children.

References

International Reflux Committee (1981) Medical versus surgical treatment of primary vesicoureteral reflux. *Pediatrics*, **67**, 392.

Task Force Report on Blood Pressure Control in Children (1987) Report of the Second Task Force on Blood Pressure Control in Children. *Pediatrics*, **79**, 1–25.

Further reading

Becker, N. and Avner, E.D. (1995) Congenital nephropathies and uropathies. *Pediat. Clin. North Am.*, **42**, 1319–42.

Chantler, C. (1993) Kidney disease in children, in *Diseases of the Kidney*, 5th edn (eds R.W. Schrier and C.W. Gottschalk), Little Brown & Co., Boston, pp. 2379–2404.

Churg, J., Habib, R. and White, R.H. (1970) Pathology of the nephrotic syndrome in children: a report for the International Study of Kidney Diseases in Children. *Lancet*, **76**, 1299–1302.

Clark, G. and Barratt, T.M. (1994) Minimal change nephrotic syndrome and focal segmental glomerulosclerosis, in *Pediatric Nephrology*, 3rd edn (eds M. Holliday, T.M. Barratt and E.D. Avner), Williams & Wilkins, Baltimore, pp. 767–87.

Habib, R. (1993) Nephrotic syndrome in the first year of life. *Pediat. Nephrol.*, 7, 347–53.

Ingelfinger, J.R. (1994) Pediatric hypertension. *Curr. Opin. Pediat.*, **6**, 198–205.

Jones, K.V. and Asscher, A.W. (1992) Urinary tract infections and vesicoureteral reflux, in *Pediatric Kidney Disease* (ed. C.M. Edelmann), Little Brown & Co., Boston, pp. 1943–92.

Lieu, T.A., Grasmeder, H.M. and Kaplan, B.S. (1991) An approach to the evaluation and treatment of microscopic hematuria. *Pediat. Clin. North Am.*, **38**, 579–92.

Robson, W.L., Leung, A.K. and Kaplan, B.S. (1993) Hemolytic uremic syndrome. *Curr. Prob. Pediat.*, **3**, 16–33.

Index

Note: Page references in **bold** refer to Figures; those in *italics* refer to Tables